Diabetes Management

Editor

IRL B. HIRSCH

MEDICAL CLINICS OF NORTH AMERICA

www.medical.theclinics.com

Consulting Editors
DOUGLAS S. PAAUW
EDWARD R. BOLLARD

January 2015 • Volume 99 • Number 1

ELSEVIER

1600 John F. Kennedy Boulevard • Suite 1800 • Philadelphia, Pennsylvania, 19103-2899

http://www.theclinics.com

MEDICAL CLINICS OF NORTH AMERICA Volume 99, Number 1
January 2015 ISSN 0025-7125, ISBN-13: 978-0-323-34178-3

Editor: Jessica McCool
Developmental Editor: Susan Showalter

Medical Clinics of North America (ISSN 0025-7125) is published bimonthly by Elsevier Inc., 360 Park Avenue South, New York, NY 10010-1710. Months of publication are January, March, May, July, September, and November. Business and editorial offices: 1600 John F. Kennedy Boulevard, Suite 1800, Philadelphia, PA 19103-2899. Periodicals postage paid at New York, NY, and additional mailing offices. Subscription prices are USD $255.00 per year (US individuals), $471.00 per year (US institutions), $125.00 per year (US Students), $320.00 per year (Canadian individuals), $612.00 per year (Canadian institutions), $200.00 per year (Canadian and foreign students), $390.00 per year (foreign individuals), and $612.00 per year (foreign institutions). To receive student/resident rate, orders must be accompanied by name of affiliated institution, date of term, and the signature of program/residency coordinator on institution letterhead. Orders will be billed at individual rate until proof of status is received. Foreign air speed delivery is included in all Clinics' subscription prices. All prices are subject to change without notice. **POSTMASTER:** Send address changes to *Medical Clinics of North America*, Elsevier Health Sciences Division, Subscription Customer Service, 3251 Riverport Lane, Maryland Heights, MO 63043. **Customer Service: Telephone: 1-800-654-2452** (U.S. and Canada); **1-314-447-8871** (outside U.S. and Canada). **Fax: 314-447-8029. E-mail: journalscustomerserviceusa@elsevier.com** (for print support); **journalsonlinesupport-usa@elsevier.com** (for online support).

Reprints. For copies of 100 or more of articles in this publication, please contact the Commercial Reprints Department, Elsevier Inc., 360 Park Avenue South, New York, NY 10010-1710. Tel.: 212-633-3874; Fax: 212-633-3820; E-mail: reprints@elsevier.com.

Medical Clinics of North America is also published in Spanish by McGraw-Hill Interamericana Editores S. A., P.O. Box 5-237, 06500 Mexico, D.F., Mexico.

Medical Clinics of North America is covered in *MEDLINE/PubMed (Index Medicus), Current Contents, ASCA, Excerpta Medica, Science Citation Index, and ISI/BIOMED.*

Printed in the United States of America.

PROGRAM OBJECTIVE

The goal of the *Medical Clinics of North America* is to keep practicing physicians up to date with current clinical practice by providing timely articles reviewing the state of the art in patient care.

LEARNING OBJECTIVES

Upon completion of this activity, participants will be able to:
1. Review updates to diabetes classification.
2. Describe insulin therapy in Type 1 and Type 2 diabetes.
3. Review screening and treatment for the primary care provider of common diabetes complications.

ACCREDITATION

The Elsevier Office of Continuing Medical Education (EOCME) is accredited by the Accreditation Council for Continuing Medical Education (ACCME) to provide continuing medical education for physicians.

The EOCME designates this enduring material for a maximum of 15 *AMA PRA Category 1 Credit*(s)™. Physicians should claim only the credit commensurate with the extent of their participation in the activity.

All other health care professionals requesting continuing education credit for this enduring material will be issued a certificate of participation.

DISCLOSURE OF CONFLICTS OF INTEREST

The EOCME assesses conflict of interest with its instructors, faculty, planners, and other individuals who are in a position to control the content of CME activities. All relevant conflicts of interest that are identified are thoroughly vetted by EOCME for fair balance, scientific objectivity, and patient care recommendations. EOCME is committed to providing its learners with CME activities that promote improvements or quality in healthcare and not a specific proprietary business or a commercial interest.

The planning committee, staff, authors and editors listed below have identified no financial relationships or relationships to products or devices they or their spouse/life partner have with commercial interest related to the content of this CME activity:

William R. Adam, PhD, MBBS, FRACP; Stephen A. Brietzke, MD; Dawn DeWitt, MD, MSc, MACP, FRACP, FRCPC; David C. Dugdale, MD, FACP; Alison B. Evert, MS, RD, CDE; Matthew P. Gilbert, DO, MPH; Sara J. Healy, MD; Kristen Helm; Brynne Hunter; Sandy Lavery; Sachin Majumdar, MD; Farah Meah, DO; Jessica McCool; Douglas S. Paauw, MD, MACP; Lindsay Parnell; Michelle D. Po, PhD; Santha Priya; Michael C. Riddell, PhD; Stuart A. Ross, MD; Elizabeth Stephens, MD; Megan Suermann; Celeste C. Thomas, MD, MS; Subbulaxmi Trikudanathan, MD, MRCP, MMSc; John R. White, Jr, PA-C, Pharm D

The planning committee, staff, authors and editors listed below have identified financial relationships or relationships to products or devices they or their spouse/life partner have with commercial interest related to the content of this CME activity:

Kathleen M. Dungan, MD, MPH is a consultant/advisor for Eli Lilly and has research grants from Merck, Novo Nordisk, Grifols and Boehringer Ingelheim.

Irl B. Hirsch, MD, has research grants from Sanofi, Novo and Halozyme; also is a consultant/advisor for Abbott and Roche.

Silvio Inzucchi, MD is a consultant/advisor for Merck, Boeringer Ingelheim, Novo Nordisk and Bristol Myers Squibb; has research grant from Takeda.

Rattan Juneja, MBBS, MD, MRCP (UK) is on speakers bureau for Astra Zeneca, Boehringer Ingelheim, Eli Lilly, Merck and Janssen.

Joshua J. Neumiller, PharmD, CDE, FASCP has research grants from Amylin Pharmaceuticals LLC, Astra-Zeneca, Johnson & Johnson, Merck & Co., Inc., and Novo Nordisk; is a consultant/advisor for Janssen Pharmaceuticals, Inc., and sanofi-aventis U.S. LLC, and is on speakers bureau for Janssen Pharmaceuticals, Inc.

Louis H. Philipson, MD, PhD, has a research grant from Pfizer, Inc.

Hugh D. Tildesley, MD, is a consultant/advisor for and has a research grant from Medtronic, Inc.

UNAPPROVED/OFF-LABEL USE DISCLOSURE

The EOCME requires CME faculty to disclose to the participants:
1. When products or procedures being discussed are off-label, unlabelled, experimental, and/or investigational (not US Food and Drug Administration (FDA) approved); and
2. Any limitations on the information presented, such as data that are preliminary or that represent ongoing research, interim analyses, and/or unsupported opinions. Faculty may discuss information about pharmaceutical agents that is outside of FDA-approved labelling. This information is intended solely for CME

and is not intended to promote off-label use of these medications. If you have any questions, contact the medical affairs department of the manufacturer for the most recent prescribing information.

TO ENROLL
To enroll in the *Medical Clinics of North America* Continuing Medical Education program, call customer service at 1-800-654-2452 or sign up online at http://www.theclinics.com/home/cme. The CME program is available to subscribers for an additional annual fee of USD $295.

METHOD OF PARTICIPATION
In order to claim credit, participants must complete the following:
1. Complete enrolment as indicated above.
2. Read the activity.
3. Complete the CME Test and Evaluation. Participants must achieve a score of 70% on the test. All CME Tests and Evaluations must be completed online.

CME INQUIRIES/SPECIAL NEEDS
For all CME inquiries or special needs, please contact elsevierCME@elsevier.com.

MEDICAL CLINICS OF NORTH AMERICA

RELATED INTEREST

Endocrinology and Metabolism Clinics of North America,
March 2014 (Vol. 43, No. 1)
Diabetes Mellitus: Associated Conditions
Leonid Poretsky and Emilia Liao, *Editors*
http://www.endo.theclinics.com/

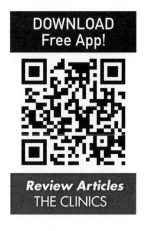

NOW AVAILABLE FOR YOUR iPhone and iPad

Contributors

CONSULTING EDITORS

DOUGLAS S. PAAUW, MD, MACP
Professor of Medicine, Division of General Internal Medicine; Rathmann Family Foundation Endowed Chair for Patient-Centered Clinical Education, Medicine Student Programs, Professor of Medicine, University of Washington School of Medicine, Seattle, Washington

EDWARD R. BOLLARD, MD, DDS, FACP
Professor of Medicine; Associate Dean of Graduate Medical Education, Designated Institutional Official (DIO), Department of Medicine, Penn State–Milton S. Hershey Medical Center, Penn State University College of Medicine, Hershey, Pennsylvania

EDITOR

IRL B. HIRSCH, MD
Professor of Medicine, University of Washington School of Medicine, Seattle, Washington

AUTHORS

WILLIAM R. ADAM, PhD, MBBS, FRACP
Professor of Medicine, Rural Health Academic Centre, Melbourne Medical School, Parkville, Graham St. Shepparton, Victoria, Australia

STEPHEN A. BRIETZKE, MD
Professor of Clinical Medicine, Division of Endocrinology, Diabetes, and Metabolism, Department of Medicine, University of Missouri-Columbia, Columbia, Missouri

DAWN DeWITT, MD, MSc, FRACP, FRCPC
Master of the American College of Physicians; Professor, Department of Medicine, University of British Columbia, Vancouver, British Columbia, Canada

DAVID C. DUGDALE, MD, FACP
Professor of Medicine, Division of Internal Medicine, Department of Medicine, University of Washington, Seattle, Washington

KATHLEEN M. DUNGAN, MD, MPH
Associate Professor of Medicine, Division of Endocrinology, Diabetes and Metabolism, The Ohio State University Wexner Medical Center, Columbus, Ohio

ALISON B. EVERT, MS, RD, CDE
Coordinator, Diabetes Education Programs, Diabetes Care Center, University of Washington Medical Center, Seattle, Washington

MATTHEW P. GILBERT, DO, MPH
Assistant Professor of Medicine, Division of Endocrinology and Diabetes, Department of Medicine, College of Medicine, The University of Vermont, Burlington, Vermont

SARA J. HEALY, MD
Division of Endocrinology, Diabetes and Metabolism, The Ohio State University Wexner Medical Center, Columbus, Ohio

SILVIO INZUCCHI, MD
Professor of Medicine; Clinical Chief, Department of Endocrinology, Yale University School of Medicine; Medical Director, Yale Diabetes Center, Yale-New Haven Hospital, New Haven, Connecticut

RATTAN JUNEJA, MBBS, MD, MRCP (UK)
Clinical Associate Professor (Adjunct), Division of Endocrinology, Indiana University School of Medicine, Indianapolis, Indiana

SACHIN MAJUMDAR, MD
Assistant Clinical Professor, Yale University School of Medicine, New Haven, Connecticut; Chief, Section of Endocrinology, Bridgeport Hospital, Yale New Haven Health System, Bridgeport, Connecticut

FARAH MEAH, DO
Endocrinology Fellow, Division of Endocrinology, Indiana University School of Medicine, Indianapolis, Indiana

JOSHUA J. NEUMILLER, PharmD, CDE, FASCP
Associate Professor, Department of Pharmacotherapy, College of Pharmacy, Washington State University, Spokane, Washington

LOUIS H. PHILIPSON, MD, PhD
Professor, Departments of Pediatrics, Section of Endocrinology, Diabetes and Metabolism, The University of Chicago; Director, Chicago Kovler Diabetes Center, Chicago, Illinois

MICHELLE D. PO, PhD
SCRIPT, Toronto, Ontario, Canada

MICHAEL C. RIDDELL, PhD
Professor and Graduate Program Director, Muscle Health Research Center, School of Kinesiology and Health Science, Bethune College, York University, Toronto, Ontario, Canada

STUART A. ROSS, MD
Faculty of Medicine, University of Calgary, Calgary, Alberta, Canada

ELIZABETH STEPHENS, MD, FACP
Endocrinology Faculty, Providence Medical Group NE-Medical Education; Affiliate Associate Professor, Department of Internal Medicine, Oregon Health and Sciences University, Portland, Oregon

CELESTE C. THOMAS, MD, MS
Assistant Professor, Department of Medicine, Section of Endocrinology, Diabetes and Metabolism, The University of Chicago, Chicago, Illinois

HUGH D. TILDESLEY, MD
Department of Endocrinology and Metabolism, St Paul's Hospital, University of British Columbia, Vancouver, British Columbia, Canada

SUBBULAXMI TRIKUDANATHAN, MD, MRCP, MMSc
Clinical Assistant Professor, Division of Metabolism, Endocrinology and Nutrition, Department of Medicine, University of Washington Medical Center, Seattle, Washington

JOHN R. WHITE Jr, PA-C, PharmD
Professor and Chair, Department of Pharmacotherapy, Washington State University, Spokane, Washington

Contents

Diabetes mellitus is a group of metabolic diseases characterized by hyperglycemia resulting from defects in insulin secretion, insulin action, or both. The goal in diagnosing diabetes mellitus is to identify those with significantly increased premature mortality and increased risk of microvascular and cardiovascular complications. This brief review shows the evolving nature of the classification of diabetes mellitus. No classification scheme is ideal, and all have some overlap and inconsistencies. Diabetes mellitus classification will continue to evolve as we work to fully understand the pathogenesis of the major forms.

Internet blood glucose monitoring systems (IBGMS) are associated with improved glycemic control in patients with type 2 diabetes (T2D) who are pharmacologically managed, using oral agents or insulin. IBGMS improves glycemic levels in patients with type 1 diabetes (T1D). IBGMS has not led to increased hypoglycemia. Mechanisms underlying IBGMS-associated glycemic improvement extend beyond optimizing insulin dose titration. The most important effects seem to be associated with increased patient self-motivation and improved patient-physician communication. IBGMS have been recommended in clinical practice guidelines, and their effectiveness and safety in trials suggest that this approach is appropriate for patients with T1D or T2D.

Monitoring of glycemic control is a key component of the diabetes treatment plan. Patients who are not meeting targets often require more intensive monitoring, ranging from frequent self-monitored glucose to continuous glucose monitoring in order to facilitate medication and lifestyle changes. However, more intensive monitoring demands more training and a structured plan for interpretation and use of the data. Better patient and provider tools to support decision-making and progress toward an artificial pancreas may help to alleviate this burden.

Hyperglycemia is the unifying metabolic abnormality for all forms of diabetes mellitus, forming the basis for its diagnosis and treatment. The strong epidemiologic associations between hyperglycemia and the complications of diabetes have given rise to the glucose hypothesis—that the complications of diabetes are caused by hyperglycemia and that they can be prevented by normalizing glucose levels. Herein the authors review the epidemiologic relationships between hyperglycemia and the complications of diabetes, the major trials of glucose lowering, and the extent to which the glucose hypothesis is supported by these studies and how this information can be translated into clinical practice.

Diabetes now affects more than 29 million Americans, and more than 9 million of these people do not know they have diabetes. In adults, type 2 diabetes accounts for about 90% to 95% of all diagnosed cases of diabetes and is the focus of this article. Lifestyle intervention is part of the initial treatment as well as the ongoing management of type 2 diabetes. Lifestyle intervention encompasses a healthful eating plan, physical activity, and often medication to assist in achievement of glucose, lipid, and blood pressure goals. Patient education and self-care practices are also important aspects of disease management.

The epidemic of type 2 diabetes mellitus has been met by evolving strategy and clinical tactics, including the generally-accepted recommendation to initiate drug therapy concurrent with therapeutic lifestyle changes. Barring contraindications, metformin should be the first drug treatment prescribed, based on considerations of cost, efficacy, and safety. When metformin monotherapy fails to produce the goal for glycemic control, add-on therapy can include a sulfonylurea, a sodium-glucose transporter type 2 inhibitor, an alpha-glucosidase inhibitor, or a thiazolidinedione. New niche therapies include colesevelam and bromocriptine mesylate. Consideration should be given to the effect of the drug therapy on cardiovascular disease.

Incretin hormones, namely glucagon-like peptide 1 (GLP-1) and gastric inhibitory peptide, have been recognized for some time as playing a key role in glucose homeostasis, with the effects of incretin hormones believed to be responsible for up to 60% of postprandial insulin release. Two predominant therapeutic strategies have been developed to augment the incretin response: (1) GLP-1 receptor agonists resistant to degradation by the enzyme dipeptidyl peptidase 4 (DPP-4); and (2) DPP-4 inhibitors. With an expanding arsenal of incretin-based therapies available, understanding the differentiating efficacy and safety profiles for available agents is important in optimizing drug selection and patient outcomes.

Diabetes is the leading cause of end-stage renal disease, blindness, and nontraumatic lower-limb amputation. The largest reductions in cardiovascular events are seen when multiple risk factors are addressed simultaneously. The benefit of aspirin as secondary prevention in patients with previous stroke or myocardial infarction has been well established. Regular, dilated eye examinations are effective in detecting sight-threatening diabetic retinopathy and have been shown to prevent blindness. The use of appropriate tools and clinical examination/inspection provides greater than 87% specificity in detecting diabetic peripheral neuropathy. Early treatment of risk factors, including hypertension, hyperglycemia, and dyslipidemia can delay or prevent diabetic nephropathy.

Polycystic ovarian syndrome (PCOS) is a complex and phenotypically heterogeneous endocrine disorder that typically presents in reproductive-aged women. Key clinical components include hyperandrogenism, menstrual irregularities, infertility, and cardiometabolic abnormalities. Definition of PCOS has been confusing and controversial because of the lack of consistent diagnostic criteria. Management choices in women with PCOS should target the phenotype and individual needs of the patient. Oral contraceptives remain the first line of treatment for hyperandrogenic symptoms and menstrual dysfunction. Lifestyle modifications and metformin improve metabolic abnormalities. Particular attention should be placed on addressing and preventing the long-term cardiometabolic implications of PCOS.

Foreword
Diabetes Management

 CrossMark

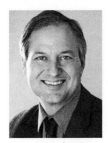

Douglas S. Paauw, MD, MACP
Consulting Editor

About 10% of the United States population has diabetes. The prevalence is expected to rise dramatically over the next 40 years due to an aging population more likely to develop type 2 diabetes, increases in minority groups that are at increased risk for type 2 diabetes, and people with diabetes living longer. It is estimated that, by 2050, 20% to 33% of the population of the United States will have diabetes.[1] This issue of *Medical Clinics of North America* focuses on current issues in the management of patients with diabetes, a field where rapid changes in management have developed over the past decade. The issue is edited by Dr Irl B. Hirsch, one of the leading diabetologists and diabetes educators in the world. This issue will update you on current approaches to monitoring and treatment of diabetes with an eye toward the future of diabetes management.

Douglas S. Paauw, MD, MACP
Division of General Internal Medicine
Department of Medicine
University of Washington School of Medicine
Seattle, WA 98195, USA

E-mail address:
DPaauw@medicine.washington.edu

REFERENCE

1. Boyle J, Thompson TJ, Gregg EW, et al. Projection of the year 2050 burden of diabetes in the US adult population: dynamic modeling of incidence, mortality, and prediabetes prevalence. Popul Health Metr 2010;8:29.

Med Clin N Am 99 (2015) xv
http://dx.doi.org/10.1016/j.mcna.2014.09.005
0025-7125/15/$ – see front matter © 2015 Elsevier Inc. All rights reserved.
medical.theclinics.com

Preface

Diabetes Management

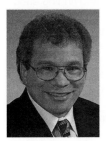

Irl B. Hirsch, MD
Editor

In 2001, a report from the Centers of Disease Control and Prevention (CDC) in Atlanta projected the number of Americans with diabetes would increase from 11 million in 2000 (prevalence 4.0%) to 29 million in 2050.[1] This 165% increase was predicted to be the greatest for those 75 years of age and older. By 2014, we can see how poor those projections for the future actually were. The most recent CDC data report that 29.1 million Americans (9.3% of the population) are diagnosed with diabetes, while 8.1 million people have diabetes and are undiagnosed.[2] What this means is that the 2001 prediction for diabetes prevalence for 2050 was surpassed in 2014! The earlier projection did correctly note the high number of older people with diabetes. For those 65 years of age or older, more than one in four have diabetes (25.9%).[2] What this means is any family practice physician, internist, geriatrician, gynecologist, oncologist, surgeon, anesthesiologist, cardiologist, rheumatologist, infectious disease specialist, and certainly endocrinologist need to stay updated on all aspects of diabetes, especially updated in understanding all evidenced-based therapies.

It would be incorrect to assume this increase in diabetes is simply an American or even North American concern. The International Diabetes Federation (IDF) reports that, while North America and the Caribbean have a prevalence of diabetes of 10%, the Middle East and North Africa, Southeast Asia, South and Central America, the Western Pacific, and Europe have prevalence rates of 11%, 9%, 8%, 8%, and 7%, respectively.[3] The overall world population of diabetes is 382 million, and this number is expected to increase by 55% by 2035 to 592 million.[3]

The burden on quality of life can be more difficult to quantitate, but mortality and economic costs are more easily captured. For example, the IDF reports that the proportion of deaths due to diabetes in people less than 60 years of age (in 2013) is 38% for North America, but as high as 76% for Africa.[3] Health care expenditures are 263 billion dollars (USD) for North and Central America, and 26 billion dollars for South America. For a world-wide public health concern with such rapid growth, deadly consequences, and unsustainable costs, one would think diabetes would be a major focus of virtually every government of the world. Unfortunately, this is not the case.

There are other issues not noted in these statistics. For example, the special needs of children and young adults with type 2 diabetes are in need of much more attention and research. This is a population that didn't exist a few years ago, and finding effective therapies may be different in these younger patients. Associated with that is the topic of pregnancy in women with pregestational type 2 diabetes. This was quite rare in decades past. Given the large number of women of child-bearing age with type 2 diabetes, nonspecialists will need to become familiar with all of the issues required to prepare these women for pregnancy. Finally, in both Europe and the United States, there is a rapidly growing population of older adults over the age of 60 with type 1 diabetes. While these individuals were few in number 30 years ago, this is now not the case, and our health care system and clinicians caring for these patients will need to adapt to this population's special needs.

Given the tremendous growing impact of diabetes in North America and around the world, it is appropriate that this issue of *Medical Clinics of North America* is devoted to diabetes. While there has been an incredible improvement in our understanding of the fundamental pathogenesis of diabetes and its complications, this issue is focused on strategies for diabetes therapies. Starting with an article of the current classification scheme, including an update of the various forms of monogenic diabetes, the reader will learn how Internet blood glucose monitoring systems can improve care. Nutrition and exercise fundamentals are reviewed as are our various biomarkers for assessing diabetes control in addition to specific glycemic targets. Much of the issue reviews how to best use both the older and the newer medications to treat diabetes, and strategies for insulin use for both type 1 and type 2 diabetes are presented. Screening and treatment of the various diabetes complications for the nonspecialist are reviewed, along with a discussion of polycystic ovarian syndrome. It is hoped that all clinicians caring for patients with diabetes can benefit from the expertise of our experienced authors.

Finally, I would like to thank Dr Douglas Paauw for inviting me to be editor of this issue, and also Mr Yonah Korngold and Mrs Jessica McCool for their assistance.

Irl B. Hirsch, MD
University of Washington School of Medicine
4245 Roosevelt Way NE, 3rd Floor
Seattle, WA 98105, USA

E-mail address:
ihirsch@uw.edu

REFERENCES

1. Boyle JP, Honeycutt AA, Narayan KM, et al. Projection of diabetes burden through 2050: impact of changing demography and disease prevalence in the U.S. Diabetes Care 2001;24:1936–40.
2. Available at: http://www.cdc.gov/diabetes/pubs/estimates14.htm. Accessed September 21, 2014.
3. Available at: http://wwwidf.org/worlddiabetesday/toolkit/gp/facts-figures. Accessed September 21, 2014.

Erratum

The article "Elbow Tendinopathy" by Michael E. Pitzer, Peter H. Seidenberg, and Dov A. Bader (Med Clin N Am 2014;98:833-849) was published with a credit given to the incorrect author. On page 835, the sentence should read: "This theory was supported by Riek et al. who discovered via computer analysis and magnetic resonance imaging that novice tennis players with improper backhand technique underwent eccentric contraction of very lengthened extensor muscles and suggested the microtrauma caused by this technique to be the cause for lateral epicondylitis.(14)" The citation at the end of the sentence was published correctly. The authors apologize for the error.

Med Clin N Am 99 (2015) xix
http://dx.doi.org/10.1016/j.mcna.2014.10.002
0025-7125/15/$ – see front matter © 2015 Elsevier Inc. All rights reserved.

Update on Diabetes Classification

Celeste C. Thomas, MD, MS[a],*, Louis H. Philipson, MD, PhD[a,b]

KEYWORDS

- Classification of diabetes mellitus • Gestational diabetes mellitus
- Latent autoimmune diabetes of adults • Monogenic diabetes
- Maturity-onset diabetes of the young • Neonatal diabetes • Secondary diabetes
- Type 1 and Type 2 diabetes mellitus

KEY POINTS

- The classification of diabetes mellitus is evolving as we work to fully understand the pathogenesis of the major forms.
- The goal of classification is to say something meaningful about the cause, natural history, genetics, heritability, clinical phenotype and optimum treatments of a disease. In the case of diabetes, this is getting harder to do rather than easier.
- Monogenic diabetes mellitus remains undiagnosed in more than 90% of the individuals who have this form of diabetes caused by one of the known gene mutations.

"The first step in wisdom is to know the things themselves; this notion consists in having a true idea of the objects; objects are distinguished and known by classifying them methodically and giving them appropriate names. Therefore, classification and name-giving will be the foundation of our science."
—*Carolus Linnaeus, 1735*

INTRODUCTION

Diabetes mellitus is a group of metabolic diseases characterized by hyperglycemia resulting from defects in insulin action, insulin secretion, or both. The chronic hyperglycemia of diabetes results in disturbances of carbohydrate, fat, and protein metabolism and is associated with long-term damage, dysfunction, and failure of various

This work was partially supported by the Chicago Diabetes Research and Training Center P30 DK020595.

[a] Department of Medicine, Section of Endocrinology, Diabetes and Metabolism, The University of Chicago, 5841 South Maryland Avenue, MC 1027, Chicago, IL 60637, USA; [b] Department of Pediatrics, Section of Endocrinology, Diabetes and Metabolism, The University of Chicago, 900 East 57th Street, Chicago, IL 60637, USA
* Corresponding author. Department of Medicine, The University of Chicago, 900 East 57th Street, Chicago, IL 60637.
E-mail address: cthomas5@bsd.uchicago.edu

http://dx.doi.org/10.1016/j.mcna.2014.08.015
0025-7125/15/$ – see front matter
medical.theclinics.com

organs, especially the eyes, kidneys, nerves, heart, and blood vessels.[1,2] The goal in diagnosing diabetes mellitus is to identify those with significantly increased premature mortality and increased risk of microvascular and cardiovascular complications. Although there are several existing useful classifications (see American Diabetes Association 2014 guidelines for example), one can envision three schema to classify the disease: (1) based on the pathophysiology, (2) based on a specific gene defect itself, or (3) based on another common phenotype. Some classifications are more appropriate for research, others for patient care. The goal of classification is to say something meaningful about the cause, natural history, genetics, heritability, clinical phenotype, and optimum therapies. In the case of diabetes, this is getting harder to do rather than easier. No classification scheme is ideal, and all have some inconsistences and overlap. Diabetes mellitus classification will continue to evolve as we work to fully understand the pathogenesis of the major forms.

DIAGNOSTIC CRITERIA FOR DIABETES MELLITUS

The World Health Organization (WHO) diagnostic criteria for diabetes mellitus include fasting plasma glucose level $\geq$126 mg/dL (7.0 mmol/L) or 2-hour plasma glucose level $\geq$200 mg/dL (11.1 mmol/L) after a 75-g oral glucose load.[1] More recently, a glycated hemoglobin level of $\geq$6.5% is recommended by WHO as the cut point for diagnosing diabetes.[3] Impaired glucose tolerance, a condition of intermediate hyperglycemia with increased risk of progression to frank diabetes, is defined as a 2-hour plasma glucose level $\geq$140 mg/dL (7.8 mmol/L) and less than 200 mg/dL (11.1 mmol/L) after a 75-g oral glucose load. Impaired fasting glucose is defined as fasting glucose level between 110 mg/dL and 125 mg/dL (6.1–6.9 mmol/L).

These categories, impaired glucose tolerance and impaired fasting glucose, as well as a glycated hemoglobin value between 5.7% and 6.4% are collectively associated with increased risk of diabetes development and are often known as prediabetes.[4]

EXISTING CLASSIFICATIONS

Until recently, the prevailing conceptual classification was that there were two primary types of diabetes mellitus: autoimmune (type 1) and nonautoimmune (type 2). Every other metabolic disorder of glucose regulation was classified into a special category of (mostly type 2 related, nonautoimmune) diabetes, such as, monogenic, gestational, steroid induced, cystic fibrosis related, postpancreatectomy, acromegaly associated, human immunodeficiency virus (HIV) associated, hepatitis C virus associated, polycystic ovary syndrome related, and ketosis prone diabetes.

Classification of diabetes mellitus has suffered from a lack of clear etiology of either type 1 or type 2. Advances in classification terminology have included the evolution of autoimmune diabetes from juvenile to insulin dependent to type 1 diabetes mellitus (T1DM). However T1DM has been further divided into antibody positive (type 1a) and antibody negative (type 1b).[5] Others have shown that the slower adult-onset forms (latent autoimmune diabetes of adults [LADA]) can also be further subdivided and may include more subtle forms of immune involvement, which furthermore may include a subset of individuals otherwise thought to have type 2 (**Fig. 1**).[6]

Type 1 Diabetes Mellitus

T1DM is generally autoimmune in etiology with, 1 of 4 autoantibodies to β-cell antigens are being positive, including islet cell antibodies, glutamic acid decarboxylase-65 antibody, insulinoma antigen-2 antibody, or insulin autoantibodies.[6,7] Autoantibodies that

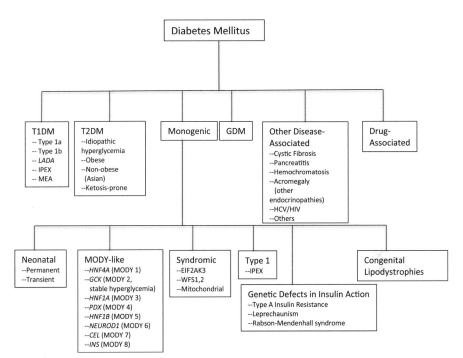

Fig. 1. Diabetes Classification.

bind to specific proteins found in the pancreatic islet cells were first described more than 30 years ago.[8] Although there is some debate as to the definition of autoimmune disease, the frequent presence of autoantibodies, reproduction of autoimmune disease in experimental animals, and experimental disease with immunopathologic lesions that parallel those in the natural disease all suggest autoimmunity.[9] However, autoimmunity is a mechanism for the manifestation of T1DM but may not be its primary cause.[10,11] The disease presents in genetically susceptible individuals, likely as a result of an environmental trigger. The immune system attacks the β-cells in the islets of Langerhans of the pancreas, destroying or damaging them sufficiently to reduce and eventually eliminate insulin production. Despite extensive research on the autoimmune nature of T1DM, questions remain regarding the timeframe and nature of β-cell destruction and dysfunction. Type 1 could almost be considered monogenic with its high linkage to human leukocyte antigen (HLA) region, but this is not the case for some nonwhite populations.[12,13] Concordance rates between monozygotic twins are approximately 50%, whereas between dizygotic twins it is approximately 10%.[14,15] Although with longer follow-up, disease may ultimately develop in discordant twins.[16] Clinical onset of T1DM is thought to result from a combination of overt β-cell loss and β-cell dysfunction. However, our understanding of how β-cell metabolic abnormalities arise during the pathogenesis of the disease remains incomplete.

Latent Autoimmune Diabetes of Adults—a Subtype of Type 1

Latent Autoimmune Diabetes of Adults (LADA) has also been called *type 1.5 diabetes,* slowly *progressive insulin-dependent diabetes mellitus, latent type 1 diabetes, youth-onset diabetes of maturity, latent-onset type 1 diabetes,* and *antibody-positive non–insulin-dependent diabetes.* In the United Kingdom Prospective Diabetes Study

(UKPDS), approximately 10% of adults with presumed type 2 diabetes mellitus (T2DM) at diagnosis had evidence of islet autoimmunity in the form of circulating islet cell antibodies or glutamic acid decarboxylase-65 antibodies.[17] Most of these adults progressed to insulin dependence within 6 years. Controversy exists as to whether LADA and adult-onset T1DM are the same clinical entity. There is epidemiologic evidence suggesting that T1DM peaks around the time of puberty and again with a lesser peak at age 40 years.[18] The Immunology of Diabetes Society[19] proposed that patients classified as having LADA be ≥30 years of age, positive for at least 1 of the 4 antibodies commonly found in T1DM, and not treated with insulin within the first 6 months after diagnosis. This final criterion of a period of insulin independence after diagnosis is intended to distinguish LADA from T1DM. One group found that the level of insulin secretion in LADA was intermediate between type 1 diabetes and type 2 diabetes.[20] This study found that fasting and stimulated C-peptide were reduced in patients with LADA compared with type 2 diabetes patients and healthy control subjects and that a rapid decline in stimulated C-peptide secretion occurred within a few years of diagnosis in LADA patients treated with oral hypoglycemic agents. In UKPDS and another European study on LADA, the highest-risk HLA phenotypes for T1DM (DR3/4 and DQ2/8) were more prevalent in LADA patients than in healthy control subjects, consistent with the known genetic predisposition to islet autoimmunity.[21,22] Epidemiologic studies suggest that LADA may account for 2% to 12% of all cases of diabetes.[6] Clinicians should maintain vigilance in identifying this entity amongst the many cases of T2DM.

Type 2 Diabetes Mellitus

T2DM is perhaps best termed *idiopathic hyperglycemia* as coined by Dr Sir Edwin Gale in 2013.[23] It is characterized by insulin resistance and relative insulin deficiency. T2DM is often associated with obesity and the metabolic syndrome, but 15% of white individuals with T2DM are nonobese. Moreover, the majority of south Asians are nonobese, suggesting that T2DM in nonobese Asians is a different entity (or entities) altogether.[24,25]

Additionally, although many obese individuals, who tend to have insulin resistance, progress to diabetes, some do not have overt diabetes. Their β-cells continue to function adequately, and they are able to maintain glucose homeostasis and compensate for increasing insulin resistance with increasing insulin secretion.

Acknowledging the limitations of human autopsy studies, pancreatic tissue from individuals with T2DM had a relatively reduced β-cell mass, whether they were lean or obese. Obese subjects without diabetes had an approximately 50% increase in relative β-cell volume.[26] Subjects with impaired fasting glucose levels also had decreased relative β-cell volume, suggesting that this is an early process and mechanistically relevant in the development of T2DM.[26]

Normally, pancreatic β-cells respond to insulin resistance, which occurs transiently at times of stress and disrupted sleep, by increasing their output of insulin to meet the needs of tissues. T2DM develops when there is a failure of the β-cell to adequately compensate for insulin resistance. Available data support a genetic predisposition to β-cell failure.[27] Multiple genetic mutations have been identified. However, in clinical practice, it is often not possible to identify a genetic abnormality, and environmental factors predominate as the underlying etiology as well as therapeutic interventions for individuals with T2DM. Two hypotheses for impaired β-cell function in T2DM include glucotoxicity, whereby chronic hyperglycemia depletes insulin secretory granules from β-cells, and lipotoxicity, in which chronic increases in free fatty acid levels decrease the conversion of proinsulin to insulin, both diminishing insulin secretion.[28]

An alternative hypothesis is the accumulation of pancreatic amyloid, which has also been associated with development and progression of T2DM.[29] Using the homeostasis model assessment to quantify β-cell function, the UKPDS found that β-cell function continued to deteriorate in association with progressively increasing hyperglycemia despite treatment.[17]

The heterogeneity of the disease process is supported by The Baltimore Longitudinal Study of Aging,[30] that concluded that fasting and postchallenge hyperglycemia may represent T2DM phenotypes with distinct natural histories in the evolution of the disease. One specific example of the unique natural histories is ketosis-prone type 2 diabetes, also known as *atypical diabetes*, *Flatbush diabetes*, and *diabetes type 1.5*, ketosis prone diabetes exemplifies the heterogeneity of the disease classified as T2DM. It was described among African Americans who presented with diabetic ketoacidosis but whose subsequent disease course more closely resembled T2DM.[31] The underlying pathogenesis is unclear. However, studies have shown a transient secretory defect of β-cells at the time of presentation with remarkable recovery of insulin-secretory capacity during the period(s) of remission.[32] Since its original description, ketosis-prone T2DM has been reported in many other ethnicities.[33–35]

Gestational Diabetes Mellitus

Hyperglycemia in pregnancy is diabetes that presents during pregnancy and resolves postpartum. It is important to distinguish gestational diabetes mellitus (GDM) from T2DM, T1DM, polycystic ovary syndrome-related diabetes, or LADA that was present prior to pregnancy whether diagnosed or undiagnosed. However, in practice all of these pre-existing or emerging forms of diabetes are often lumped together.

Contributing factors to the development of true GDM include (1) the physiologic insulin resistance of late pregnancy induced by human placental lactogen and tumor necrosis factor-α and (2) lower insulin secretion for the degree of insulin resistance, often secondary to genetic predisposition for β-cell failure.

Most women who have GDM have evidence for β-cell dysfunction related to chronic insulin resistance, but a small number do not. Some of these women may have autoimmune β-cell dysfunction (T1DM or LADA) and some may have a monogenic form of diabetes (maturity-onset diabetes of the young [MODY] 3, 2, 1, and less often 5), which may have a young age at onset and mild hyperglycemia (MODY 2), so it may be detected during routine pregnancy screening.

The Hyperglycemia and Adverse Pregnancy Outcome (HAPO) study[36] and others showed that the risk of adverse pregnancy outcomes increases continuously with increases in maternal glycemia, whether evaluated using fasting glucose concentrations, post-oral glucose tolerance test (OGTT) glucose concentrations, or glycosylated hemoglobin.

Primary outcomes in the blinded HAPO cohort were birth weight greater than the 90th percentile, primary cesarean section delivery, clinically defined neonatal hypoglycemia, and cord C-peptide greater than the 90th percentile. Secondary outcomes included preeclampsia, preterm delivery, shoulder dystocia/birth injury, hyperbilirubinemia, and intensive neonatal care.

After reviewing the results of the HAPO study and others, the International Association of Diabetes and Pregnancy Study Group recommended the following definition of GDM be used in clinical practice: fasting plasma glucose ≥92 mg/dL (5.1 mmol/L), 1-hour post 75-g glucose load plasma glucose value ≥180 mg/dL (10.0 mmol/L), and 2-hour post 75-g glucose load plasma glucose value ≥153 mg/dL (8.5 mmol/L).[37] The ADA initially endorsed the International Association of Diabetes and Pregnancy Study Group guidelines and then suggested use of those guidelines or the older American

College of Obstetrics and Gynecology approach in 2014.[2] The American College of Obstetrics and Gynecology approach involves 2-step testing. The first step is a 50-g glucose challenge. Those individuals that meet or exceed the screening threshold with a blood glucose of 140 mg/dL or greater then undergo a 100-g, 3-hour OGTT.[38]

Monogenic Diabetes

Monogenic diabetes is potentially the most important class for clinicians to consider as a possible etiology, as most causes can be determined down to a single base change in DNA or a deletion/insertion of a methylation defect. Although many of these highly penetrant causes were first discovered in the 1990s, more than 94% of MODY cases remain undiagnosed in the United States.[39] There are 2 basic subtypes: neonatal and MODY-like. Classification is increasingly complicated by the realization that the full expression of phenotypes owing to highly penetrant genes is not yet known. For example, although mutations in *FOXP3* cause IPEX (immune dysregulation, polyendocrinopathy, enteropathy, X-linked) syndrome, an early-onset, antibody-positive form of monogenic T1DM without other syndromic findings may appear first and obscure the existence of syndromic diabetes.

Neonatal diabetes mellitus (NDM) is defined as diabetes mellitus with onset before approximately 6 months of age. Some forms might better be termed *congenital diabetes* (Greeley SA, personal communication, 2009). The term encompasses diabetes of any etiology, but it is recognized that diabetes diagnosed before age 6 months is almost always monogenic in nature, although it can be (rarely) autoimmune.[40] NDM subtypes include transient NDM (TNDM) and permanent NDM (PNDM). TNDM often develops within the first few weeks of life and resolves by a few months of age. However, relapse occurs in adolescence or adulthood in approximately 50% of cases. TNDM is most frequently caused by abnormalities in the imprinted region of chromosome 6q24, leading to overexpression of paternally derived genes. Mutations in the genes *KCNJ11* and *ABCC8*, which encode the 2 subunits of the adenosine triphosphate–sensitive potassium channel on the β-cell membrane, can cause TNDM or PNDM. Importantly, diabetes secondary to mutations in *KCNJ11* and *ABCC8* often responds to sulfonylureas. Mutations in other genes critical to β-cell function and regulation, and in the insulin gene itself, also cause NDM. In approximately 40% of NDM cases, the genetic cause remains unknown.[40] The population prevalence of PNDM was recently studied and estimated to be 1 in 250,000 in youth less than 20 years of age.[41]

MODY describes a heterogeneous group of disorders caused by mutations in genes important for β-cell development, function and regulation, glucose sensing, and in the insulin gene itself.[27,42] MODY should be suspected and recognized if a type 2 diabetes–like condition occurs in 2 to 3 or more generations in an autosomal dominant pattern of inheritance. However, de novo cases certainly occur. Mutations in at least 8 different genes can cause MODY.[43] The natural history varies based on the underlying genetic defect.

Mutations in *HNF1A* (MODY 3) are the most common cause of MODY, responsible for 52% of monogenic diabetes in a large UK series, and in a US cohort, 27 of 49 MODY mutations identified (55%) were in the *HNF1A* gene.[39,44] *HNF1A* encodes a transcription factor important for pancreatic development and β-cell differentiation and function. The mutation is highly penetrant, and diabetes develops by age 25 years in more than 60% of mutation carriers.[45] Sulfonylureas are the treatment of choice in *HNF1A* diabetes. In one study, 70% of individuals with a genetic diagnosis of *HNF1A* diabetes successfully switched from insulin to sulfonylurea treatment and remained off insulin for a median of 39 months with relatively good glycemic control.[46]

HNF4A (MODY 1) also encodes a transcription factor important for pancreatic development and β-cell differentiation and function. *HNF4A* mutations account for approximately 10% of MODY.[44] *HNF4A* mutations cause a similar clinical phenotype as *HNF1A* mutations characterized by progressive insulin deficiency, diabetes onset before age 25 years, and a response to relatively low-dose sulfonylurea therapy. *HNF1A* mutations were identified in 8 of 49 (16%) MODY mutations found in a study of 586 American youth with diabetes mellitus.[39]

Glucokinase catalyzes the first step in glycogen storage and glycolysis, phosphorylation of glucose to glucose-6-phosphate. Glucokinase acts as the glucose sensor in β-cells and liver linking insulin secretion to increases in serum glucose. Heterozygous inactivating mutations in *GCK* (MODY 2) increase the set point for insulin secretion in response to increased blood sugar, causing a stable, mild fasting hyperglycemia. Complications are extremely rare, and generally glucokinase-related diabetes does not require any therapy. Importantly, treatment with insulin or oral hypoglycemic agents does not change overall glycemia.[47] Family history often reveals borderline diabetes or gestational diabetes in parents and grandparents. Women with *GCK* mutations are commonly treated with insulin during pregnancy to avoid fetal macrosomia. However, the optimal treatment of *GCK* hyperglycemia during pregnancy is uncertain.[48] With weight gain or obesity and aging, the average blood sugars may increase, but recent work continues to suggest that individuals with *GCK* hyperglycemia do not progress to diabetes complications development.[47]

Mutations in *HNF1B* (MODY 5) most often cause developmental renal disease, particularly renal cysts. *HNF1B* mutations can also cause isolated diabetes or diabetes associated with kidney disease (renal cysts and diabetes syndrome). Urogenital tract anomalies and atrophy of the pancreas may also occur.

MODY caused by mutations in *PDX*, *NEUROD1*, *CEL*, and *INS* (also a rare cause of type 1b diabetes) is very rare. Overall, 10% to 20% of patients with a classic MODY phenotype do not have a mutation in any of the known MODY genes.[48]

Mitochondrial diabetes is also monogenic in etiology and can be discriminated from MODY based on maternal transmission and, in those with maternally inherited diabetes and deafness syndrome, bilateral hearing impairment in most carriers. The disease associates with a range of mutations in mitochondrial DNA, with the most common (maternally inherited diabetes and deafness) an A3434G mutation.[49] This mutation is estimated to account for 0.2% to 2% of diabetes cases with high penetrance, as greater than 85% of carriers will have diabetes during their lifetime.[50] Diabetes associated with Wolfram syndrome (WFS1 and WFS2) is also monogenic in etiology. Cystic fibrosis–related diabetes (CFRD) could also be considered a monogenic form of the disease (see later discussion).

SECONDARY DIABETES MELLITUS
Pancreatic Disease Processes

Cystic fibrosis
Cystic fibrosis related diabetes (CFRD) is the most common secondary complication of cystic fibrosis. Patients with cystic fibrosis, even those with normal glucose tolerance, tend to have decreasing insulin secretion over time. One study found that patients with cystic fibrosis who are 8 years and older have delayed and eventually diminished insulin secretion in response to oral and intravenous stimuli and increased glucose concentrations compared with controls.[51] Insulin sensitivity is generally

normal or only slightly decreased, except in the settings of acute illness or glucocorticoid treatment when insulin resistance can be severe.[52]

Initially, the disorder was thought to be caused by damage to the endocrine pancreas after scarring and fibrosis of the exocrine pancreas. However, histopathology studies have found that patients with cystic fibrosis with CFRD do not necessarily have more pancreatic fibrosis at autopsy than patients with cystic fibrosis without CFRD. More recent evidence suggests that the cystic fibrosis transmembrane conductance regulator (CFTR) defect itself might be involved in impaired insulin secretion.[52]

Chronic pancreatitis

Chronic pancreatitis is a disease characterized by pancreatic inflammatory and fibrotic injury, resulting in irreversible parenchymal damage. The condition is associated with many genetic mutations and polymorphisms that predispose to disease along with environmental triggers.[53] Development of diabetes mellitus in chronic pancreatitis mainly occurs from the destruction of islet cells by pancreatic inflammation. In some tropical countries there is an idiopathic variety of early-onset, chronic, calcific, nonalcoholic pancreatitis that is associated with malnutrition that has been termed *tropical chronic pancreatitis*.[54] A WHO study group termed the associated diabetes *fibrocalculous pancreatic diabetes*.[55] Persons with secondary diabetes from chronic pancreatitis are often misclassified as having T2DM and, if treated with sulfonylureas, are at increased risk of hypoglycemia given the diminished action of glucagon.

Hereditary hemochromatosis

Hereditary hemochromatosis was originally described as a triad of diabetes, cirrhosis, and skin pigmentation. Recent studies show the prevalence of diabetes to be 13% to 22% and impaired glucose tolerance 18% to 30%.[56,57] The pathophysiology of diabetes associated with hereditary hemochromatosis is controversial, with evidence suggesting that both insulin deficiency and insulin resistance are contributing factors. Similar disease processes are seen in patients with transfusion iron overload, especially beta thalassemia major.

Pancreatic neoplasia

Most diabetes associated with pancreatic cancer is diagnosed either concomitantly with the cancer or during the 2 years before the cancer is found.[58] Glucose intolerance is present in 80% of cases of pancreatic neoplasia and diabetes in approximately 50%.[59] This and other data suggest that recently developed glucose intolerance or diabetes may be a consequence of pancreatic cancer, and for some patients, recent onset of glucose intolerance or diabetes may be an early sign of pancreatic cancer. Several studies have found that diabetes in pancreatic cancer patients is characterized by peripheral insulin resistance.[60] Insulin resistance is also found in nondiabetic or glucose-intolerant pancreatic cancer patients, although to a lesser degree.[61]

Result of Surgery/Trauma

Postpancreatectomy

Pancreatectomy for chronic pancreatitis results in secondary diabetes. Islet autotransplantation after the pancreatectomy offers some patients a chance for insulin independence.[62]

Drug Associated

Many medications are associated with derangements in glucose metabolism via different mechanisms. Some drugs impair insulin secretion and may not cause diabetes by themselves but may precipitate diabetes in individuals with preexisting insulin resistance. Certain toxins such as Vacor (a rat poison), streptozotocin, and intravenous pentamidine can permanently destroy pancreatic β-cells. Also many drugs and hormones impair insulin action. The following medications are some of the more commonly used drugs associated with the development of diabetes.

Glucocorticoids

One of the most distressing side effects for patients treated long term with glucocorticoids is weight gain, often with abnormal fat deposition. In humans treated with glucocorticoids, the accumulation of adipocytes occurs primarily in the visceral fat and interscapular depots, leading to characteristic truncal obesity and dorsocervical fat pad or "buffalo hump." This occurs through effects of glucocorticoids on differentiation of preadipocytes into mature adipocytes. Glucocorticoids also induce insulin resistance, hyperglycemia, and hyperlipidemia. Although increases in visceral fat contribute to the insulin resistance that occurs with glucocorticoid therapy, direct actions of glucocorticoids on muscle, liver, and other tissues also play a role. Glucocorticoids have been found to inhibit several steps in the insulin-signaling network through several different mechanisms. In skeletal muscle, glucocorticoids cause insulin resistance by decreasing transcription of IRS-1, while increasing transcription of 2 proteins that counter insulin action, protein tyrosine phosphatase type 1B (PTP1B) and p38MAPK. A similar increase in transcription of p38MAPK is observed in the liver.[63]

Atypical antipsychotics

Although clozapine, olanzapine, and other atypical antipsychotic drugs (APDs) have fewer extrapyramidal side effects, they have serious metabolic side effects such as substantial weight gain, intra-abdominal obesity, and hyperglycemia[64] with a predominant type 2 phenotype when overt diabetes develops. Accumulated data from both clinical and animal studies suggest that increasing appetite and food intake as well as delayed satiety signaling are key behavioral changes related to APD-induced weight gain. Less well understood is the extent to which changes of resting metabolic rate, decreased activity and sedation affect weight gain associated with this class of medications. Analysis of the US Food and Drug Administration Adverse Event database also showed that adjusted report ratios for type 2 diabetes were the following: olanzapine, 9.6 (95% confidence interval [CI], 9.2–10.0); risperidone, 3.8 (95% CI, 3.5–4.1); quetiapine, 3.5 (95% CI, 3.2–3.9); clozapine, 3.1 (95% CI, 2.9–3.3); ziprasidone, 2.4 (95% CI, 2.0–2.9); aripiprazole, 2.4 (95% CI, 1.9–2.9); and haloperidol, 2.0 (95% CI, 1.7–2.3), which suggests differential risks of diabetes across various APDs but also a class effect.[65]

Calcineurin inhibitors/mammalian target of rapamycin inhibitors

Some immunosuppressive medications used to prevent and treat rejection of transplanted organs contribute to glucose dysregulation and the development of new-onset diabetes mellitus after transplantation. The development of diabetes in transplant recipients receiving prednisolone has been reported to be as high as 46%, although this study used capillary blood glucose rather than venous for making the diagnosis.[66] Calcineurin inhibitors (e.g., cyclosporine and tacrolimus) have also been associated with an increased risk for diabetes after transplantation. Clinical studies indicate that the risk for diabetes was found to be up to 5 times higher with tacrolimus 1 year after kidney transplantation compared with cyclosporine.[67] Sirolimus and everolimus, mammalian targets of rapamycin inhibitors, have also been associated with higher incidence of new-onset diabetes mellitus after transplantation especially when used in combination with calcineurin inhibitors.[68]

Human immunodeficiency virus/acquired immunodeficiency syndrome antiretroviral therapy

HIV protease inhibitors reversibly inhibit the insulin-responsive glucose transporter, Glut 4, leading to peripheral insulin resistance and impaired glucose tolerance.[69] Additional data suggest that therapeutic levels of protease inhibitors are sufficient to impair glucose sensing by β-cells.[70] Another class of drugs used in the treatment of HIV/acquired immunodeficiency syndrome is nucleoside analogs (reverse transcriptase inhibitors). It was previously thought that nucleoside reverse transcriptase inhibitors were less likely to cause metabolic abnormalities. However, a 2008 study, which analyzed 130,151 person-years of exposure, showed that these drugs increase the risk of diabetes as well.[70] Proposed mechanisms include insulin resistance, lipodystrophy, and mitochondrial dysfunction. More recently, less metabolically toxic agents are being used for initial treatment of HIV.[71]

Others Thiazide diuretics, hydroxymethylglutaryl-CoA reductase inhibitors, nicotinic acid, and diazoxide, mechanisms underlying the diabetogenic influence of hydroxymethylglutaryl-CoA reductase inhibitors (also known as statins), are incompletely understood. Simvastatin and atorvastatin have been found to decrease insulin secretion in β-cells.[72] Diazoxide is rarely used today except in cases of hyperinsulinism. It opens potassium channels resulting in hyperpolarization of insulin-secreting cells, preventing or diminishing insulin secretion (**Box 1**).

Endocrinopathies

Counter-regulatory hormones, including glucagon, epinephrine, cortisol, and growth hormone, antagonize insulin action. Excess amounts of these hormones found in glucagonoma, pheochromocytoma, Cushing's syndrome, and gigantism/acromegaly respectively, can cause diabetes. This generally occurs in individuals with preexisting defects in insulin secretion, and hyperglycemia typically resolves when the hormone excess is corrected. Separately, somatostatinoma and aldosteronoma-induced hypokalemia can contribute to the development of diabetes by inhibiting insulin secretion. Hyperglycemia generally resolves after successful removal of the tumor.

Human Immunodeficiency Virus Associated

Distinct from medication side effects, the natural history of HIV infection is also associated with the development of diabetes.[73] Viral factors that contribute to

---

Box 1
Drug-associated diabetes mellitus

Glucocorticoids

Diazoxide

Calcineurin/mammalian targets of rapamycin inhibitors

Atypical antipsychotics

Antiretroviral agents

Thiazide diuretics

Nicotinic acid

Statins

β-adrenergic agonists

Others

diabetes risk include an increase in viral burden of 0.5 log over a 6-month period, a lower CD4 count, and longer duration of HIV infection.[73] The increased accumulation of visceral fat, with wasting of subcutaneous fat, noted in these patients, creates higher levels of inflammatory cytokines such as tumor necrosis factor α. This leads to diabetes or impaired glucose tolerance by increasing insulin resistance (**Box 2**).

INTERNATIONAL STATISTICAL CLASSIFICATION OF DISEASES–9 AND –10 CODING FOR DIABETES MELLITUS

Another attempt at classification of diabetes mellitus has been presented in the Clinical Modification of the International Statistical Classification of Diseases and Related Health Problems (ICD-10-CM) (10th revision), provided by the Centers for Medicare and Medicaid Services and the National Center for Health Statistics, for medical coding and reporting in the United States.[74] The ICD-10-CM is based on the International Statistical Classification of Diseases (ICD)-10, the statistical classification of disease published by the World Health Organization.[75] In the ICD-9 guide,[76] diabetes mellitus is given the code group "250.XX" but excluded from this are gestational diabetes (648.8), hyperglycemia not otherwise specified (790.29), neonatal diabetes mellitus (775.1), nonclinical diabetes (790.29), and secondary diabetes (249.0–249.9). T1DM is indicated by 250.1X and T2DM by 250.0X. However, ICD-10 focuses on the degree of control of diabetes with 5 major categories:

- E08, Diabetes mellitus caused by underlying condition
- E09, Drug- or chemical-induced diabetes mellitus
- E10, T1DM
- E11, T2DM
- E13, Other specified diabetes mellitus

E13 includes a variety of syndromes: diabetes mellitus caused by genetic defects of β-cell function, diabetes mellitus caused by genetic defects in insulin action, postpancreatectomy diabetes mellitus, postprocedural diabetes mellitus, secondary diabetes mellitus not elsewhere classified. It will be interesting to see if this scheme proves useful.

Box 2
Other genetic syndromes (that may be associated with diabetes mellitus)
Down syndrome (T1DM and T2DM)
Klinefelter syndrome
Turner syndrome
Huntington chorea
Friedreich ataxia
Prader-Willi syndrome
Myotonic dystrophy
Porphyria
Laurence-Moon-Biedl syndrome
Others

SUMMARY

This article highlights the difficulties in creating a definitive classification of diabetes mellitus in the absence of a complete understanding of the pathogenesis of the major forms. This brief review shows the evolving nature of the classification of diabetes mellitus. No classification scheme is ideal, and all have some overlap and inconsistencies. The only diabetes in which it is possible to accurately diagnose by DNA sequencing, monogenic diabetes, remains undiagnosed in more than 90% of the individuals who have diabetes caused by one of the known gene mutations. The point of classification, or taxonomy, of disease, should be to give insight into both pathogenesis and treatment. It remains a source of frustration that all schemes of diabetes mellitus continue to fall short of this goal.

REFERENCES

1. World Health Organization: World Health Organization, International Diabetes Federation, editors. Definition and diagnosis of diabetes mellitus and intermediate hyperglycemia. Report of a WHO/IDF Consultation. Geneva (Switzerland): WHO Press; 2006.
2. American Diabetes Association. Diagnosis and classification of diabetes mellitus. Diabetes Care 2014;37(Suppl 1):S81–90.
3. World Health Organization. Use of glycated haemoglobin (HbA1c) in diagnosis of diabetes mellitus: abbreviated report of a WHO consultation. WHO Press; 2011.
4. American Diabetes Association. Standards of medical care in diabetes–2013. Diabetes Care 2012;36(Suppl 1):S11–66. http://dx.doi.org/10.2337/dc13-S011.
5. Atkinson MA, Eisenbarth GS, Michels AW. Type 1 diabetes. Lancet 2013;383: 69–82.
6. Naik RG, Brooks-Worrell BM, Palmer JP. Latent autoimmune diabetes in adults. J Clin Endocrinol Metab 2009;94(12):4635–44. http://dx.doi.org/10.1210/jc. 2009-1120.
7. Arvan P, Pietropaolo M, Ostrov D, et al. Islet autoantigens: structure, function, localization, and regulation. Cold Spring Harb Perspect Med 2012;2(8). pii: a007658.
8. Bottazzo GF, Florin-Christensen A, Doniach D. Islet-cell antibodies in diabetes mellitus with autoimmune polyendocrine deficiencies. Lancet 1974;2(7892): 1279–83.
9. Rose NR, Bona C. Defining criteria for autoimmune diseases (Witebsky's postulates revisited). Immunol Today 1993;14(9):426–30. http://dx.doi.org/10.1016/ 0167-5699(93)90244-F.
10. Atkinson MA, Bluestone JA, Eisenbarth GS, et al. How does type 1 diabetes develop? The notion of homicide or β-cell suicide revisited. Diabetes 2012; 60(5):1370–9.
11. Maganti A, Evans-Molina C, Mirmira RG. From immunobiology to β-cell biology: the changing perspective on type 1 diabetes. Islets 2014;6(1):e28778-1–5. http://dx.doi.org/10.4161/isl.28778.
12. Noble JA, Johnson J, Lane JA, et al. HLA Class II genotyping of african american type 1 diabetic patients reveals associations unique to african haplotypes. Diabetes 2013;62(9):3292–9.
13. Valdes AM, Erlich HA, Carlson J, et al. Use of class I and class II HLA loci for predicting age at onset of type 1 diabetes in multiple populations. Diabetologia 2012;55(9):2394–401. http://dx.doi.org/10.1007/s00125-012-2608-z.

14. Redondo MJ, Fain PR, Krischer JP, et al. Expression of beta-cell autoimmunity does not differ between potential dizygotic twins and siblings of patients with type 1 diabetes. J Autoimmun 2004;23(3):275–9. http://dx.doi.org/10.1016/j.jaut.2004.07.001.

15. Melanitou E, Fain P, Eisenbarth GS. Genetics of type 1A (immune mediated) diabetes. J Autoimmun 2003. http://dx.doi.org/10.1016/S0896-8411(03)00097-0.

16. Kyvik KO. Concordance rates of insulin dependent diabetes mellitus: a population based study of young Danish twins. BMJ 1995;311:913–7.

17. UK prospective diabetes study 16: overview of 6 years' therapy of type II diabetes: a progressive disease. U.K. Prospective Diabetes Study Group. Diabetes 1995;44(11):1249–58.

18. Karjalainen J, Salmela P, Ilonen J. A comparison of childhood and adult type I diabetes mellitus. N Engl J Med 1989;320(14):881–6.

19. Fourlanos S, Dotta F, Greenbaum CJ, et al. Latent autoimmune diabetes in adults (LADA) should be less latent. Diabetologia 2005. http://dx.doi.org/10.1007/s00125-005-1960-7.

20. Gottsäter A, Landin-Olsson M, Fernlund P, et al. β-cell function in relation to islet cell antibodies during the first 3 Yr after clinical diagnosis of diabetes in type ii diabetic patients. Diabetes Care 1993;16(6):902–10. http://dx.doi.org/10.2337/diacare.16.6.902.

21. Turner R, Stratton I, Horton V, et al. UKPDS 25: autoantibodies to islet-cell cytoplasm and glutamic acid decarboxylase for prediction of insulin requirement in type 2 diabetes. Lancet 1997;350(9087):1288–93. http://dx.doi.org/10.1016/S0140-6736(97)03062-6.

22. Tuomi T, Carlsson A, Li H, et al. Clinical and genetic characteristics of type 2 diabetes with and without GAD antibodies. Diabetes 1999;48(1):150–7. http://dx.doi.org/10.2337/diabetes.48.1.150.

23. Gale E. Is type 2 diabetes a category error? Lancet 2013;381(9881):1956–7.

24. Mohan V, Amutha A, Ranjani H, et al. Associations of β-cell function and insulin resistance with youth-onset type 2 diabetes and prediabetes among Asian Indians. Diabetes Technol Ther 2013;15(4):315–22. http://dx.doi.org/10.1089/dia.2012.0259.

25. Mitsui R, Fukushima M, Nishi Y, et al. Factors responsible for deteriorating glucose tolerance in newly diagnosed type 2 diabetes in Japanese men. Metabolism 2006;55(1):53–8. http://dx.doi.org/10.1016/j.metabol.2005.07.006.

26. Butler AE, Janson J, Bonner-Weir S, et al. β-cell deficit and increased β-Cell apoptosis in humans with type 2 diabetes. Diabetes 2003;52(1):102–10. http://dx.doi.org/10.2337/diabetes.52.1.102.

27. Bell GI, Polonsky KS. Diabetes mellitus and genetically programmed defects in β-cell function. Nature 2001;414(6865):788–91. http://dx.doi.org/10.1038/414788a.

28. Del Prato S. Role of glucotoxicity and lipotoxicity in the pathophysiology of Type 2 diabetes mellitus and emerging treatment strategies. Diabet Med 2009;26(12):1185–92.

29. Epstein FH, Höppener J, Ahrén B. Islet amyloid and type 2 diabetes mellitus. N Engl J Med 2000. http://dx.doi.org/10.1056/NEJM200008103430607.

30. Meigs JB, Muller DC, Nathan DM, et al. The natural history of progression from normal glucose tolerance to type 2 diabetes in the Baltimore Longitudinal Study of Aging. Diabetes 2003;52(6):1475–84.

31. Winter WE, Maclaren NK, Riley WJ. Maturity-onset diabetes of youth in black Americans. N Engl J Med 1987;316(6):285–91.

32. Mauvais-Jarvis F, Sobngwi E, Porcher R, et al. Ketosis-prone type 2 diabetes in patients of Sub-Saharan African origin clinical pathophysiology and natural history of β-cell dysfunction and insulin resistance. Diabetes 2004;53(3): 645–53. http://dx.doi.org/10.2337/diabetes.53.3.645.

33. Umpierrez GE, Smiley D, Kitabchi AE. Narrative review: ketosis-prone type 2 diabetes mellitus. Ann Intern Med 2006;144(5):350–7. http://dx.doi.org/10.7326/0003-4819-144-5-200603070-00011.

34. Tanaka K, Moriya T, Kanamori A, et al. Analysis and a long-term follow up of ketosis-onset Japanese NIDDM patients. Diabetes Res Clin Pract 1999;44(2): 137–46. http://dx.doi.org/10.1016/S0168-8227(99)00023-6.

35. Tan KC, Mackay IR, Zimmet PZ, et al. Metabolic and immunologic features of Chinese patients with atypical diabetes mellitus. Diabetes Care 2000. http://dx.doi.org/10.2337/diacare.23.3.335.

36. Lowe LP, Metzger BE, Dyer AR, et al. Hyperglycemia and Adverse Pregnancy Outcome (HAPO) Study Associations of maternal A1C and glucose with pregnancy outcomes. Diabetes 2012;35(3):574–80.

37. International Association of Diabetes and Pregnancy Study Groups Consensus Panel, Metzger BE, Gabbe SG. International association of diabetes and pregnancy study groups recommendations on the diagnosis and classification of hyperglycemia in pregnancy. Diabetes Care 2010;33(3): 676–82.

38. Gynecologists ACOOA, Committee on Practice Bulletins—Obstetrics. ACOG Practice Bulletin No. 137. Gestational Diabetes Mellitus. Obstet Gynecol 2013; 122(2 Pt 1):406–16.

39. Pihoker C, Gilliam LK, Ellard S. Prevalence, characteristics and clinical diagnosis of maturity onset diabetes of the young due to mutations in HNF1A, HNF4A, and glucokinase: results from the SEARCH for Diabetes in Youth. J Clin Endocrinol Metab 2013. http://dx.doi.org/10.1210/jc.2013-1279.

40. Greeley S, Naylor RN, Philipson LH, et al. Neonatal diabetes: an expanding list of genes allows for improved diagnosis and treatment. Curr Diab Rep 2011. http://dx.doi.org/10.1007/s11892-011-0234-7.

41. Shankar RK, Pihoker C, Dolan LM, et al. Permanent neonatal diabetes mellitus: prevalence and genetic diagnosis in the SEARCH for Diabetes in Youth Study. Pediatr Diabetes 2012;14:174–80. http://dx.doi.org/10.1111/pedi.12003.

42. Fajans SS, Bell GI, Polonsky KS. Molecular mechanisms and clinical pathophysiology of maturity-onset diabetes of the young. N Engl J Med 2001. http://dx.doi.org/10.1056/nejmra002168.

43. Naylor RN, Greeley S, Bell GI. Genetics and pathophysiology of neonatal diabetes mellitus. J Diabetes Investig 2011. http://dx.doi.org/10.1111/j.2040-1124.2011.00106.x.

44. Shields BM, Hicks S, Shepherd MH, et al. Maturity-onset diabetes of the young (MODY): how many cases are we missing? Diabetologia 2010;53(12):2504–8. http://dx.doi.org/10.1007/s00125-010-1799-4.

45. Lango Allen H, Johansson S, Ellard S, et al. Polygenic risk variants for type 2 diabetes susceptibility modify age at diagnosis in monogenic HNF1A diabetes. Diabetes 2009;59(1):266–71. http://dx.doi.org/10.2337/db09-0555.

46. Shepherd M, Shields B, Ellard S, et al. A genetic diagnosis of HNF1A diabetes alters treatment and improves glycaemic control in the majority of insulintreated patients. Diabet Med 2009;26(4):437–41. http://dx.doi.org/10.1111/j.1464-5491.2009.02690.x.

47. Steele AM, Shields BM, Wensley KJ, et al. Prevalence of vascular complications among patients with glucokinase mutations and prolonged, mild hyperglycemia. JAMA 2014. http://dx.doi.org/10.1001/jama.2013.283980.
48. Naylor RN, Philipson LH. Who should have genetic testing for maturity-onset diabetes of the young? Clin Endocrinol (Oxf) 2011;75:422–6.
49. Maassen JA, Hart LM, van Essen E, et al. Mitochondrial Diabetes Molecular Mechanisms and Clinical Presentation. Diabetes 2004;53(suppl 1):S103–9. http://dx.doi.org/10.2337/diabetes.53.2007.S103.
50. Maassen JA, 't Hart LM, Janssen GM, et al. Mitochondrial diabetes and its lessons for common Type 2 diabetes. Biochem Soc Trans 2006;34(5):819. http://dx.doi.org/10.1042/BST0340819.
51. Battezzati A, Mari A, Zazzeron L, et al. Identification of insulin secretory defects and insulin resistance during oral glucose tolerance test in a cohort of cystic fibrosis patients. Eur J Endocrinol 2011;165(1):69–76.
52. Ode KL, Moran A. New insights into cystic fibrosis-related diabetes in children. Lancet Diabetes Endocrinol 2013;1(1):52–8.
53. Gupte AR, Forsmark CE. Chronic pancreatitis. Curr Opin Gastroenterol 2014; 30(5):500–5. http://dx.doi.org/10.1097/MOG.0000000000000094.
54. Papita R, Nazir A, Anbalagan VP, et al. Secular trends of fibrocalculous pancreatic diabetes and diabetes secondary to alcoholic chronic pancreatitis at a Tertiary Care Diabetes Centre in South India. JOP 2012;13(2):205–9. http://dx.doi.org/10.6092/1590-8577/608.
55. Khatib OM. Guidelines for the prevention, management and care of diabetes mellitus. World Health Organization: WHO Press; 2006.
56. Hatunic M, Finucane FM, Brennan AM, et al. Effect of iron overload on glucose metabolism in patients with hereditary hemochromatosis. Metabolism 2010. http://dx.doi.org/10.1016/j.metabol.2009.08.006.
57. McClain DA, Abraham D, Rogers J, et al. High prevalence of abnormal glucose homeostasis secondary to decreased insulin secretion in individuals with hereditary haemochromatosis. Diabetologia 2006. http://dx.doi.org/10.1007/s00125-006-0200-0.
58. Gullo L, Pezzilli R. Diabetes and the risk of pancreatic cancer. N Engl J Med 1994;331(2):81–4.
59. Pannala R, Basu A, Petersen GM, et al. New-onset diabetes: a potential clue to the early diagnosis of pancreatic cancer. Lancet Oncol 2009;10(1):88–95. http://dx.doi.org/10.1016/S1470-2045(08)70337-1.
60. Permert J, Ihse I, Jorfeldt L, et al. Pancreatic cancer is associated with impaired glucose metabolism. Eur J Surg 1993;159(2):101–7.
61. Muniraj T, Chari ST. Diabetes and pancreatic cancer. Minerva Gastroenterologica e Dietologica 2014;1–22.
62. Bramis K, Gordon-Weeks AN, Friend PJ, et al. Systematic review of total pancreatectomy and islet autotransplantation for chronic pancreatitis. Br J Surg 2012; 99(6):761–6. http://dx.doi.org/10.1002/bjs.8713.
63. Ferris HA, Kahn CR. New mechanisms of glucocorticoid-induced insulin resistance: make no bones about it. J Clin Invest 2012;122(11):3854–7.
64. Deng C. Effects of antipsychotic medications on appetite, weight, and insulin resistance. Endocrinol Metab Clin North Am 2013. http://dx.doi.org/10.1016/j.ecl.2013.05.006.
65. Baker RA, Pikalov A, Tran QV, et al. Atypical antipsychotic drugs and diabetes mellitus in the US Food and Drug Administration Adverse Event database: a

systematic Bayesian signal detection analysis. Psychopharmacol Bull 2009; 42(1):11–31.

66. Yates CJ, Fourlanos S, Colman PG, et al. Screening for new-onset diabetes after kidney transplantation: limitations of fasting glucose and advantages of after-noon glucose and glycated hemoglobin. Transplantation 2013;96(8):726–31.

67. Khong MJ, Chong CP. Prevention and management of new-onset diabetes mellitus in kidney transplantation. Neth J Med 2014;72(3):127–34.

68. Teutonico A, Schena PF, Di Paolo S. Glucose metabolism in renal transplant recipients: effect of calcineurin inhibitor withdrawal and conversion to sirolimus. J Am Soc Nephrol 2005;16(10):3128–35. http://dx.doi.org/10.1681/ASN.2005 050487.

69. Koster JC, Remedi MS, Qiu H, et al. HIV protease inhibitors acutely impair glucose-stimulated insulin release. Diabetes 2003;52(7):1695–700.

70. De Wit S, Sabin CA, Weber R, et al. Incidence and risk factors for new-onset diabetes in HIV-infected patients the data collection on adverse events of anti-HIV drugs (D:A:D) Study. Diabetes Care 2008;31(6):1224–9. http://dx.doi. org/10.2337/dc07-2013.

71. Nix LM, Tien PC. Metabolic syndrome, diabetes, and cardiovascular risk in HIV. Curr HIV/AIDS Rep 2014. http://dx.doi.org/10.1007/s11904-014-0219-7.

72. Corrao G, Ibrahim B, Nicotra F, et al. Statins and the risk of diabetes: evidence from a large population-based cohort study. Diabetes 2014. http://dx.doi.org/10. 2337/dc13-2215.

73. Kalra S, Kalra B, Agrawal N. Understanding diabetes in patients with HIV/AIDS. Diabetol Metab Syndr 2011;3(1):2.

74. Centers for Medicare and Medicaid (CMS), National Center for Health Statistics. ICD-10-CM Official Guidelines for Coding and Reporting - 2014. US Department of Health and Human Services 2014.

75. World Health Organization. International statistical classification of diseases and related health problems. WHO Press; 2004.

76. Centers for Medicare and Medicaid (CMS), National Center for Health Statistics. ICD-9-CM Official Guidelines for Coding and Reporting - 2011. US Department of Health and Human Services 2011.

Internet Blood Glucose Monitoring Systems Provide Lasting Glycemic Benefit in Type 1 and 2 Diabetes

A Systematic Review

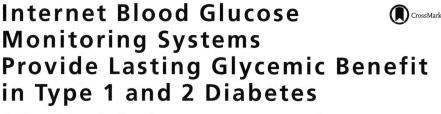

Hugh D. Tildesley, MD[a],*, Michelle D. Po, PhD[b], Stuart A. Ross, MD[c]

KEYWORDS

- Diabetes • Glycemic control • Hypoglycemia • Self-monitoring of blood glucose
- Internet medicine • Internet blood glucose monitoring system

KEY POINTS

- Internet blood glucose monitoring systems (IBGMS) result in glycemic improvement in patients with type 1 or 2 diabetes, including those with poorly controlled glycemia at baseline.
- IBGMS help decrease glycemic levels without increasing the risk of hypoglycemia.
- Other benefits, seen in some studies of IBGMS, include improvements in cardiovascular risk markers and quality of life outcomes.
- Glycemic improvements with IBGMS are not limited to patients on insulin or to those who increase their frequency of glucose self-monitoring as a result of the intervention.
- Glycemic improvements likely result from a combination of factors, including increased patient motivation and increased communication between patient and health care provider.

INTRODUCTION

Effective glycemic control is associated with reduced risk of complications of type 1 diabetes (T1D) and type 2 diabetes (T2D).[1–4] In controlled clinical trials, even when

Disclosures: H.D. Tildesley uses Internet blood glucose monitoring routinely in managing patients with diabetes. M.D. Po and S.A. Ross declare that they have no financial or other competing interest in the topics discussed here.

[a] Department of Endocrinology and Metabolism, St Paul's Hospital, University of British Columbia, Room 410, 1033 Davie Street, Vancouver, British Columbia V6E 1M7, Canada; [b] SCRIPT, 2010 Yonge St, Toronto, ON M4N 2K4, Canada; [c] University of Calgary, 2500 University Dr NW, Calgary, AB T2N 1N4, Canada
* Corresponding author.
E-mail address: hdtildesley@gmail.com

Med Clin N Am 99 (2015) 17–33
http://dx.doi.org/10.1016/j.mcna.2014.08.019
0025-7125/15/$ – see front matter

the early glycemic control is lost at a later point, patients who establish and maintain good control early in the course of their disease may enjoy reduced risk of macrovascular and microvascular complications of diabetes over a period of years to decades.[3–5] For this reason, current treatment guidelines emphasize the need for timely introduction of lifestyle and, if necessary, pharmacologic interventions, to bring patients to appropriate glycemic targets within months of diagnosis.[6] Despite this guidance, and despite clear evidence that effective glycemic control can prevent diabetic complications, only half of North American patients achieve the standard glycemic target of hemoglobin A_{1c} (HbA_{1c}) level less than 7%.[7–9]

For patients with T1D and insulin-using patients with T2D, American Diabetes Association (ADA) and Canadian Diabetes Association (CDA) treatment guidelines support regular self-monitoring of blood glucose (SMBG), which allows the patient to titrate insulin doses, evaluate their success in reaching glycemic targets, and gauge their risk of hypoglycemia.[6,10] However, the clinical usefulness and cost-effectiveness of SMBG in controlling glycemic levels in non–insulin-using patient with T2D is less clear. A recent meta-analysis showed that regular SMBG in this patient population was associated with a statistically significant but quantitatively minor glycemic benefit.[11] Uncertainty about the role of SMBG outside the context of insulin dose adjustment is reflected in the 2014 ADA guidelines; these guidelines recommend SMBG as a part of a broader educational context, and to help guide treatment decisions for non–insulin-using, as well as insulin-using, patients.[10]

We have proposed elsewhere[12–14] that increased patient-physician communication, in the form of ongoing Internet-based contact, could increase the effectiveness of SMBG as a means to improve diabetes management in combination with regular care. In this article, a systematic review of Internet blood glucose monitoring systems (IBGMS) is provided, which facilitate regular health care provider review and feedback regarding a patient's SMBG results. In such systems (**Fig. 1**), patients carry out regular glucose monitoring and upload the resulting data to a secure Web site. From there, the data are reviewed by a health care professional, who provides feedback on the results, offers encouragement, and, as appropriate, recommends changes to the patient's monitoring practices, insulin titration, or diet.

In this article, the efficacy, safety and other outcomes are evaluated from numerous small studies comparing patients using IBGMS with other patients with more

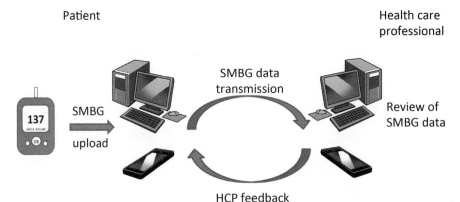

Fig. 1. IBGMs. All Internet-based interventions considered in this review include the following: (1) patient's SMBG, (2) uploading and transmitting the SMBG data to a health care professional (HCP), (3) the HCP reviewing and submitting feedback to the patient.

traditional patterns of physician contact. IBGMS is consistently associated with significant improvement in glycemic control, with no evident safety concerns. Several hypotheses to explain the benefits of this intervention in patients are then considered, with various treatment histories. The evidence is examined that, given the prevalence of personal computers and mobile devices in contemporary society, IBGMS offer a potentially cost-effective and time-sparing approach to diabetes management.

METHODS

We performed PubMed searches in March, 2014, using the following terms to find research articles reporting IBGMS trials: Internet + diabetes, Web-based + diabetes, telemedicine + diabetes, and telehealth + diabetes. Additional articles were chosen by examining the reference lists of relevant reviews. Forward searching using Web of Science identified works in which key articles were cited.

Publications on T1D or T2D were included in this analysis if they reported randomized controlled trials of standard practice versus IBGMS, which were defined as systems with 3 components: Web-based uploading of patients' SMBG data, regular review of the data by a health care professional, and digital or telephonic feedback. Studies were excluded if they included only adolescent patients or if they did not report HbA_{1c} as an outcome. No formal evaluation of levels of evidence was conducted.

SELF-MONITORING OF BLOOD GLUCOSE LEVELS ON INTERNET BLOOD GLUCOSE MONITORING SYSTEMS

It was anticipated that patients using IBGMS might monitor their glucose more frequently than other patients.

We identified 6 randomized controlled trials that reported SMBG frequency in both the IBGMS and control groups. In the 3 T1D studies identified,[15–17] there were no significant differences in SMBG frequency between patients in IBGMS and control groups. In the 3 T2D studies identified, patients on IBGMS self-monitored significantly more often than patients on conventional care: 55.7 times/mo versus 14.9 times/mo, $P<.001$,[18] 23.8 times/mo versus 12.7 times/mo, significance not reported[19] and 34 times/mo versus 22 times/mo, $P = .024$.[20]

SHORT-TERM AND LONGER-TERM GLYCEMIC CONTROL WITH INTERNET BLOOD GLUCOSE MONITORING SYSTEMS IN TYPE 2 DIABETES

We identified 9 randomized controlled IBGMS trials that enrolled type 2 patients and 4 studies that enrolled patients with either T1D or T2D (**Table 1**). All but 1 of these studies[21] showed significantly improved HbA_{1c} level in the IBGMS group compared with the control group, as seen either in a significant difference in glycosylated hemoglobin change (ΔHbA_{1c}) between groups or in a significant decrease in HbA_{1c} level in the IBGMS group but not the control group.

Of the 12 T2D studies, 7[18,20,22–26] enrolled 50% or more non–insulin-using patients, suggesting that IBGMS is effective in non-insulin-using patients. In the 1 study that failed to find a significant improvement in HbA_{1c} level with IBGMS in the total patient population, a subanalysis of non–insulin-using patients nevertheless showed a significant decline in HbA_{1c} level in the IBGMS group relative to controls: mean HbA_{1c} level decreased from 6.95% to 6.66% in the IBGMS group compared with 7.21% to 7.2% in the control group ($P = .02$). In 3 studies, some patients were treated with diet and exercise alone, with no pharmacotherapy for diabetes.[18,25,27] However, because these

Table 1
Randomized controlled studies of IBGMS versus conventional care: glycemic, cardiovascular risk, and quality of life outcomes

Study	Participants (Intervention vs Usual Care)	Treatments in Use	Duration (mo)	Description of IBGMS (Method of Upload; Review; Feedback)	Mean HbA1c Levels in IBGMS, from Baseline to Follow-Up (%)	Mean HbA1c Levels in Control Group, from Baseline to Follow-Up (%)	P Value, Δ HbA1c Levels Between Groups	CVD Outcomes at Follow-Up in IBGMS Compared with Control Group	QOL at Follow-Up in IBGMS Compared with Control Group
T2D									
Shea et al,[25] 2009; Trief et al,[46] 2007	≥55, 352 vs 353	65% OHA alone, 14% insulin alone, 15% insulin + OHA, 5% diet alone	60	Home telemedicine unit; nurse managers (diabetologists consulted when needed); Web-based	7.43–7.09, NR	7.45–7.38, NR	<.001	Significant improvement in SBP, DBP	No significant difference in depression or diabetes distress
Stone et al,[28] 2010	64 vs 73	76% OHA, 79% insulin (breakdown of OHA alone and insulin alone not reported)	6	Wireless glucometer; nurse under supervision of an endocrinologist; phone	9.6–7.9	9.4–8.6	<.001	Significant improvement in LDL	
Ralston et al,[24] 2009	30 vs 35	Diet, OHAs or insulin (38% used insulin)	12	Web-based; diabetes case manager; e-mail	8.2–7.3, P = .01	7.9–8.1, NR	<.01	No significant CVD benefits identified	
Kim et al,[20] 2007	25 vs 26	67% OHA, 31% insulin	12	Web-based; diabetic educator or professor; text message	8.09–7.04, P<.05	7.59–7.70, NS	.011	No significant CVD benefits identified	
Cho et al,[18] 2006	40 vs 40	69% OHA, 12% insulin only, 10% OHA + insulin, 9% exercise/diet	30	Web-based; clinical investigator, daily; Web-based	7.7–6.7, P<.05	7.5–7.4, NS	.022	Significant improvement in triglycerides	

Study	N	Medication	Duration (mo)	Intervention	HbA1c (intervention)	HbA1c (control)	P	CVD outcomes	QOL outcomes
Kwon et al,[19] 2004	51 vs 50	NR	3	Web-based; endocrinology fellow; Web-based	7.59–6.94, P<.001	7.19–7.62, NR	<.05		
Tildesley et al,[14] 2010; Tildesley et al,[13] 2011	24 vs 23	Insulin	6	Web-based; endocrinologist; Web-based	8.8–7.6, P<.001	8.5–8.4, P = .51	<.05	Significant improvement in total cholesterol and LDL	
Kim et al,[22] 2008	Obese 18 vs16	68% OHA, 32% insulin	12	Web-based; diabetic educator or professor; both by phone and Web-based	8.16–6.67, P<.05	7.66–8.19, NS	NR		
Yoon and Kim,[26] 2008	25 vs 26	69% on OHA only, 31% insulin	12	Web-based; endocrinologist/professor; text message	8.09–6.77, P<.05	7.59–8.4, P<.05	NR	No significant CVD benefits identified	
Bujnowska-Fedak et al,[21] 2011	50 vs 50	50% insulin, 50% noninsulin	6	Wireless glucometer; physician; phone	7.6–7.4, NR	7.6–7.4, NR	NS	No significant CVD benefits identified	No significant QOL differences
T1D and T2D									
Bond et al,[27] 2007; Bond et al,[41] 2010	≥60 y old 36 vs 31	49% insulin, 45% insulin + OHA, 6% diet and exercise	6	Web-based; nurse; e-mail or instant messaging	7.0–6.4, NR	7.1–7.0, NR	.01	Significant improvements in total cholesterol, HDL, SBP	Significant improvements in depression (CES-D), QOL (PAID)
Harno et al,[40] 2006	101 vs 74	NR	12	Glucometer; diabetes team; text message	7.8–7.3, NR	8.2–7.8, NR	<.05	Significant improvements in total cholesterol, LDL, TG, DBP	

(continued on next page)

Table 1 (*continued*)

Study	Participants (Intervention vs Usual Care)	Treatments in Use	Duration (mo)	Description of IBGMS (Method of Upload; Review; Feedback)	Mean HbA$_{1c}$ Levels in IBGMS, from Baseline to Follow-Up (%)	Mean HbA$_{1c}$ Levels in Control Group, from Baseline to Follow-Up (%)	P Value, Δ HbA$_{1c}$ Levels Between Groups	CVD Outcomes at Follow-Up in IBGMS Compared with Control Group	QOL at Follow-Up in IBGMS Compared with Control Group
McMahon et al,[23] 2005	HbA$_{1c}$ ≥9% 52 vs 52	51% on OHA, 49% on insulin	12	Web-based; nurse, physician; Web-based	−1.6 reduction from baseline, P<.001	−1.2 reduction from baseline, P<.001	<.05	Significant improvements in HDL, TG, SBP	
Tjam et al,[29] 2006	34 vs 19	NR	12	Web-based; nurse; Web-based	6.7–6.5, P = .045	6.8–6.8, P = .88	NR		
T1D only									
Charpentier et al,[15] 2011	61 vs 59	Insulin	6	cell-phone; physician; phone; Additional: Diabeo Decision-support software	9.11–8.41, NR	8.91–9.1, NR	<.001		No significant differences by DQOL and Diabetes Health Profile
Kirwan et al,[30] 2013	36 vs 36	Insulin	6	Smartphone app; diabetes educator; text message	9.08–7.8, P<.001	8.47–8.58, NS	<.001		No significant differences by DQOL
Montori et al,[16] 2004	16 vs 16	Insulin	6	Direct upload from glucometer; nurse (supervised by endocrinologist; phone call)	9.1–7.8, NR	8.8–8.2, NR	.03		
Jansa et al,[36] 2006	16 vs 14	Insulin	12	Glucometer through phone line; nurse; phone (teleconsultations took the place of in-person visits)	8.4–7.6, P = .008	8.9–7.6, P = .001	NS		No significant differences by DQOL

Gomez et al,[47] 2002	10 (crossover design)	Insulin	14	PDA; physicians and nurses; PDA-based	8.4–7.9, NR	8.1–8.15, NR	.053	Significant improvements in DQOL global score and DQOL satisfaction with life subscale
Benhamou et al,[32] 2007	15 vs 15	Continuous subcutaneous insulin infusion	6	PDA/cell; investigator; text message	8.31–8.18, $P = .17$	8.22–8.34, $P = .33$	.097	Significant improvements in perceived frequency of hyperglycemic episodes on DTSQ and social relations on DQOL
Rossi et al,[17] 2013	63 vs 64	Insulin	6	Cell phone; physician; text message; Additional: automatic dosage calculation based on carb intake	8.4–7.9, <.0001	8.4–7.9, <.0001	.73	No significant CVD benefits identified
McCarrier et al,[48] 2009	25 vs 16	Insulin	12	Web-based; nurse; e-mail	7.99–7.62, NS	8.05–8.16, NS	.16	
Biermann et al,[35] 2002	27 vs 16	Insulin	8	Web-based; physician; phone (teleconsultations took the place of in-person visits)	8.3–7.1, NR	8.0–6.8, NR	NS	

Abbreviations: CES-D, Centre for Epidemiological Studies Depression scale; CVD, cardiovascular disease; DBP, diastolic blood pressure; DQOL, diabetes-specific quality of life questionnaire; DTSQ, diabetes treatment satisfaction questionnaire; HDL, high-density lipoprotein; LDL, low-density lipoprotein; NR, not reported; NS, nonsignificant; OHA, oral hypoglycemic agent; PAID, problem areas in diabetes; PDA, personal digital assistant (a small handheld computer); QOL, quality of life; SBP, systolic blood pressure; TG, triglycerides.

patients represented a small proportion of the study populations ($\sim$7–9%), and no subgroup analyses were performed, the effectiveness of IBGMS in patients relying on lifestyle modification alone to control their T2D cannot be evaluated.

Most studies were short, with follow-up between 3 and 12 months. Significant reductions in HbA_{1c} level with IBGMS were observed in as little as 3 months.[14,19,22,23,26] Two longer-term studies showed that the glycemic benefit of IBGMS can be maintained over several years. Cho and colleagues[18] reported that intervention patients experienced a decrease in HbA_{1c} level from a mean of 7.7% to 6.7% (P<.05) after 30 months, compared with 7.5% to 7.4% (not significant) in controls. The large-scale The Informatics for Diabetes Education and Telemedicine (IDEATel) trial also showed that IBGMS can deliver long-term glycemic benefit. After a 5-year follow-up, patients in the Internet intervention arm showed a mean decrease in HbA_{1c} level from 7.43% to 7.09%, compared with 7.45% to 7.38% in the conventional care arm; the change from baseline was significantly different between groups.[25] Both these studies had 70% to 78% non–insulin-using patients, suggesting that IBGMS can facilitate long-term glycemic control in individuals with T2D, independent of any benefits related to insulin dose titration.

Although these studies showed significant decline in HbA_{1c} level within 3 months of IBGMS use, this short-term intervention may not be sufficient to effect lasting glycemic control. Tildesley and colleagues[13] reported that mean HbA_{1c} levels in insulin-using patients with T2D decreased significantly, from 8.8% to 7.6% (P<.001) after a 6-month follow-up. However, after patients in the intervention group were returned to conventional care, HbA_{1c} levels returned to baseline within 6 months. Thus, ongoing patient-physician communication may be required to maintain the benefits of IBGMS.

INTERNET BLOOD GLUCOSE MONITORING SYSTEMS IN WELL AND POORLY CONTROLLED TYPE 2 DIABETES

Studies focusing on patients with higher HbA_{1c} level at baseline have shown some of the most remarkable improvements in glycemic control with IBGMS. Of 6 T2D studies featuring mean baseline HbA_{1c} level 8% or greater (1 with insulin only[14]; 5 with oral agents with or without insulin[20,22–24,28]), the mean decrease in HbA_{1c} level ranged from 1.05% to 1.7%, with the largest decrease seen in the study with the highest baseline HbA_{1c} level.[28]

In addition, patients with T2D who are at or near their glycemic target seem to maintain or improve their degree of glycemic control with IBGMS. Thus, in a study of both T1D and T2D, with patients on a variety of therapies, mean HbA_{1c} level declined from 7.0% to 6.4% in the Internet intervention group, whereas the control group HbA_{1c} level declined nonsignificantly from 7.1% to 7.0%.[27] Two studies that carried out a subanalysis of patients with baseline HbA_{1c} level less than 7.0% both showed a significant difference between intervention and control groups with regard to follow-up HbA_{1c} level.[18,19] Moreover, in the IBGMS study with the best glycemic control at baseline, HbA_{1c} level decreased significantly from a mean of 6.7% to 6.5% (P = .045) in the IBGMS group, versus 6.8% to 6.8% (not significant) in the control group.[29] Hence, baseline glycemic control does not seem to be a limitation in patient selection for IBGMS.

INTERNET BLOOD GLUCOSE MONITORING SYSTEMS IN WELL AND POORLY CONTROLLED TYPE 1 DIABETES

Although Internet interventions in T1D do not result in the same widespread improvement as seen in T2D studies, IBGMS result in a consistent trend toward greater

HbA_{1c} level reduction. This improvement reached statistical significance in some T1D trials, namely those in which patients experienced poor glycemic control at baseline.

Of the 9 identified trials of T1D, 3 showed a glycemic benefit for IBGMS compared with conventional care.[15,16,30] All of the studies that showed a significant glycemic benefit in the intervention arm had a mean baseline HbA_{1c} level of 8.4% or greater, whereas all the studies that failed to show a significant benefit of IBGMS use had a mean baseline HbA_{1c} level of 8.4% or less. As in comparable studies in T2D, greater change in HbA_{1c} level with IBGMS occurs in patients with poorly controlled disease.

HYPOGLYCEMIA AND INTERNET BLOOD GLUCOSE MONITORING SYSTEMS

Insulin and some oral agents decrease glycemic exposure at the cost of heightening patients' risk of overall and serious hypoglycemia.[1,2] This dose-limiting toxicity is important clinically, because of the intrinsic adverse effects of hypoglycemia, and also because of its psychological effect, whereby fear of hypoglycemia delays treatment implementation and reduces treatment adherence.[31]

Several studies reporting overall and severe hypoglycemic episodes rates showed no significant change in either outcome with IBGMS use.[15,16,20,23,32] This finding is interesting in itself, given that frequency of SMBG commonly increases with the introduction of IBGMS (see earlier discussion). Because biochemically defined hypoglycemia commonly goes unnoticed by patients,[33,34] it might have been expected that mild hypoglycemia would be detected in IBGMS patients at an increased rate. However, no study has reported such an effect. Rather, studies have reported nonsignificant trends toward a lower hypoglycemia rate or, in 2 cases, a significant decrease in the frequency of moderately severe[17] and severe hypoglycemia.[21] Crucially, this apparent increase in treatment safety with IBGMS was seen in insulin-using[16,17,32,35,36] as well as non–insulin-using patients,[20,21,23] and in studies of patients with poor baseline glycemic control, in which changes in HbA_{1c} level with treatment were particularly striking.

Because use of IBGMS increases monitoring by a health care professional, this intervention is expected to address these psychological barriers to effective pharmacotherapy. In 1 T1D study, patients with IBGMS reported an improved fear of hypoglycemia dimension of the Diabetes-Specific Quality of Life Scale Questionnaire compared with control patients, but this difference did not reach statistical significance ($P = .06$).[17] Given the apparent decline in hypoglycemia incidence in patients using IBGMS, we speculate that broader implementation will help to alleviate fear of hypoglycemia in both health professionals and patients.

IMPROVED GLYCEMIA IN INTERNET BLOOD GLUCOSE MONITORING SYSTEMS: SOME POTENTIAL MECHANISMS

We hypothesized that improved glycemic control seen in IBGMS interventions could arise in part because of increased insulin doses or increased frequency SMBG, which, in some studies of T1D or T2D, correlates with decreased HbA_{1c} level.[37–39]

Improved HbA_{1c} level with IBGMS does not seem to be primarily a consequence of increased insulin doses. As noted earlier,[18,20,22–26] the benefit of IBGMS is not restricted to insulin-using patients. Moreover, among 4 studies reporting insulin dose data, none identified significant differences in insulin dose, comparing baseline and follow-up or between treatment arms.[14–16,36] Thus, it seems that improvement in HbA_{1c} level with IBGMS is largely independent of insulin dose adjustments. This conclusion is consistent with the finding that treatment modification was the least frequent type of feedback for patients to receive by means of IBGMS, with encouragement being the most frequent type of feedback.[18] Therefore, support and encouragement to increase frequency of SMBG and improve diet and exercise may be more important factors to explain the benefits of IBGMS, compared with any effect on insulin doses.

The beneficial effect of SMBG as an explanation of IBGMS outcomes is more difficult to rule out. SMBG frequency is expected to increase with IBGMS; as noted earlier, several studies have documented this effect.[18,19] However, other studies confirming the efficacy of IBGMS have found no increase in SMBG frequency.[15,16] Moreover, even in studies in which SMBG frequency increased, no correlation has been found between patients' SMBG frequency and improvement in HbA_{1c} level. These studies suggest that although SMBG may contribute to better glycemic control, increased SMBG alone does not explain the glycemic benefits of IBGMS.

In addition to a possible effect of increased SMBG frequency, patients using IBGMS often report increased self-motivation, because of being followed more closely by their health care provider. The number of data uploads from a given patient may offer a quantitative measure of this self-motivation, and this measurement seems to correlate well with IBGMS efficacy. Thus, McMahon and colleagues[23] identified a significant association between data upload frequency and improvement in HbA_{1c} level (decreases of –2.1% and –1.0% in the highest and lowest tertiles, respectively; $P<.02$). Another study, not reaching statistical significance, reported a similar trend.[24]

We propose that glycemic improvements seen in patients on IBGMS result from a combination of factors that stem from increased self-motivation and increased patient-physician communication. Such factors may include improved diet, increased exercise, and, in some cases, increased frequency of SMBG or more effective use of medications.

CARDIOVASCULAR RISK FACTOR CHANGE WITH INTERNET BLOOD GLUCOSE MONITORING SYSTEMS

Decreased risk of cardiovascular (CV) disease is expected in individuals achieving improved HbA_{1c} levels.[3,4] To evaluate whether IBGMS affected patients' CV risk, we examined risk marker changes in various studies of IBGMS. Lipid measures were reported in 12 studies,[14,17–20,23–25,27,28,40] of which 6 showed improvements to at least 1 lipid measure compared with conventional care.[14,18,23,27,28,40] Similarly, of the 7 IBGMS studies reporting blood pressure data,[17,23,25,27,28,40] 4 showed improvements in either systolic or diastolic blood pressure, compared with conventional care.[23,25,27,40] Although these findings are suggestive, longer-term follow-up studies involving more patients may be needed to confirm the CV benefits of IBGMS.[3,4]

QUALITY OF LIFE AND PATIENT SATISFACTION WITH INTERNET BLOOD GLUCOSE MONITORING SYSTEMS

Three studies reported significantly improved quality of life (QOL) in the Internet intervention group, compared with control groups,[17,32,41] and 5 reported no significant difference.[15,21,30]

Of the 3 showing QOL benefits, 1[41] reported a significant improvement in HbA_{1c} levels compared with controls, 1 showed a trend to improvement in HbA_{1c} levels compared with controls,[32] and 1 showed significant improvement in both intervention and control arms, but there was no significance between the groups.[17] This finding suggests that patients may experience benefits from IBGMS beyond those detected by clinical measures. In a study in which HbA_{1c} level change was not significantly different between the IBGMS and control arms, 85% of patients in the intervention arm believed that the Internet intervention was better than conventional care. Reasons cited included better surveillance of SMBG data by the physician and faster intervention in the case of problems.[35]

COST-EFFECTIVENESS OF INTERNET BLOOD GLUCOSE MONITORING SYSTEMS

No formal pharmacoeconomic studies have been published assessing the cost-effectiveness of IBGMS in widespread implementation. However, some of the randomized controlled studies discussed earlier report comparisons of costs between intervention and control groups.

Cost outcomes have varied substantially over time, with dramatically lower costs seen in recent years, as personal mobile devices became ubiquitous and became a popular platform for Internet medicine. Thus, in the IDEATel study, which started in 2000, health care costs increased 71% to 116% in the intervention group compared with the control group.[42] The costs associated with the intervention arm, more than $8000 per patient per year, were driven mainly by the cost of a specialized home telemedicine unit and associated training and demonstrating costs.[42] However, as early as 2003, Jansa and colleagues[36] reported that, in the absence of technical problems, IBGMS use was associated with a decrease in health care provider costs of €40 (~$55 US) per case over 12 months, because of decreased lengths of appointments in the intervention group.

With more recent Internet-based interventions using patients' Internet-connected personal computers or data-connected cellular phones, Internet intervention costs will likely decrease dramatically. A study that recruited patients who owned iPhones to use the free *Glucose Buddy* app for SMBG tracking estimated an intervention cost of $8.08 AUD (~$7.50 US) per patient over the 6-month study.[30] This modest cost covered the salary of the certified diabetes educator, who spent 5 minutes per patient per week reviewing cases and sending feedback.

From a health care provider's perspective, the automatic uploading of patients' SMBG data increases accuracy of data interpretation by showing the uploaded data in table and graph formats and saves time by automatically incorporating data into electronic medical records. Furthermore, IBGMS Internet or cell phone feedback can potentially replace appointments for dosage adjustments, thus decreasing overall health care costs and freeing up clinic resources.

For patients, IBGMS use has the potential to reduce the number of appointments for dose adjustments or routine follow-up, resulting in decreased travel time. Taking into account travel time and time off work, Biermann and colleagues[35] calculated a savings of €650 (~$900 US) for patients in their intervention, compared with control patients. In this study, physicians followed up with patients by phone every 2 to 4 weeks, compared with monthly in-person visits in the control group. Jansa and colleagues[36] estimated the cost savings of teleconferences instead of in-person visits at €396 (~$548 US) over 12 months. In that study, the intervention group attended 9 teleconferences and 3 hospital appointments versus 12 hospital appointments in the control group.

Long-term cost-benefit analyses, especially in widespread implementations of IBGMS, are needed to show that improved HbA_{1c} level from IBGMS translate to reduced use of health care resources.[43] In principle, such savings could be substantial, because sustained annual cost savings per patient have been reported at $685 to $950 for patients achieving a decrease in HbA_{1c} level of 1% or more.[11] As noted earlier, this level of glycemic improvement is commonly reported in studies of IBGMS.[44]

WIDESPREAD IMPLEMENTATION OF INTERNET BLOOD GLUCOSE MONITORING SYSTEMS

IBGMS is emerging as the standard of care for patients with diabetes in the Canadian province of British Columbia. In this jurisdiction, family physicians, general internists, and endocrinologists are now remunerated for reviewing patient glucose reports. Patients are asked to upload their SMBG data every 2 weeks through a choice of platforms. The patient's physician then reviews the readings and sends feedback via e-mail.

A total of 1200 patients have been enrolled, and outcome data on the first 409 patients showed significant improvement of HbA_{1c} levels after 3 to 9 months of follow-up (**Fig. 2**). Glycemic control improved significantly after introduction of IBGMS in patients with T1D and baseline HbA_{1c} level 6.9% or greater. Similarly, patients with T2D, treated with insulin or oral agents, showed significant improvement in HbA_{1c} level.[44] As was previously reported in a clinical trial, individuals who used the IBGMS frequently (frequent uploaders) experienced greater improvement in glycemic control, relative to infrequent uploaders.[23]

These real-world findings generally agree with results from randomized controlled trials, in that IBGMS seems effective in T2D, irrespective of baseline glycemia or mode of treatment, as well as in T1D for patients with poor glycemic control. Moreover, more frequent use of the system to upload of SMBG data (presumably reflecting greater patient self-motivation) was associated with improved HbA_{1c} levels.

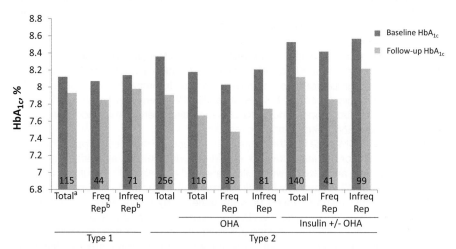

Fig. 2. Mean HbA_{1c} level at baseline and follow-up in patients with IBGMS who upload their blood glucose data frequently (Freq Rep) versus infrequently (Infreq Rep). When patients with HbA_{1c} level less than 6.9% were excluded, patients with T1D showed a significant improvement in HbA_{1c} level at follow-up ($P<.01$). Total T2D, T2D on OHA only, and T2D patients on insulin ± OHA all showed significant decreases in HbA_{1c} level at follow-up (all $P<.001$). $P = .05$ for frequent reporters compared with infrequent reporters for each type of diabetes. [a] Excluding patient HbA_{1c} level less than 6.9%; [b] excluding patient HbA_{1c} level less than 7.4%. OHA, oral hypoglycemic agent. (*Data from* Tildesley HD, Conway ME, Ross SA, et al. Review of the effect of internet therapeutic intervention in patients with type 1 and type 2 diabetes. Diabetes Care 2014;37(2):e31–2.)

> **Box 1**
> **Sample messages to patients**
>
> High in the AM; please increase evening metformin to 750 mg at supper. Let's see if there is any shift in 2 weeks.
>
> Your lunch value is excellent, but supper is showing variability. Please work on having supper at the same time each day, which should improve consistency, and report again in 2 weeks. Thanks.
>
> Your sugar levels are a little high at lunch and supper. Try a carb ratio of 10:1 at breakfast and lunch. Please report again in 2 weeks. Thanks

PRACTICAL TIPS FOR EFFECTIVE INTERNET BLOOD GLUCOSE MONITORING SYSTEMS

One key to efficient implementation of IBGMS is the use of clear and standardized reports of patient glucose levels. Reports should clearly indicate time of day, average glucose levels, range and standard deviation (SD) of glucose values. They should be organized so that raw data, as well as summary data, can be accessed easily. As a general rule, testing frequency should be such that there are at least 10 values for a given time of day across the reporting period, for instance 10 before breakfast measurements within 2 weeks, or else the statistics may be less accurate to their true values. Most glucose meters and some insulin pumps and sensors are designed to facilitate the uploading and transmission of stored data.

One rule of thumb is to first check the SD of glucose levels by time of day. In general, if the SD is less than 50 mg/dL (<2.8 mmol/L for measurements in SI units), the data can be used for determining appropriate therapeutic changes. If the SD is increased, therapeutic changes should be delayed until the patient is able to provide more consistent values. Larger SD values are related to meal timing, meal content, timing of medications, or possibly, major stresses, which result in less focus on diabetes self-management. Possible causes could include major life events such as the death of a family member, recent unemployment, or development of a mental health disorder; for such situations, the cause of stress should be addressed directly, often with the aid of a mental health professional. The next step is to decide if average values are at target by time of day; if not, medications are adjusted according to their onset and duration of action and effect.

With practice, reports can be reviewed efficiently, allowing a health professional to offer clear guidance in a concise text or e-mail message to the patient. Typically, such a message suggests changes in diet (eg, carbohydrate ratio for specific meals) or in the timing or dose of insulin or an oral agent. The patient should always be asked to follow up at a specified time (eg, 2 weeks later) to discuss the outcomes of these changes (**Box 1**).

SUMMARY AND FUTURE PERSPECTIVES

Telehealth (Internet-based and telephone-based) interventions have been increasingly discussed in recent clinical practice guidelines. The CDA 2013 Clinical Practice Guidelines recommend that technologically based home blood glucose monitoring systems be integrated into self-management education interventions, to improve glycemic control.[6] Likewise, the ADA 2013 Standards of Medical Care Position Statement indicates that telehealth can help provide self-management education and support.[10]

We have argued here that IBGMS is broadly useful in patients with T1D and T2D, in large part because it improves communication between patients and their health care providers. Widespread rollout of IBGMS is ongoing in some locations, and experience from these nascent programs should answer lingering questions about the benefits and cost-effectiveness of the approach. The findings are encouraging. Since 2011, the Canadian province of British Columbia has reimbursed endocrinologists for the review of IBGMS data.

Although a cost analysis of this IBGMS implementation is not available, a health professional is typically able to review patient data and send feedback to the patient via e-mail in just a few minutes per case, performed every 2 to 4 weeks. Most recently, the United Kingdom has undertaken a 30-month study called *HeLP-Diabetes* (Healthy Living for People with type 2 Diabetes). The study will be conducted in 2 inner city London boroughs, in which there are ~14,000 potential users of *HeLP-Diabetes*,[45] making this the largest IBGMS program yet designed. Data from this study are eagerly awaited.

Available study data on IBGMS support the clinical usefulness of this approach to diabetes management, with improved glycemic control in all types of diabetes patients and no increase in hypoglycemia risk. IBGMS seems to be well accepted by patients and to involve minimal time commitment from the health professional, with some evidence of health care cost savings and reduced burden on clinical resources. IBGMS thus warrants consideration, both for widespread implementation and for insurance coverage.

ACKNOWLEDGMENTS

The authors wish to thank John Ashkenas, PhD (SCRIPT, Toronto, Canada) for editorial assistance. H.D. Tildesley gratefully acknowledges the Endocrine Research Society for financial support for this project.

REFERENCES

1. The effect of intensive treatment of diabetes on the development and progression of long-term complications in insulin-dependent diabetes mellitus. The Diabetes Control and Complications Trial Research Group. N Engl J Med 1993;329(14): 977–86.
2. Intensive blood-glucose control with sulphonylureas or insulin compared with conventional treatment and risk of complications in patients with type 2 diabetes (UKPDS 33). UK Prospective Diabetes Study (UKPDS) Group. Lancet 1998; 352(9131):837–53.
3. Holman RR, Paul SK, Bethel MA, et al. 10-year follow-up of intensive glucose control in type 2 diabetes. N Engl J Med 2008;359(15):1577–89.
4. Nathan DM, Cleary PA, Backlund JY, et al. Intensive diabetes treatment and cardiovascular disease in patients with type 1 diabetes. N Engl J Med 2005;353(25): 2643–53.
5. Nathan DM, DCCT/EDIC Research Group. The diabetes control and complications trial/epidemiology of diabetes interventions and complications study at 30 years: overview. Diabetes Care 2014;37(1):9–16.
6. Cheng AY, Lau DC. The Canadian Diabetes Association 2013 clinical practice guidelines–raising the bar and setting higher standards! Can J Diabetes 2013; 37(3):137–8.
7. Braga M, Casanova A, Teoh H, et al. Treatment gaps in the management of cardiovascular risk factors in patients with type 2 diabetes in Canada. Can J Cardiol 2010;26(6):297–302.

8. Hoerger TJ, Segel JE, Gregg EW, et al. Is glycemic control improving in US adults? Diabetes Care 2008;31(1):81–6.
9. Ali MK, Bullard KM, Saaddine JB, et al. Achievement of goals in US diabetes care, 1999-2010. N Engl J Med 2013;368(17):1613–24.
10. American Diabetes Association. Standards of medical care in diabetes–2014. Diabetes Care 2014;37(Suppl 1):S14–80.
11. Malanda UL, Welschen LM, Riphagen II, et al. Self-monitoring of blood glucose in patients with type 2 diabetes mellitus who are not using insulin. Cochrane Database Syst Rev 2012;(1):CD005060.
12. Ross SA, Tildesley HD, Ashkenas J. Barriers to effective insulin treatment: the persistence of poor glycemic control in type 2 diabetes. Curr Med Res Opin 2011;27(Suppl 3):13–20.
13. Tildesley HD, Mazanderani AB, Chan JH, et al. Efficacy of A1c reduction using internet intervention in patients with type 2 diabetes treated with insulin. Can J Diabetes 2011;35(3):250–3.
14. Tildesley HD, Mazanderani AB, Ross SA. Effect of Internet therapeutic intervention on A1C levels in patients with type 2 diabetes treated with insulin. Diabetes Care 2010;33(8):1738–40.
15. Charpentier G, Benhamou PY, Dardari D, et al. The Diabeo software enabling individualized insulin dose adjustments combined with telemedicine support improves HbA1c in poorly controlled type 1 diabetic patients: a 6-month, randomized, open-label, parallel-group, multicenter trial (TeleDiab 1 Study). Diabetes Care 2011;34(3):533–9.
16. Montori VM, Helgemoe PK, Guyatt GH, et al. Telecare for patients with type 1 diabetes and inadequate glycemic control: a randomized controlled trial and meta-analysis. Diabetes Care 2004;27(5):1088–94.
17. Rossi MC, Nicolucci A, Lucisano G, et al. Impact of the "diabetes interactive diary" telemedicine system on metabolic control, risk of hypoglycemia, and quality of life: a randomized clinical trial in type 1 diabetes. Diabetes Technol Ther 2013; 15(8):670–9.
18. Cho JH, Chang SA, Kwon HS, et al. Long-term effect of the Internet-based glucose monitoring system on HbA1c reduction and glucose stability: a 30-month follow-up study for diabetes management with a ubiquitous medical care system. Diabetes Care 2006;29(12):2625–31.
19. Kwon HS, Cho JH, Kim HS, et al. Establishment of blood glucose monitoring system using the internet. Diabetes Care 2004;27(2):478–83.
20. Kim C, Kim H, Nam J, et al. Internet diabetic patient management using a short messaging service automatically produced by a knowledge matrix system. Diabetes Care 2007;30(11):2857–8.
21. Bujnowska-Fedak MM, Puchala E, Steciwko A. The impact of telehome care on health status and quality of life among patients with diabetes in a primary care setting in Poland. Telemed J E Health 2011;17(3):153–63.
22. Kim SI, Kim HS. Effectiveness of mobile and internet intervention in patients with obese type 2 diabetes. Int J Med Inform 2008;77(6):399–404.
23. McMahon GT, Gomes HE, Hickson Hohne S, et al. Web-based care management in patients with poorly controlled diabetes. Diabetes Care 2005;28(7): 1624–9.
24. Ralston JD, Hirsch IB, Hoath J, et al. Web-based collaborative care for type 2 diabetes: a pilot randomized trial. Diabetes Care 2009;32(2):234–9.
25. Shea S, Weinstock RS, Teresi JA, et al. A randomized trial comparing telemedicine case management with usual care in older, ethnically diverse, medically

underserved patients with diabetes mellitus: 5 year results of the IDEATel study. J Am Med Inform Assoc 2009;16(4):446–56.

26. Yoon KH, Kim HS. A short message service by cellular phone in type 2 diabetic patients for 12 months. Diabetes Res Clin Pract 2008;79(2):256–61.

27. Bond GE, Burr R, Wolf FM, et al. The effects of a web-based intervention on the physical outcomes associated with diabetes among adults age 60 and older: a randomized trial. Diabetes Technol Ther 2007;9(1):52–9.

28. Stone RA, Rao RH, Sevick MA, et al. Active care management supported by home telemonitoring in veterans with type 2 diabetes: the DiaTel randomized controlled trial. Diabetes Care 2010;33(3):478–84.

29. Tjam EY, Sherifali D, Steinacher N, et al. Physiological outcomes of an internet disease management program vs. in-person counselling: a randomized, controlled trial. Can J Diabetes 2006;30(4):397–405.

30. Kirwan M, Vandelanotte C, Fenning A, et al. Diabetes self-management smartphone application for adults with type 1 diabetes: randomized controlled trial. J Med Internet Res 2013;15(11):e235.

31. Cryer PE. Hypoglycaemia: the limiting factor in the glycaemic management of type I and type II diabetes. Diabetologia 2002;45(7):937–48.

32. Benhamou PY, Melki V, Boizel R, et al. One-year efficacy and safety of Web-based follow-up using cellular phone in type 1 diabetic patients under insulin pump therapy: the PumpNet study. Diabetes Metab 2007;33(3):220–6.

33. Chico A, Vidal-Rios P, Subira M, et al. The continuous glucose monitoring system is useful for detecting unrecognized hypoglycemias in patients with type 1 and type 2 diabetes but is not better than frequent capillary glucose measurements for improving metabolic control. Diabetes Care 2003;26(4):1153–7.

34. Weber KK, Lohmann T, Busch K, et al. High frequency of unrecognized hypoglycaemias in patients with type 2 diabetes is discovered by continuous glucose monitoring. Exp Clin Endocrinol Diabetes 2007;115(8):491–4.

35. Biermann E, Dietrich W, Rihl J, et al. Are there time and cost savings by using telemanagement for patients on intensified insulin therapy? A randomised, controlled trial. Comput Methods Programs Biomed 2002;69(2):137–46.

36. Jansa M, Vidal M, Viaplana J, et al. Telecare in a structured therapeutic education programme addressed to patients with type 1 diabetes and poor metabolic control. Diabetes Res Clin Pract 2006;74(1):26–32.

37. Hirsch IB, Bode BW, Childs BP, et al. Self-monitoring of blood glucose (SMBG) in insulin- and non-insulin-using adults with diabetes: consensus recommendations for improving SMBG accuracy, utilization, and research. Diabetes Technol Ther 2008;10:419–39.

38. Karter AJ, Parker MM, Moffet HH, et al. Longitudinal study of new and prevalent use of self-monitoring of blood glucose. Diabetes Care 2006;29(8):1757–63.

39. Strowig SM, Raskin P. Improved glycemic control in intensively treated type 1 diabetic patients using blood glucose meters with storage capability and computer-assisted analyses. Diabetes Care 1998;21(10):1694–8.

40. Harno K, Kauppinen-Makelin R, Syrjalainen J. Managing diabetes care using an integrated regional e-health approach. J Telemed Telecare 2006;12(Suppl 1):13–5.

41. Bond GE, Burr RL, Wolf FM, et al. The effects of a web-based intervention on psychosocial well-being among adults aged 60 and older with diabetes: a randomized trial. Diabetes Educ 2010;36(3):446–56.

42. Moreno L, Dale SB, Chen AY, et al. Costs to medicare of the informatics for diabetes education and telemedicine (IDEATel) home telemedicine demonstration: findings from an independent evaluation. Diabetes Care 2009;32(7):1202–4.

43. Malanda UL, Bot SD, Nijpels G. Self-monitoring of blood glucose in noninsulin-using type 2 diabetic patients: it is time to face the evidence. Diabetes Care 2013;36(1):176–8.
44. Tildesley HD, Conway ME, Ross SA, et al. Review of the effect of internet thera-peutic intervention in patients with type 1 and type 2 diabetes. Diabetes Care 2014;37(2):e31–2.
45. Ross J, Stevenson F, Dack C, et al. Evaluating the implementation of HeLP-Diabetes within NHS services: study protocol. BMC Health Serv Res 2014;14:51.
46. Trief PM, Teresi JA, Izquierdo R, et al. Psychosocial outcomes of telemedicine case management for elderly patients with diabetes: the randomized IDEATel trial. Diabetes Care 2007;30(5):1266–8.
47. Gomez EJ, Hernando ME, Garcia A, et al. Telemedicine as a tool for intensive management of diabetes: the DIABTel experience. Comput Methods Programs Biomed 2002;69(2):163–77.
48. McCarrier KP, Ralston JD, Hirsch IB, et al. Web-Based Collaborative Care for Type 1 Diabetes: A Pilot Randomized Trial. Diabetes Technol Ther 2009;11(4): 211–7.

Monitoring Glycemia in Diabetes

Sara J. Healy, MD, Kathleen M. Dungan, MD, MPH*

KEYWORDS

- Glucose monitor • Self-monitored blood glucose • Continuous glucose monitoring
- HbA1c

KEY POINTS

- Hemoglobin A1C (HbA1c) is the most important global measure of glucose control but must be interpreted with caution in some circumstances.
- Capillary glucose self-monitoring should be performed in patients requiring complex insulin regimens and in patients who are properly trained to interpret and use the results for adjusting therapy.
- Professional continuous glucose monitoring requires little training and may be useful for patients with type 1 or type 2 diabetes who are not meeting glucose targets.
- Personal continuous glucose monitoring may be beneficial for adults and children with type 1 diabetes who can demonstrate near-daily use. As technology advances, however, its use will likely expand.

INTRODUCTION

Monitoring of glycemia has evolved substantially since the first home glucose monitor became available in the late 1970s. Since then, monitoring of glycemic control has become an indispensable component of any diabetes therapeutic regimen, whether it consists of periodic hemoglobin A1C (HbA1c) measurement or continuous interstitial glucose monitoring. This article highlights the advantages, disadvantages, indications, and implementation of approaches for monitoring glycemia.

MARKERS OF GLUCOSE CONTROL
Hemoglobin A1c

HbA1c is a stable hemoglobin variant formed by nonenzymatic attachment of glucose to the beta chain of hemoglobin and reflects mean glycemia during the previous

Disclosures: K.M. Dungan reports research support from Novo Nordisk, Merck, AstraZeneca, and advisory board for Eli Lilly. S.J. Healy has nothing to disclose.
Division of Endocrinology, Diabetes and Metabolism, The Ohio State University Wexner Medical Center, 5th Floor McCampbell Hall, 1581 Dodd Drive, Columbus, OH 43210, USA
* Corresponding author.
E-mail address: kathleen.dungan@osumc.edu

3 months. Although the average lifespan of an erythrocyte is 120 days, more recent glycemic levels contribute more to the HbA1c level.[1] The Diabetes Control and Complications Trial (DCCT) and the United Kingdom Prospective Diabetes Study demonstrated that HbA1c has strong predictive value for diabetes complications. HbA1c may be used to diagnose diabetes (cutoff point ≥6.5% for diagnosis) and monitor overall control 2 to 4 times per year. Point-of care testing for HbA1c is recommended to facilitate timely treatment changes.

Correlating hemoglobin A1c with average plasma glucose

The National Glycohemoglobin Standardization Program began in 1996 to standardize HbA1c results to those of the DCCT.[2] The internationalA1c-Derived Average Glucose trial[3] derived an average glucose level from HbA1c based on data from frequent self-monitored blood glucose (SMBG) and continuous glucose monitoring (CGM) in 507 adults with type 1, type 2, and no diabetes, most of whom were non-Hispanic whites (**Table 1**). There were no significant differences among racial and ethnic groups between HbA1c and mean glucose, although there was a trend among African or African American compared with non-Hispanic white groups. There are no current recommendations for different interpretations of HbA1c in these groups, although this is widely debated.[4]

Limitations of hemoglobin A1c and alternative markers of glycemia

HbA1c does not indicate the degree of glucose fluctuations or hypoglycemia and, because it only provides an estimate of average glucose levels, it cannot direct specific treatment changes targeted to any glucose pattern, particularly among patients who are receiving insulin therapy. Also, hemoglobinopathies and clinically silent hemoglobin variants, as well as disorders affecting erythrocyte turnover, may cause spurious results.[5] Inaccuracies due to hemoglobin variants may be assay-dependent, whereas those due to erythrocyte turnover are not.[6] Factors affecting HbA1c are listed in **Box 1**. HbA1c values that are inconsistent with the clinical presentation should be further investigated with SMBG or CGM. Alternative markers of glycemic control, such as fructosamine, glycated albumin, and 1,5-anhydroglucitol, may also be considered. These tests are useful for reflecting shorter term changes in glycemia or as alternate glucose markers in the setting of discrepant HbA1c and glucose testing. Longitudinal data are becoming available for their use in predicting diabetes diagnosis and complications, but the evidence for their use is not nearly as robust

Table 1
Correlation of hemoglobin A1c and estimated average glucose

A1c (%)	Estimated Average Glucose	
	mg/dL	mmol/L
6	126 (100–152)	7.0 (5.5–8.5)
7	154 (123–185)	8.6 (6.8–10.3)
8	183 (147–217)	10.2 (8.1–12.1)
9	212 (170–249)	11.8 (9.4–13.9)
10	240 (193–282)	13.4 (10.7–15.7)
11	269 (217–314)	14.9 (12.0–17.5)
12	298 (240–347)	16.5 (13.3–19.3)

Data in parentheses are 95% CIs.
Data from Refs.[3,4,57]

Box 1
Factors affecting hemoglobin A1c
Factors affecting HbA1c interpretation (not assay-dependent)
Alterations of red blood cell lifespan and its treatment
• Anemia (iron deficiency, B12 deficiency)
• Erythrocyte destruction: splenectomy or splenomegaly, hemoglobinopathy, hemolysis
• Red blood cell transfusion
• Chronic liver disease
• Chronic kidney disease
Factors affecting HbA1c Measurement (assay dependent)[a]
• Carbamylated hemoglobin, hemoglobinopathies, hemoglobin F, hemoglobin variants
• Hyperbilirubinemia
• Alcoholism
• Medications: large doses of aspirin, chronic opiate use
• Hypertriglyceridemia
[a] Specific assays available at http://www.ngsp.org.

as for HbA1c.[4,7,8] Each marker has advantages and disadvantages that may be leveraged in individual situations. Early data suggest that a combination of markers may provide a more complete picture of glucose control and complication risk but this requires confirmation before routine use can be recommended.[7–9]

SELF-MONITORED BLOOD GLUCOSE

SMBG was introduced in the 1980s and its benefit has been reasonably established in insulin-treated patients. SMBG allows the patient to identify hypoglycemia and hyperglycemia; get immediate feedback about the effect of food choices, stress, activity, and insulin dosing on glucose levels; and determine whether medication adjustment is needed. Self-monitoring of glucose can identify recurrent hypoglycemia or hyperglycemia even in the setting of an acceptable HbA1c.[10] The frequency and timing of SMBG depends on several factors, particularly on whether a patient is meeting treatment goals or a requiring complex insulin regimen. The routine measurement of postprandial glucose levels or glycemic variability remains controversial but may be useful for patients who fail to meet HbA1c targets. Glycemic variability is a strong predictor of severe hypoglycemia and thus may be used to target the intensity of treatment interventions.[11]

Self-Monitored Blood Glucose in Patients Requiring Insulin

Previous studies in type 1 diabetes have associated increased frequency of SMBG with lower HbA1c and fewer complications.[12,13] American Diabetes Association (ADA) guidelines recommend frequent SMBG in most patients with type 1 diabetes or on intensive insulin regimens such as multiple-dose insulin or insulin pump therapy. SMBG should be performed before meals and snacks, occasionally postprandial, at bedtime, before exercise, when low glucose is suspected, after treating low glucose, and before critical tasks such as driving.[4] Although needs vary by individual, testing may be required 6 to 8 times per day.

Self-Monitored Blood Glucose in Nonintensive Insulin Regimens and in Patients Not Treated with Insulin

There is less evidence regarding SMBG in patients on nonintensive insulin regimens, such as patients with type 2 diabetes on basal insulin, and in patients not treated with insulin. The ADA states that SMBG results may be helpful to guide treatment decisions and/or self-management for patients using less frequent insulin injections or noninsulin therapies.[4] The International Diabetes Federation (IDF) guideline noted a limited evidence base regarding optimal SMBG regimens in noninsulin-treated T2DM but generally agreed that it may not be necessary to perform SMBG on a daily basis.[14] A recent meta-analysis of 2552 subjects in 6 randomized controlled trials found that SMBG in subjects with noninsulin-treated type 2 diabetes reduces HbA1c by 0.25% at 6 months compared with no self-monitoring.[15] There was no effect from cointervention, such as extent of education or baseline HbA1c. A Cochrane review found that the effect of SMBG on glycemic control in patients not using insulin with a diabetes duration of 1 year or more is low for up to 6 months after initiation (mean HbA1c reduction of 0.3%) and subsides after 12 months (nonsignificant mean HbA1c reduction of 0.1%).[16] There was no evidence that SMBG affects patient satisfaction, general well-being, or general health-related quality of life.[16] However, these findings were based on highly selective data and the 12-month conclusion was based on just 2 trials, 1 of which had a limited sample size of 22 subjects.[17] Recent randomized controlled trials that have incorporated robust educational, behavioral, and/or therapeutic interventions in response to blood glucose values have demonstrated larger reductions in HbA1c.[18–20]

Accuracy of Glucose Monitors

The Food and Drug Administration (FDA) currently approves glucose monitors if they meet the analytical accuracy criteria as defined by the International Organization for Standardization (ISO) 15,197, adapted in 2003, which states that 95% of glucose results must be within 15 mg/dL of the reference for glucose less than 75 mg/dL and within 20% of the reference for glucose greater than 75 mg/dL. Soon manufacturers may have to meet the ISO benchmark of 95% of values less than 100 mg/dL within plus or minus 15 mg/dL and greater than 100 mg/dL within plus or minus 15% of the reference range.[21] The new benchmarks also may stipulate that 99% of readings must fall within zones A and B of the error grid analysis, indicating little or no effect on clinical action or outcome. However, the FDA has not yet adopted these standards. Many but not all meters currently meet the 2003 standards.[22,23]

Implementation of Self-Monitored Blood Glucose

The 4 most formidable types of barriers to the appropriate use of SMBG are knowledge barriers, human factors barriers, logbook barriers, and economic barriers.[20] Patient acceptance may be improved through more recent advances such as a decrease in sample amount, alternate site testing, and elimination of the need for coding. Patients with disabilities may benefit from features such as preloaded strips and audio reporting.

ADA guidelines recommend that "patients receive ongoing instruction and regular evaluation of SMBG technique and SMBG results, as well as their ability to use SMBG data to adjust therapy."[4] The IDF guideline for patients with noninsulin-treated T2DM states that "SMBG should be used only when individuals with diabetes (and/or their caregivers) and/or their health care providers have the knowledge, skills, and willingness to incorporate SMBG monitoring and therapy adjustment into their diabetes care plan in order to attain agreed treatment goals."[14] Performing periodic focused SMBG over short periods of time may help identify glucose patterns that reflect daily glycemic control (**Fig. 1**).[14,24] A structured SMBG program improves glycemic control and facilitates more timely and aggressive treatment changes.[19]

Patient and Provider Decision Support

Decision support tools may improve the use of glucose monitoring data and facilitate patient or provider changes in therapy. Downloading meters provides more complete and accurate data than paper logs alone.[25] In addition, the use of pattern management software improves health care provider efficiency and accuracy in identifying needed therapeutic adjustments.[26,27] Bolus calculators are known to substantially improve dosing accuracy and glycemic control in outpatients with type 1 diabetes.[28–30] An integrated approach containing a bolus calculator, automated advice for insulin dose adjustments, and communication with the healthcare provider may provide the best HbA1c reduction.[31] Telemedicine approaches have received increasing attention as a means of providing cost-effective care.[32] Smart phone applications may organize SMBG data, some allow insulin or other diabetes education, and a few provide a bolus calculator. However, their safety and usability have not been extensively studied.[33]

CONTINUOUS GLUCOSE MONITORING

SMBG may miss important fluctuations in glucose that are easily identifiable using CGM. CGM data may be used to help patients manage glucose trends in real time or retrospectively. A system is categorized according to whether it is owned by a health care provider and features only retrospective data (professional CGM) or it provides real-time (RT) data (personal CGM or RT-CGM).

A	Before breakfast	After breakfast	Before lunch	After lunch	Before dinner	After dinner	Bedtime
Week 1							
Day 1: Sunday	x	x	x	x	x	x	x
Day 2: Thursday	x	x	x	x	x	x	x
Week 2							
Day 1: Monday	x	x	x	x	x	x	x
Day 2: Friday	x	x	x	x	x	x	x
Week 3							
Day 1: Tuesday	x	x	x	x	x	x	x
Day 2: Saturday	x	x	x	x	x	x	x

B	Before breakfast	After breakfast	Before lunch	After lunch	Before dinner	After dinner	Bedtime
Day 1	x	x					
Day 2			x	x			
Day 3					x	x	
Day 4	x	x					

Fig. 1. Two possible schemes for focused SMBG. (*A*) Periodic 7-point glucose profile obtained once or twice per week. (*B*) Paired readings before meals and after meals sampled throughout the week. (*Data from* International Diabetes Federation Clinical Practice Guidelines: Self-monitoring of blood glucose in noninsulin-treated type 2 diabetes. 2009; and Schnell O, Alawi H, Battelino T, et al. Addressing schemes of self-monitoring of blood glucose in type 2 diabetes: a European perspective and expert recommendation. Diabetes Technol Ther 2011;13:959–65.)

Professional Continuous Glucose Monitoring

Professional CGM provides the glucose results after they have been collected in a download, allowing the health care provider to obtain unbiased glucose patterns during typical everyday life. The Endocrine Society recommendations for professional CGM are shown in **Table 2**. Professional CGM is more readily reimbursed than personal CGM. Currently, the dedicated professional system (Medtronic *i*Pro2, Medtronic, Inc., Minneapolis, MN) and several personal CGM systems (Dexcom G4 Platinum, Dexcom, Inc., San Diego, CA, Freestyle Navigator II, Alameda, CA, [not available in the U.S.]) can be operated in a blinded fashion to provide professional glucose data. The *i*Pro2 is wireless and requires minimal patient interaction or training. The mean absolute relative difference from the reference standard is reported to be 9.9% to 10.1% overall and is lower in the hypoglycemic range (40–80 mg/dL).[34] It is recommended that patients keep a separate diet, activity, symptom, and insulin diary during professional CGM to assist with interpretation.

Personal Continuous Glucose Monitoring (Real-Time Continuous Glucose Monitoring)

Personal CGM devices display the current glucose as well as trend arrows every few minutes. All personal CGM devices can be downloaded for retrospective review of data (**Fig. 2**). RT-CGM warns the patient of impending (projected alarm) or actual (threshold alarm) glucose levels outside of prespecified targets.

In 2008, the Juvenile Diabetes Research Foundation Continuous Glucose Monitoring Study demonstrated 0.53% (P<.01) greater HbA1c reduction among 322 adults and children with type 1 diabetes randomized to RT-CGM compared with usual care.[35] The sensor-augmented pump therapy for A1C reduction (STAR3) study

Table 2 Professional society recommendations for use of continuous glucose monitoring			
	Endocrine Society	**ADA**	**AACE**
Professional CGM	Adults and pediatric patients with DM to • Detect nocturnal hypoglycemia dawn phenomenon or postprandial hyperglycemia • Assist in management of DM therapies	—	—
Personal CGM	Adults, children, and adolescents with T1DM demonstrating near-daily use; there were no recommendations for against use for children <age 8	• T1DM >age 25 on intensive insulin regimens • Younger groups demonstrating adherence	T1DM and 1 of the following: • Frequent hypoglycemia or hypoglycemia unawareness • Elevated HbA1c • Excessive glucose variability • Preconception or pregnancy • Younger patients demonstrating near-daily use

Abbreviations: AACE, American Association of Clinical Endocrinologists; DM, Diabetes mellitus; T1DM, type 1 diabetes mellitus.

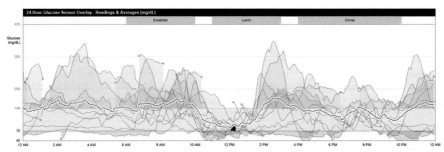

Fig. 2. Retrospective download of Personal CGM. This daily glucose overlay during the period of monitoring shows a pattern of hypoglycemia that is most pronounced in the late morning and afternoon, and overnight hypoglycemia.

randomized 485 adults and children to sensor-augmented pump therapy or multiple daily injections per day and reported a treatment difference in HbA1c of 0.6% (P<.001).[36] In both studies, HbA1c reduction was only significant among subjects who consistently used the device, generally those who were older. Meta-analyses have found more modest HbA1c reductions and reported better results among older patients using insulin pumps who had better adherence.[37] Severe hypoglycemia rates did not differ. However, the quality of most studies are limited due to small sample size, lack of blinding, lack of sufficient data to compare hypoglycemia rates, and inclusion of obsolete technology.[38,39] Subjects with a history of severe hypoglycemia were often excluded. Studies that specifically enrolled subjects at risk for hypoglycemia and used blinded CGM to assess it did show improvement in hypoglycemia.[40,41] Generic quality of life scores generally do not improve with RT-CGM but treatment-specific measures, particularly fear of hypoglycemia, and, to a lesser extent, measures of convenience, efficacy, and performance, may be improved.[42]

Guidelines and Selection of Subjects

Clinical trials have shown that HbA1c reduction is directly associated with sensor use greater than 6 days per week.[37,38,43,44] Adherence is higher in subjects older than age 25, those who perform glucose self-monitoring more than 5 times per day, and those with early CGM values between 70 to 180 mg/dL. Professional society recommendations are shown in **Table 2**.[4,45,46] These guidelines will need to be updated as new technology becomes available.

Real-Time Continuous Glucose Monitoring

RT-CGM technologies generally provide real-time glucose readings every 1 to 5 minutes. Over time, accuracy with CGM has improved substantially but remains an important limiting factor for widespread adoption of use.[47–49] Structured education programs should be completed before considering RT-CGM. Patients should be adequately informed of the benefits and, just as important, the limitations of this technology. Patients must be aware that sensor readings can deviate from actual blood glucose measurements, particularly during rapid glucose changes such as those which occur after a meal or during exercise. Patients should be instructed to verify sensor readings before taking action on meal boluses or treatment of hypoglycemia. Alarm thresholds should be set to maximize patient adherence, keeping in mind that the sensitivity for detecting hypoglycemia drops significantly as the threshold is lowered below 70 mg/dL. Algorithms for using RT-CGM data in real-time may improve quality of life and HbA1c reduction[50] as well as facilitate patient self-adjustment.[51]

Toward Closed-Loop Insulin Delivery

It should be emphasized that most prospective randomized controlled trials enroll highly motivated subjects. It is less clear whether RT-CGM can be useful for patients in the real-world setting, in which there are fewer resources for training, and less motivated patients may be overwhelmed with the additional data.[52,53] Closed-loop insulin delivery (the artificial pancreas) holds promise for automating insulin delivery in response to CGM data and potentially will allow more patients to take advantage of CGM. Recently, low-glucose threshold-suspend technology has been implemented as the first step toward an artificial pancreas. In a study of 247 subjects with type 1 diabetes and documented nocturnal hypoglycemia who were randomized to sensor-augmented pump with or without a low-glucose threshold-suspend feature, there was a lower frequency of nocturnal hypoglycemia in the low-glucose threshold-suspend group and no difference in frequency of diabetic ketoacidosis.[54] Progress toward a fully automated closed loop system is likely to progress incrementally, with overnight closed loop and hyperglycemia minimizer features as future steps.

FUTURE CONSIDERATIONS: SUMMARY

There are emerging noninvasive methods to measure glucose, including measuring glucose in exhaled breath[55] and glucose measurement in tears.[56] These approaches require further study. As current glycemic monitoring strategies evolve and more sophisticated approaches become available, additional study will be needed to assess accuracy, implementation strategies, efficacy, patient satisfaction, and cost-effectiveness.

REFERENCES

1. Goldstein DE, Little RR, Lorenz RA, et al. Tests of glycemia in diabetes. Diabetes Care 2004;27:1761–73.
2. Little RR, Rohlfing CL, Sacks DB. Status of hemoglobin A1c measurement and goals for improvement: from chaos to order for improving diabetes care. Clin Chem 2011;57:205–14.
3. Nathan DM, Kuenen J, Borg R, et al. Translating the A1C assay into estimated average glucose values. Diabetes Care 2008;31:1473–8.
4. American Diabetes Association. Standards of medical care in diabetes–2014. Diabetes Care 2014;37(Suppl 1):S14–80.
5. Gallagher EJ, Le Roith D, Bloomgarden Z. Review of hemoglobin A(1c) in the management of diabetes. J Diabetes 2009;1:9–17.
6. Little RR, Roberts WL. A review of variant hemoglobins interfering with hemoglobin A1c measurement. J Diabetes Sci Technol 2009;3:446–51.
7. Selvin E, Rawlings AM, Grams M, et al. Fructosamine and glycated albumin for risk stratification and prediction of incident diabetes and microvascular complications: a prospective cohort analysis of the Atherosclerosis Risk in Communities (ARIC) study. Lancet Diabetes Endocrinol 2014;2:279–88.
8. Nathan DM, McGee P, Steffes MW, et al. Relationship of glycated albumin to blood glucose and HbA1c values and to retinopathy, nephropathy, and cardiovascular outcomes in the DCCT/EDIC study. Diabetes 2014;63:282–90.
9. Dungan KM. Predicting outcomes and assessing control with alternate glycemic markers. Diabetes Technol Ther 2012;14:749–52.

10. Dailey G. Assessing glycemic control with self-monitoring of blood glucose and hemoglobin A(1c) measurements. Mayo Clin Proc 2007;82:229–35 [quiz: 236].

11. Kilpatrick ES, Rigby AS, Goode K, et al. Relating mean blood glucose and glucose variability to the risk of multiple episodes of hypoglycaemia in type 1 diabetes. Diabetologia 2007;50:2553–61.

12. Miller KM, Beck RW, Bergenstal RM, et al. Evidence of a strong association between frequency of self-monitoring of blood glucose and hemoglobin A1c levels in T1D exchange clinic registry participants. Diabetes Care 2013;36: 2009–14.

13. Ziegler R, Heidtmann B, Hilgard D, et al. Frequency of SMBG correlates with HbA1c and acute complications in children and adolescents with type 1 diabetes. Pediatr Diabetes 2011;12:11–7.

14. International Diabetes Federation Clinical Practice Guidelines: self-monitoring of blood glucose in non-insulin treated type 2 diabetes. Brussels: International Diabetes Federation; 2009.

15. Farmer AJ, Perera R, Ward A, et al. Meta-analysis of individual patient data in randomised trials of self monitoring of blood glucose in people with non-insulin treated type 2 diabetes. BMJ 2012;344:e486.

16. Malanda UL, Welschen LM, Riphagen II, et al. Self-monitoring of blood glucose in patients with type 2 diabetes mellitus who are not using insulin. Cochrane Database Syst Rev 2012;(1):CD005060.

17. Schnell O, Alawi H, Battelino T, et al. Self-monitoring of blood glucose in type 2 diabetes: recent studies. J Diabetes Sci Technol 2013;7:478–88.

18. Weinger K, Beverly EA, Lee Y, et al. The effect of a structured behavioral intervention on poorly controlled diabetes: a randomized controlled trial. Arch Intern Med 2011;171:1990–9.

19. Polonsky WH, Fisher L, Schikman CH, et al. Structured self-monitoring of blood glucose significantly reduces A1C levels in poorly controlled, noninsulin-treated type 2 diabetes: results from the structured testing program study. Diabetes Care 2011;34:262–7.

20. Klonoff DC, Blonde L, Cembrowski G, et al. Consensus report: the current role of self-monitoring of blood glucose in non-insulin-treated type 2 diabetes. J Diabetes Sci Technol 2011;5:1529–48.

21. In vitro diagnostic test systems—requirements for blood-glucose monitoring systems for self-testing in managing diabetes mellitus. ISO 15197:2013. Geneva: International Organization for Standardization; 2013.

22. Freckmann G, Schmid C, Baumstark A, et al. System accuracy evaluation of 43 blood glucose monitoring systems for self-monitoring of blood glucose according to DIN EN ISO 15197. J Diabetes Sci Technol 2012;6:1060–75.

23. Freckmann G, Baumstark A, Schmid C, et al. Evaluation of 12 blood glucose monitoring systems for self-testing: system accuracy and measurement reproducibility. Diabetes Technol Ther 2014;16:113–22.

24. Schnell O, Alawi H, Battelino T, et al. Addressing schemes of self-monitoring of blood glucose in type 2 diabetes: a European perspective and expert recommendation. Diabetes Technol Ther 2011;13:959–65.

25. Given JE, O'Kane MJ, Coates VE, et al. Comparing patient generated blood glucose diary records with meter memory in type 2 diabetes. Diabetes Res Clin Pract 2014;104(3):358–62.

26. Katz LB, Dirani RG, Li G, et al. Automated glycemic pattern analysis can improve health care professional efficiency and accuracy. J Diabetes Sci Technol 2013;7:163–6.

27. Parkin CG, Davidson JA. Value of self-monitoring blood glucose pattern analysis in improving diabetes outcomes. J Diabetes Sci Technol 2009;3: 500–8.

28. Shashaj B, Busetto E, Sulli N. Benefits of a bolus calculator in pre- and post-prandial glycaemic control and meal flexibility of paediatric patients using continuous subcutaneous insulin infusion (CSII). Diabet Med 2008;25: 1036–42.

29. Maurizi AR, Lauria A, Maggi D, et al. A novel insulin unit calculator for the management of type 1 diabetes. Diabetes Technol Ther 2011;13:425–8.

30. Ziegler R, Cavan DA, Cranston I, et al. Use of an insulin bolus advisor improves glycemic control in multiple daily insulin injection (MDI) therapy patients with suboptimal glycemic control: first results from the ABACUS trial. Diabetes Care 2013;36:3613–9.

31. Charpentier G, Benhamou PY, Dardari D, et al. The Diabeo software enabling individualized insulin dose adjustments combined with telemedicine support improves HbA1c in poorly controlled type 1 diabetic patients: a 6-month, randomized, open-label, parallel-group, multicenter trial (TeleDiab 1 study). Diabetes Care 2011;34:533–9.

32. Del Prato S, Nicolucci A, Lovagnini-Scher AC, et al. Telecare provides comparable efficacy to conventional self-monitored blood glucose in patients with type 2 diabetes titrating one injection of insulin glulisine-the ELEONOR study. Diabetes Technol Ther 2012;14:175–82.

33. Demidowich AP, Lu K, Tamler R, et al. An evaluation of diabetes self-management applications for Android smartphones. J Telemed Telecare 2012; 18:235–8.

34. Welsh JB, Kaufman FR, Lee SW. Accuracy of the Sof-sensor glucose sensor with the iPro calibration algorithm. J Diabetes Sci Technol 2012;6:475–6.

35. Tamborlane WV, Beck RW, Bode BW, et al. Continuous glucose monitoring and intensive treatment of type 1 diabetes. N Engl J Med 2008;359:1464–76.

36. Bergenstal RM, Tamborlane WV, Ahmann A, et al. Effectiveness of sensor-augmented insulin-pump therapy in type 1 diabetes. N Engl J Med 2010;363: 311–20.

37. Langendam M, Luijf YM, Hooft L, et al. Continuous glucose monitoring systems for type 1 diabetes mellitus. Cochrane Database Syst Rev 2012;(1):CD008101.

38. Yeh HC, Brown TT, Maruthur N, et al. Comparative effectiveness and safety of methods of insulin delivery and glucose monitoring for diabetes mellitus: a systematic review and meta-analysis. Ann Intern Med 2012;157:336–47.

39. Pickup JC. The evidence base for diabetes technology: appropriate and inappropriate meta-analysis. J Diabetes Sci Technol 2013;7:1567–74.

40. Pickup JC, Freeman SC, Sutton AJ. Glycaemic control in type 1 diabetes during real time continuous glucose monitoring compared with self monitoring of blood glucose: meta-analysis of randomised controlled trials using individual patient data. BMJ 2011;343:d3805.

41. Battelino T, Phillip M, Bratina N, et al. Effect of continuous glucose monitoring on hypoglycemia in type 1 diabetes. Diabetes Care 2011;34:795–800.

42. Rubin RR, Peyrot M. Health-related quality of life and treatment satisfaction in the sensor-augmented pump therapy for A1C Reduction 3 (STAR 3) trial. Diabetes Technol Ther 2012;14:143–51.

43. Beck RW, Buckingham B, Miller K, et al. Factors predictive of use and of benefit from continuous glucose monitoring in type 1 diabetes. Diabetes Care 2009;32: 1947–53.

44. Buse JB, Dailey G, Ahmann AA, et al. Baseline predictors of A1C reduction in adults using sensor-augmented pump therapy or multiple daily injection therapy: the STAR 3 experience. Diabetes Technol Ther 2011;13:601–6.
45. Klonoff DC, Buckingham B, Christiansen JS, et al. Continuous glucose monitoring: an Endocrine Society Clinical Practice Guideline. J Clin Endocrinol Metab 2011;96:2968–79.
46. Blevins TC, Bode BW, Garg SK, et al. Statement by the American Association of Clinical Endocrinologists Consensus Panel on continuous glucose monitoring. Endocr Pract 2010;16:730–45.
47. Keenan DB, Mastrototaro JJ, Zisser H, et al. Accuracy of the Enlite 6-day glucose sensor with guardian and Veo calibration algorithms. Diabetes Technol Ther 2012;14:225–31.
48. Christiansen M, Bailey T, Watkins E, et al. A new-generation continuous glucose monitoring system: improved accuracy and reliability compared with a previous-generation system. Diabetes Technol Ther 2013;15:881–8.
49. Luijf YM, Mader JK, Doll W, et al. Accuracy and reliability of continuous glucose monitoring systems: a head-to-head comparison. Diabetes Technol Ther 2013; 15:722–7.
50. Jenkins AJ, Krishnamurthy B, Best JD, et al. An algorithm guiding patient responses to real-time-continuous glucose monitoring improves quality of life. Diabetes Technol Ther 2011;13:105–9.
51. Buckingham B, Xing D, Weinzimer S, et al. Use of the DirecNet applied treatment algorithm (DATA) for diabetes management with a real-time continuous glucose monitor (the FreeStyle Navigator). Pediatr Diabetes 2008;9:142–7.
52. Norgaard K, Scaramuzza A, Bratina N, et al. Routine sensor-augmented pump therapy in type 1 diabetes: the INTERPRET study. Diabetes Technol Ther 2013; 15:273–80.
53. Juvenile Diabetes Research Foundation Continuous Glucose Monitoring Study Group. Effectiveness of continuous glucose monitoring in a clinical care environment: evidence from the Juvenile Diabetes Research Foundation continuous glucose monitoring (JDRF-CGM) trial. Diabetes Care 2010;33:17–22.
54. Bergenstal RM, Klonoff DC, Garg SK, et al. Threshold-based insulin-pump interruption for reduction of hypoglycemia. N Engl J Med 2013;369:224–32.
55. Roberts K, Jaffe A, Verge C, et al. Noninvasive monitoring of glucose levels: is exhaled breath the answer? J Diabetes Sci Technol 2012;6:659–64.
56. Zhang J, Hodge W, Hutnick C, et al. Noninvasive diagnostic devices for diabetes through measuring tear glucose. J Diabetes Sci Technol 2011;5:166–72.
57. Estimated average glucose, eAG. Available at: http://professional.diabetes.org/GlucoseCalculator.aspx. Accessed May 19, 2014.

Glycemic Targets
What is the Evidence?

Silvio Inzucchi, MD[a,b,*], Sachin Majumdar, MD[a,c]

KEYWORDS

- Glycemic targets • Diabetes • Microvascular • Macrovascular • Glycemic control

KEY POINTS

- The available evidence supports targeting near-normal glucose levels for the prevention and reduction of the microvascular complications of diabetes.
- Although there is a strong relationship between glucose levels and macrovascular disease in diabetes, the evidence for preventing and reducing the macrovascular complications of diabetes by glucose lowering is limited.
- Glycemic targets must be individualized and based on patient specific factors that balance the benefits of therapy with its harms.

THE GLUCOSE HYPOTHESIS

Ants, bees, and ancient physicians recognized a sweet taste in the urine of individuals afflicted by a condition of polyuria and wasting. With the attachment of the Latin term, *mellitus*, diabetes was forever linked to a disorder of glucose metabolism. Although many other metabolic abnormalities exist in diabetes, its diagnosis and, to a large degree, its management are unified through the presence of hyperglycemia. In 1943, Dr Eliot Joslin[1] observed that life expectancy after the onset of diabetes had increased from less than 5 years to greater than 14 years with the introduction of insulin therapy, and more patients were living long enough to suffer from its complications. These complications have been divided into 2 general categories: (1) microvascular: retinopathy, nephropathy, and neuropathy; and (2) macrovascular, affecting the coronary, cerebral, and peripheral vascular systems. The central question is whether the obvious abnormality of diabetes (ie, hyperglycemia) is responsible for these complications. This is the basis of the glucose hypothesis: that hyperglycemia is their direct cause and that, by normalizing systemic glucose levels, these morbidities can be prevented.

[a] Department of Endocrinology, Yale University School of Medicine, New Haven, CT; [b] Medical Director, Yale Diabetes Center, Yale-New Haven Hospital, New Haven, CT; [c] Section of Endocrinology, Bridgeport Hospital, Yale New Haven Health System, Bridgeport, CT
* Corresponding author. Department of Endocrinology, Yale University School of Medicine, New Haven, CT
E-mail address: silvio.inzucchi@yale.edu

Med Clin N Am 99 (2015) 47–67
http://dx.doi.org/10.1016/j.mcna.2014.08.018
0025-7125/15/$ – see front matter © 2015 Elsevier Inc. All rights reserved.
medical.theclinics.com

GLUCOSE AND MICROVASCULAR DISEASE

Diabetes is the leading cause of retinopathy, end-stage renal disease, and peripheral neuropathy in the United States.[2–4] These conditions also occur in nondiabetic individuals but their excess occurrence in diabetes and relationship to hyperglycemia are specific enough to be considered disease defining.[5–7]

In a 15-year cohort study of nondiabetic individuals, the cumulative incidence of retinopathy was 14% and was linked to baseline age, blood pressure, and the presence of chronic kidney disease.[8] In comparison, in a cohort of type 1 and 2 diabetics, the incidence of retinopathy over a 10-year period ranged from 67% to 89%.[9] The Wisconsin Epidemiologic Study of Diabetic Retinopathy reported a 97% cumulative incidence of any degree of retinopathy over a period of 25 years in type 1 diabetic patients.[10] Although this was not an intervention study, the most powerful predictor of retinopathy progression was glycemic control (**Fig. 1**). Findings are similar for microalbuminuria, with prevalence rates of 2.6% to 6.6% in nondiabetic populations compared with 13.8% to 16.4% for those with diabetes, with progression to overt proteinuria at rates of 36% to 44% over 10 years.[9,11] Neuropathy is similarly associated with both diabetes and glycemic control (**Fig. 2**).[12,13]

But at what levels of glycemia do microvascular complications occur and is there a threshold? Several studies show that the prevalence of retinopathy increases from less than 5% to greater than 10% as fasting glucose levels exceed 120 to 126 mg/dL and the 2-hour glucose level during an oral glucose tolerance test (OGTT) exceeds 195 to 207 mg/dL.[6,14,15] For example, a Finnish study showed a transition point around a fasting glucose of approximately120 mg/dL (**Fig. 3**).[16] The prevalence of retinopathy has also been reported in individuals ranging from normal to diabetic, and a threshold hemoglobin A_{1c} (HbA_{1c}) of approximately 6.2% was able to identify those at higher risk for retinopathy in one analysis (**Fig. 4**).[14,17] Several large population studies suggest a more continuous relationship

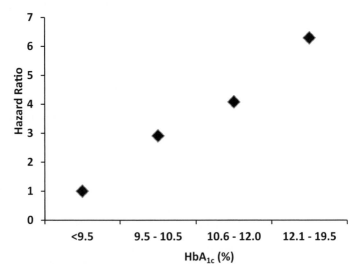

Fig. 1. Hazard ratios for the progression of proliferative retinopathy according to HbA_{1c} category in the Wisconsin Epidemiologic Study of Diabetic Retinopathy. (*Data from* Klein R, Knudston MD, Lee KE, et al. The Wisconsin epidemiologic study of diabetic retinopathy XXII: the twenty-five-year progression of retinopathy in persons with type 1 diabetes. Ophthalmology 2008;115:1859–68.)

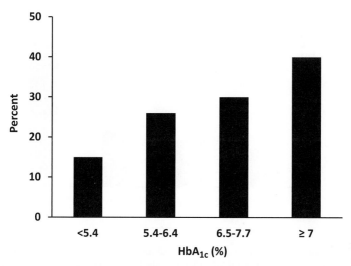

Fig. 2. Prevalence of neuropathy according to HbA$_{1c}$ category in the EURODIAB study. (*Data from* Tesfaye S, Stevens LK, Stephenson JM, et al, EURODIAB IDDM Study Group. Prevalence of diabetic peripheral neuropathy and its relation to glycaemic control and potential risk factors: the EURODIAB IDDM Complications Study. Diabetologia 1996;39:1377–84.)

without a clear threshold although rates of moderate retinopathy rose with fasting glucose concentrations greater than 112 mg/dL, with greater increases above concentrations of 128 to 140 mg/dL.[18]

Epidemiologic associations between glycemia and microvascular disease are strong but cannot determine whether the relationship is causal. Basic investigations have been helpful in identifying the effects of elevated glucose in tissues where microvascular disease occurs, primarily involving protein glycation, basement membrane

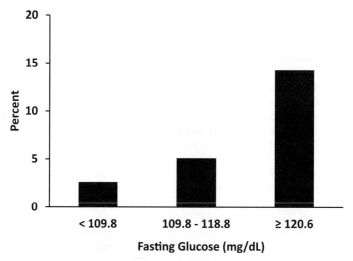

Fig. 3. Prevalence of retinopathy according to fasting glucose values in a Finnish population. (*Data from* Rajala U, Laakso M, Qiao Q, et al. Prevalence of retinopathy in people with diabetes, impaired glucose tolerance, and normal glucose tolerance. Diabetes Care 1998;21:1664–9.)

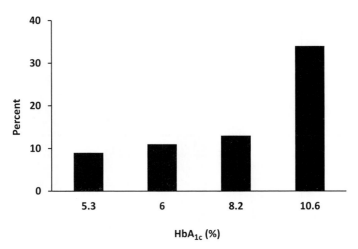

Fig. 4. Prevalence of retinopathy according to diabetes status. HbA_{1c} categories representing nondiabetic (5.3%) impaired glucose metabolism (6%), newly diagnosed diabetes (8.2%), and established diabetes (10.6%). (*Data from* Van Leiden HA, Dekker JM, Moll, AC, et al. Blood pressure, lipids, and obesity are associated with retinopathy: the Hoorn Study. Diabetes Care 2002;25:1320–5.)

expansion, and endothelial injury, but are beyond the scope of this review.[19] If the glucose hypothesis is correct, however, these complications should be preventable or perhaps even reversible by normalizing glucose levels.

GLUCOSE AND MACROVASCULAR DISEASE

Cardiovascular disease (CVD)—and not microvascular complications—is the leading cause of death in individuals with diabetes, with a prevalence 2- to 3-fold greater than in the general population. Not surprisingly, CVD is also a major contributor to the health care costs of this disease.[20–22]

Diabetes has a clear influence on cardiovascular (CV) risk—independently and through interactions with traditional risk factors. In the Multiple Risk Factor Intervention Trial, the presence of diabetes conferred a 3- to 4-fold increase of CV death that was further compounded by additional risk factors.[21] A Finnish study raised the notion that diabetes is a coronary disease risk equivalent, meaning that individuals with diabetes, without preexisting coronary heart disease (CHD), have the same risk of subsequent myocardial infarction (MI) as those in whom it is already established.[23] Follow-up at 18 years showed that diabetic individuals without preexisting CHD had risks of CHD mortality similar to those with established heart disease, but when both conditions were present mortality was approximately 3-fold greater than with either condition alone (**Fig. 5**).[24] Other investigations, however, have refuted this claim of diabetes as a CHD risk equivalent and one explanation for the discordant findings may be variation in glycemic control.[25,26] In older subjects with type 2 diabetes mellitus followed for an average of 7.4 years, CV mortality increased according to fasting glucose across quintiles from approximately 16% mortality for those with levels less than 121 mg/dL to approximately 33% for those with levels greater than 180 mg/dL.[27] In a 6-year Swedish registry study of type 2 diabetics, fatal CV events occurred in 7.6%, 8.9%, and 11.2% of subjects with mean HbA_{1c} levels of 6.5%, 7.5%, and 8.5%, respectively.[28] Similar data also exist for type 1 diabetes mellitus, showing

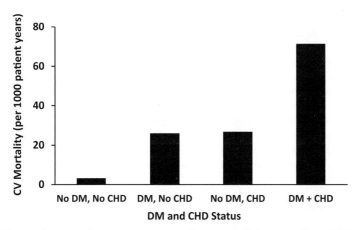

Fig. 5. CV mortality according to presence or absence of diabetes mellitus (DM), coronary heart disease (CHD) or both, at baseline. (*Data from* Juutilainen A, Lehto S, Ronnemaa T, et al. Type 2 diabetes as a "coronary heart disease equivalent". Diabetes Care 2005;28:2901–7.)

lower CV risk with HbA$_{1c}$ levels of 7.2% versus 9.0%.[29] Still, it is not clear from these studies whether glucose is directly responsible for the higher risk or whether it is more of a marker.

Fasting glucose, the response to an OGTT, and HbA$_{1c}$ can predict risk of CVD.[30–34] This risk increases with degrees of glycemia that are either within or slightly above the normal range, for example, fasting glucose greater than 101 mg/dL or HbA$_{1c}$ greater than 5% (**Fig. 6**).[30–32] Twenty-year follow-up of several large studies has even

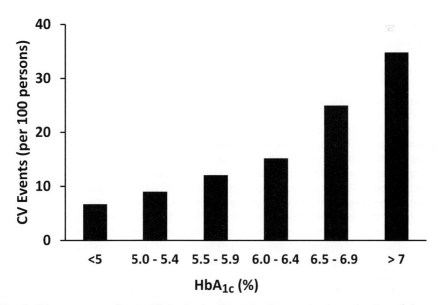

Fig. 6. CV events according to HbA$_{1c}$ in the European Prospective Investigation of Cancer (EPIC)-Norfolk study. (*Data from* Khaw KT, Wareham N, Luben R, et al. Glycated hemoglobin, diabetes, and mortality in men in Norfolk cohort of European Prospective Investigation of Cancer and Nutrition (EPIC-Norfolk). BMJ 2001;322:1–6.)

shown elevated CVD and mortality in nondiabetic individuals with glucose levels ranging from 100 to 169 mg/dL after 2-hour OGTT compared with levels less than 100 mg/dL.[35] Glucose tolerance also corresponds to a significant increase in the prevalence of peripheral vascular disease, particularly with 2-hour levels greater than 200 mg/dL.[6,36,37] The bulk of the data suggest no specific threshold as exists with microvascular disease and, although basic science supports a role for hyperglycemia in promoting atherosclerosis, its origins and progression are influenced by an interplay of factors, including dyslipidemia, hypertension, inflammation, insulin resistance, and genetics. These factors make the independent effect of glucose on atherogenesis more difficult to discern, contrasting with microvascular disease, which predominantly involves injury to a single endothelial layer and seems primarily driven by hyperglycemia.[19,38]

Given all the uncertainty regarding the precise effects of hyperglycemia on vascular diseases, particularly as it relates to treatment targets, clinical trials of glucose-lowering therapies have constituted the necessary test of the glucose hypothesis for both microvascular and macrovascular complications. Herein lies the bulk of the knowledge on this fundamentally important clinical question in diabetes care.

LARGE RANDOMIZED CLINICAL TRIALS TESTING GLYCEMIC TARGETS ON CLINICAL ENDPOINTS
Diabetes Control and Complications Trial

The Diabetes Control and Complications Trial (DCCT) set out to determine whether achieving near-normal glucose levels with intensive insulin therapy could prevent the onset and progression of the vascular and neurologic complications of type 1 diabetes mellitus.[39] Retinopathy was selected as a principal outcome and 2 major questions were asked: (1) Can intensive therapy prevent the development of retinopathy (primary prevention)? and (2) Can intensive therapy prevent the progression of early retinopathy (secondary prevention)? Other vascular and neurologic outcomes were also studied.

Enrollment occurred from 1983 to 1989 with 1441 patients entering the study and 1398 completing it in 1993. It was terminated after an average follow-up of 6.5 years because of significant differences in endpoints. Nonrandomized follow-up is available for an additional 18 years after treatment assignments ended.[39,40] The average age of patients entering the study was 27 years and there were 2 major study groups, those with recently diagnosed with type 1 diabetes mellitus (mean approximately 2.6 years) with no baseline retinopathy (n = 726) and those with a longer-duration type 1 diabetes mellitus (mean approximately 8.8 years) with early retinopathy (n = 715). Each group was randomized to either intensive glucose control, defined as 3 or more insulin injections per day or continuous subcutaneous insulin infusion, where both basal and prandial insulin replacement was targeted, or a conventional regimen, consisting of 1 or 2 insulin injections per day. Glycemic targets for the intensive group were premeal glucose levels of 70 to 120 mg/dL, postmeal less than 180 mg/dL, and HbA$_{1c}$ less than or equal to 6%. Conventional therapy goals were merely to avoid symptomatic hyperglycemia, hypoglycemia, and ketonuria and maintain normal weight and, in adolescents, growth.

Over approximately 9 years, the mean HbA$_{1c}$ levels were 9.1% for the conventional group and 7.2% for the intensive group.[39,40] The relative risk reductions (RRRs) in retinopathy were 76% (95% CI, 62–85; P<.001) and 54% (95% CI, 39–66; P<.001) in the primary and secondary intervention cohorts. Reductions in nephropathy (urinary albumin excretion [UAE] >40 mg/d) were 34% (95% CI, 2–56; P = .04) and 43% (95% CI,

21–58; $P = .01$) in the primary and secondary intervention cohorts, and those for neuropathy were 69% (95% CI, 24–87; $P = .006$) and 57% (95% CI, 29–73; $P \leq .001$). When the entire study population was analyzed according to HbA_{1c}, retinopathy rates were dependent on glycemic control and independent of treatment assignment, with all individuals maintaining HbA_{1c} levels of 6.5% to 7.49% having low rates of retinopathy and those with HbA_{1c} levels of 8.5% to 9.49% having higher rates—supporting the hypothesis that glucose was the determining factor.[41] CV events were insignificant. The major side effects of intensive therapy were weight gain and hypoglycemic events, with 62 versus 19 severe episodes of hypoglycemia (per 100 patient years) in the intensive versus conventional group.

After the trial, conventionally treated subjects were trained in intensive therapy and both groups returned to the care of their individual providers. They were also asked to participate in an observational study, the Epidemiology of Diabetes Interventions and Complications (EDIC) study, with follow-up now available to 18 years post-trial.[40] During the EDIC study, the mean HbA_{1c} levels for the original conventional and intensive groups were similar at approximately 8%, and, despite loss of the initial differences in HbA_{1c}, there were significant reductions in all clinically meaningful endpoints, such as advanced retinopathy, nephropathy, and CV events, for those originally assigned to intensive therapy.[40,42–44] CV benefits became significant after a mean follow-up of 17 years, when the average age of participants was 45 years in EDIC study year 11, and significant reductions in microvascular events persisted at 18 and 24 years (**Figs. 7–9**).[40,42,44] It was estimated from the EDIC experience that a 10% relative decrease in HbA_{1c} was associated with a 20% risk reduction in CV events.[42] The EDIC study also reported on a musculoskeletal condition associated with diabetes, cheiroarthropathy, or periarticular thickening of the skin of the hands, resulting in significant disability.[43] At EDIC years 18 and 19, it was present in 64% and 68% of intensive and conventional subjects, respectively, and was proportional to diabetes duration and glycemic control and associated with the presence of microvascular complications.

The DCCT showed that achieving near-normal glucose levels in young adults with type 1 diabetes mellitus can prevent microvascular complications, supporting the glucose hypothesis and establishing intensive therapy as the standard of care for this form of the disease. EDIC suggested that initial intensive therapy has long-term health benefits despite later deterioration in glucose control, giving rise to the somewhat theoretic terms, *metabolic memory* and *legacy effect*.

United Kingdom Prospective Diabetes Study

The United Kingdom Prospective Diabetes Study (UKPDS) is the largest and longest trial to study the relationship between glucose control and patient outcomes in individuals with newly diagnosed type 2 diabetes mellitus.[45–47] The major aims of the study were to determine whether achieving near-normal fasting glucose levels (<108 mg/dL) improves morbidity and mortality and if there are advantages to using various treatment modalities, such as insulin, sulfonylurea, or metformin.

Enrollment began in 1977 with 5 centers, and additional were ones added in 1982 and 1987, with recruitment ending in 1991. The trial concluded in 1997 and follow-up data are available until 2007.[48] The initial randomization included 4209 newly diagnosed diabetics referred from local general practitioners and excluded those with MI within the last year, any major vascular event, or severe retinopathy.[46] After a 3-month dietary run-in period, individuals with glucose levels of 108 to 270 mg/dL were randomized to either intensive therapy with either a sulfonylurea or insulin, aiming for fasting glucose levels less than 108 mg/dL, or to dietary therapy, aiming for fasting

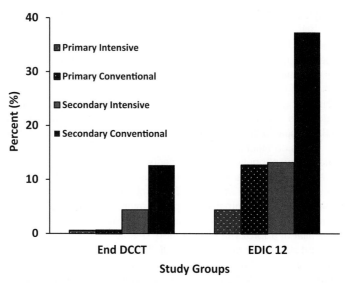

Fig. 7. Prevalence of proliferative retinopathy at the end of DCCT and at EDIC year 12 according to cohort, primary prevention and secondary prevention, and treatment intervention, intensive versus conventional. (*Data from* Diabetes Control and Complications Trial/ Epidemiology of Diabetes Interventions and Complications Research Group. Prolonged effect of intensive therapy on the risk of retinopathy complications in patients with type 1 diabetes mellitus: 10 years after the diabetes control and complications trial. Arch Ophthalmol 2008;126(12):1707–15.)

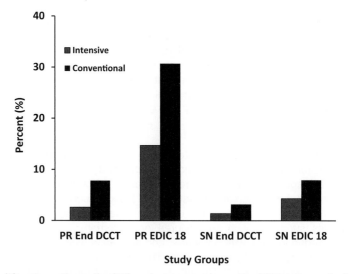

Fig. 8. Proliferative retinopathy (PR) and severe nephropathy (SN) at the end of the DCCT and at EDIC year 18 in combined primary and secondary intervention cohorts, by intensive versus conventional therapy. Severe nephropathy defined as albumin excretion ratio (AER) greater than 300 mg/d or end-stage renal disease. (*Data from* Nathan DM. The diabetes control and complications trial/epidemiology of diabetes interventions and complications study at 30 years: overview. Diabetes Care 2014;37:9–16.)

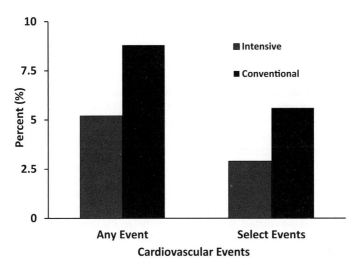

Fig. 9. CV events at EDIC year 11 according to original treatment assignment. Any event: death from CVD, nonfatal acute MI, silent MI, revascularization, angina, or nonfatal cerebrovascular event. Select events: nonfatal MI, stroke, and death from CV disease. (*Data from* The Diabetes Control and Complications Trial/Epidemiology of Diabetes Interventions and Complications (DCCT/EDIC) Study Research Group. Intensive diabetes treatment and cardiovascular disease in patients with type 1 diabetes. N Engl J Med 2005;353:2643–53.)

glucose less than 270 mg/dL and the absence of hyperglycemic symptoms. For intensive therapy, the sulfonylureas used were chlorpropamide, glibenclamide, and glipizide, with dosing adjusted to achieve glycemic targets. Insulin-treated patients began with once-daily basal insulin, such as ultralente or isophane (ie, NPH) insulin. If daily doses were more than 14 units per day or premeal or bedtime glucose values were greater than 126 mg/dL, regular human insulin was added for meals and home glucose monitoring was encouraged. In a small substudy within the UKPDS, overweight subjects (>120% ideal body weight) were additionally randomized to intensive therapy with metformin (instead of sulfonylurea or insulin). Study protocols were later modified in an effort to maintain glucose control by adding insulin or metformin to sulfonylurea therapy.[47,49] Conventional group participants were randomized to insulin, sulfonylurea, or metformin if they became symptomatic or if fasting glucose levels exceeded 270 mg/dL.

Intensive therapy with sulfonylureas or insulin resulted in a difference in HbA_{1c} of approximately 0.9% over 10 years with median HbA_{1c} values of 7% and 7.9%, respectively, compared with conventional therapy.[46] Microvascular outcomes were reduced by 25% (RRR) (95% CI, 0%–40%; $P = .009$), and there was a trend toward reduced risk of MI by 16% (RRR) (95% CI, 0%–29%; $P = .052$). In obese subjects randomized to metformin, a difference in HbA_{1c} of 0.6% was maintained between intensive and conventional groups (7.4% vs 8.0%) over a median of 10.7 years, and there were RRRs of 36% in the aggregate endpoint of all-cause mortality (95% CI, 9–55; $P = .011$), 32% in any diabetes-related endpoint (95% CI, 13–47; $P = .002$), 42% in diabetes-related death (95% CI, 9–63; $P = .017$), and 39% in MI (95% CI, 11–59; $P = .01$). There were no significant reductions in microvascular endpoints,[47] likely a reflection of the higher mean HbA_{1c} in this group (7.4%) or reduced power to detect differences, based on the small study sample, with only 342 patients randomized to metformin.

When all subjects were stratified according to glycemic control, similar to the type 1 diabetes mellitus patients in DCCT, there was a clear relationship between glycemic control and microvascular complications. When HbA_{1c} was compared across tertiles from less than 6.2%, to 6.2% to 7.4%, to greater than or equal to 7.5%, the relative risks (RRs) of developing new retinopathy were 1.4 (95% CI, 1.1–1.8) and 2.5 (95% CI, 2.0–3.2) for the second and third tertiles, and for those with preexisting retinopathy, RRs of progression were 4.1 (95% CI, 3.1–5.6) and 8.1 (95% CI, 6.3–10.5) for the second and third tertiles.[50] An analysis of complications according to HbA_{1c} estimated that for every 1% reduction in HbA_{1c} the risk reductions in microvascular endpoints, MI, and diabetes-related death were 37%, 14%, and 21%, respectively.[51]

As with DCCT, nonrandomized follow-up study of the original UKPDS cohort was arranged. Shortly after the trial ended in 1997, differences in HbA_{1c} were lost between the 2 groups and over the next 10 years HbA_{1c} was maintained at approximately 8%, and despite this, there were persistent reductions in complications, including overall mortality and diabetes-related death in groups originally assigned to intensive therapy.[48] At a median follow-up of 16.8 years, those initially treated more intensively with insulin or sulfonylureas had RRRs of 24% (95% CI, 11–36; P = .001) in microvascular disease. Also, because the accumulation of more events over time, a statistically significant, although still modest, 15% relative reduction in MI was observed (95% CI, 3–26; P = .01). For those originally randomized to metformin, there were significant reductions in MI (RRR 33%; 95% CI, 11–49; P = .005) but, again, no benefit in microvascular endpoints, at a median follow-up of 17.7 years.

The UKPDS had several major findings regarding glucose lowering: (1) achieving near-normal glucose levels in newly diagnosed type 2 diabetics can reduce the microvascular complications of diabetes; (2) for those able to maintain tighter glycemic control, complication rates were lower; (3) in obese subjects, metformin reduced macrovascular events and mortality, suggesting a glucose-independent benefit of metformin on macrovascular disease; (4) monotherapies failed to maintain glycemic control over time, largely due to declining β-cell function, yet (5) the impact of initial intensive therapy had long-term benefits on micro- and macrovascular disease that were apparent 15 to 20 years later—despite deterioration in glucose control.

Kumamoto Study

The Kumamoto study was a randomized clinical trial with a similar design to DCCT and sought to answer 2 main questions in adults with previously diagnosed type 2 diabetes mellitus: (1) Will intensive insulin therapy prevent microvascular complications in those without preexisting complications (primary prevention) and (2) Will intensive insulin therapy prevent the progression of early microvascular complications (secondary prevention)?

The small study was done in Japan at a single university center and consisted of just 110 adult diabetic patients with an average age of 49 and diabetes duration of 6 to 10 years.[52] Initial HbA_{1c} levels were approximately 9% and patients were divided into 2 groups of 55 each: those with no retinopathy or nephropathy (UAE <30 mg/ 24 h) and those with early retinopathy and microalbuminuria (UAE <300 mg/24 h). Each group of 55 subjects was then randomly assigned to intensive versus conventional insulin therapy. Intensive therapy consisted of 3 or more injections of insulin daily with rapid-acting insulin for meals and intermediate insulin at bedtime and aimed for fasting glucose concentrations of less than 140 mg/dL, 2-hour postprandial glucose less than 200 mg/dL, HbA_{1c} less than 7%, and mean amplitude of glycemic excursions of less than 100 mg/dL. Visits to clinics were made biweekly to achieve and maintain goals. Conventional therapy consisted of 1 to 2 injections of intermediate-acting insulin and aimed to achieve fasting glucose concentrations of less than 140 mg/dL and absence of symptomatic hyper- or hypoglycemia.

Follow-up data for the Kumamoto study have been reported at 6 and 8 years.[52,53] Over 8 years, the mean HbA$_{1c}$ and fasting glucose levels in the intensive group were 7.2% and 122 mg/dL compared with 9.4% and 162 mg/dL in the conventional group.[53] Intensive glycemic control resulted in significant reductions in the development and progression of microvascular complications. In the primary prevention cohort, the risk reductions in retinopathy and nephropathy at 8 years were 68% and 74% but were reported as events per 100 patient years, with 1.9 versus 6.0 (P = .022) for retinopathy, and 1.4 versus 5.4 (P = .029) for nephropathy, for intensive versus conventional treatment. In the secondary prevention group, the risk reductions in retinopathy and nephropathy progression were 57% and 60%, respectively. The results were reported as 3.0 versus 7.0 events/100 patient years (P = .023) and 2.0 versus 5.0 events/100 patient years (P = .043) for intensive versus conventional treatment.

When data from the primary and secondary prevention cohorts were combined and microvascular complications were analyzed according to degree of glycemic control, there was, as with DCCT and UKPDS, a continuous relationship between increasing complication risk and glycemia. Retinopathy and nephropathy did not progress, however, in patients who maintained the following parameters: fasting glucose less than 110 mg/dL, 2-hour postprandial glucose less than 180 mg/dL, and HbA$_{1c}$ less than 6.5%.

Overall, the Kumamoto study is similar to DCCT and UKPDS in supporting the glucose hypothesis and the notion of tight glycemic control for preventing the microvascular complications of diabetes.

Action to Control Cardiovascular Risk in Diabetes, Action in Diabetes and Vascular Disease: Preterax and Diamicron Modified-Release Controlled Evaluation, and Veterans Affairs Diabetes Trial

The Action to Control Cardiovascular Risk in Diabetes (ACCORD) trial, Action in Diabetes and Vascular Disease: Preterax and Diamicron Modified-Release Controlled Evaluation (ADVANCE) trial, and Veterans Affairs Diabetes Trial (VADT) were designed to determine whether achieving near-normal glucose levels could reduce macrovascular events in individuals with established type 2 diabetes mellitus with high CV risk.[54–57]

ACCORD randomized 10,251 patients to intensive therapy aiming for HbA$_{1c}$ levels of less than 6% versus 7% to 7.9% (**Table 1**).[54] Approximately 35% of the participants had experienced a prior CV event; the remainder had at least 2 additional CVD risk factors. The primary outcome was first occurrence of nonfatal MI or nonfatal stroke or death from CV causes. Over an average follow-up of 3.5 years, the study was stopped because of increased mortality in the intensive group. Although nonfatal MI was significantly reduced (3.6% vs 4.6%; P = .004), overall mortality and fatal CV events were significantly increased with intensive treatment (5% vs 4%, and 2.6% vs 1.8%, respectively; $P \leq .05$ for both). Subgroup analyses identified increased mortality in the intensively treated patients who failed to lower HbA$_{1c}$ rather than, as initially suspected, directly due to hypoglycemia, suggesting other factors associated with the inability to achieve glycemic targets with intensive therapy were responsible.[58] Nonetheless, severe hypoglycemic events also predicted mortality in both treatment groups, with, if anything, worse outcomes in the conventional group,[59] suggesting that hypoglycemia may have identified a group of more vulnerable patients with other confounding factors influencing their outcomes—independent of treatment

Table 1
Comparison of selected characteristics between major diabetes trials

	ACCORD	ADVANCE	VADT	DCCT[a]	UKPDS-I-SU[b]	UKPDS-MET[b]	Kumamato[a]
Mean age (y)	62 ± 7	66 ± 6	60 ± 9	27	54 ± 9	53 ± 8	48 ± 12
Duration DM (y)	10	8	11.5	2.6	New dx	New dx	6.5
Baseline HbA$_{1c}$ (%)	8.3	7.5	9.4	8.8	9	9	9.1
Prior CV event (%)	35	32	40	None	Excluded	Excluded	Excluded
Study duration (y)	3.5	5	5.6	6.5	10	10.7	8
Int vs std HbA$_{1c}$ (%)	6.4 vs 7.5	6.5 vs 7.3	6.9 vs 8.4	7.2 vs 9.1	7 vs 7.9	7.4 vs 8.0	7.2 vs 9.4
Microvascular benefit	—	Nephropathy	Nephropathy	Yes	Yes	No	Yes
Macrovascular benefit	↓Nonfatal MI (ARR 1%)	No	No	No / Yes (in EDIC)	No / Yes (10-y FU)	Yes	—
Major harms	↑Mortality (ARI 1%)	Hypoglycemia	Hypoglycemia	Hypoglycemia	Hypoglycemia	Low rates hypoglycemia	Low rates hypoglycemia

Abbreviations: ARE, absolute risk increase; ARR, absolute risk reduction; DM, diabetes mellitus; FU, follow up; Int, intensive; std, standard therapy HbA$_{1c}$ goals.
[a] These are the primary prevention group data.
[b] UKPDS-I-SU is the insulin-sulfonylurea study and UKPDS-MET is the metformin study.

assignment. There was a trend toward benefit with intensive control for those without prior CV events whose baseline HbA_{1c} levels were less than 8%, suggesting that aggressive glycemic reductions may be safer (and more effective) in patients without preexisting CV disease but riskier (and ineffective) once atherosclerosis is overt.

ADVANCE randomized 11,140 patients to compare CV outcomes between intensive therapy aiming to achieve HbA_{1c} levels of less than 6.5% versus 7% (see **Table 1**).[55] At baseline, 32% of the participants had experienced a prior CV event, and others had at least one CV risk factor or had microvascular disease. The primary outcomes were composites of macro- and microvascular outcomes (CV death, nonfatal MI and stroke, new or worsening nephropathy or retinopathy). After a median follow-up of 5 years when HbA_{1c} levels were 6.5% versus 7.3%, there were no significant differences in macrovascular events or mortality. A significant reduction in nephropathy was found, however, mainly in the form of macroalbuminuria, progressing in 2.9% of the intensive versus 4.1% of the standard control group ($P \leq .001$). Overall, new or worsening nephropathy occurred in 4.1% of intensive versus 5.2% in the standard group ($P = .006$). There were no differences in retinopathy, but this was defined by its more advanced forms, such as proliferative retinopathy and diabetes-related blindness. The frequency of severe hypoglycemia was low but significantly different, occurring in 2.7% of the intensive and 1.5% of the standard groups ($P \leq .0001$).

Post-trial follow-up at a median of 5.4 years was recently reported for ADVANCE.[56] Similar to DCCT and UKPDS differences in glycemic control between treatment groups were lost after the study ended, but unlike the earlier studies there was no evidence of emerging CV benefits and there was only a suggestion of persisting benefits on nephropathy reduction, which may reflect benefits carried forward from the original trial.

The VADT randomized 1791 patients to intensive therapy aiming for an absolute reduction in HbA_{1c} of 1.5% between the intensive and standard groups (see **Table 1**).[57] More than 95% of participants were men, and they were at high CV risk, with approximately 40% having experienced a previous macrovascular event. The VADT participants had a longer duration of disease (11.5 years) and a higher HbA_{1c} (9.4%) that the other trials. The primary outcome was time to first occurrence of any one of a composite of CV endpoints (MI; stoke; CV death; CHF; the need for intervention on cardio-, cerebral-, or peripheral vascular disease; or amputation for ischemic gangrene). After a median follow-up of 5.6 years during which mean HbA_{1c} levels were 6.9% versus 8.4%, no differences were found in CV events or mortality. The only significant differences were in reductions of albuminuria, and, when reported as any increase in albuminuria, there was progression in 9.1% of the intensive versus 13.8% in the standard group ($P = .01$). There were no differences in clinically significant or proliferative retinopathy. Serious adverse events were more common in the intensive group, occurring in 24.1% versus 17.6% ($P = .05$), with many of these due to hypoglycemia, of which severe episodes were the strongest predictors of death at 90 days. Subgroup analysis suggested CV benefits for tighter control in individuals with lower coronary artery calcification scores at baseline and shorter diabetes duration.[60,61]

ADVANCE, ACCORD, and VADT did not show a benefit of tight glycemic control for reducing composite macrovascular events in type 2 diabetes mellitus, although there was evidence for reduced progression of nephropathy and perhaps nonfatal MI. The results of ACCORD, however, have specifically raised concerns for harm associated with tight glycemic control, particularly in those with pre-established CVD.

Compared with DCCT, UKPDS, and their respective observational studies, these trials differed in ways that may have obscured benefits in the intensive groups while increasing risk for adverse events because of tighter control. (1) Glycemic targets were substantially lower in all treatment groups with intensively managed patients approaching the euglycemic range and standard therapy groups having HbA_{1c} levels closer to those achieved in the tight control groups from older studies which could (see **Table 1**) have minimized differences between groups. However, allowing for looser control (eg, HbA_{1c} approximately 9% vs lower) was not possible due to ethical concerns, given the known benefits of tighter control on microvascular events. Reduced targets also meant more hypoglycemia, and, despite the data indicating that hypoglycemia was not the direct cause of events in these studies, it still may have attenuated any benefit from improved glycemia. (2) Study durations, including the post-trial follow-up for ADVANCE, were also shorter, whereas major differences in macrovascular events were seen after only 10 years or more in UKPDS and DCCT—and mainly in their follow-up studies (see **Table 1**). Moreover, certain differences in microvascular endpoints may have gone undetected, because study durations may have been too short to observe differential effects, in, for example, retinopathy. (3) Patients were older, had longer durations of poorly controlled diabetes, were at higher CV risk, and were on more-intensive blood pressure and lipid-lowering regimens, all factors that could have minimize changes in CV outcomes. (4) Finally, direct harm from certain pharmacologic agents used in these later trials may have masked the benefits from glucose control, a discussion beyond the scope of this review.

RECONCILING THE EVIDENCE: ANSWERS FROM META-ANALYSES

Several meta-analyses have examined the relationship between tight glycemic control and macrovascular outcomes.[62–64] One that included ADVANCE, ACCORD, VADT, UKPDS, and Prospective Pioglitazone Clinical Trial in Macrovascular Events suggested a 17% reduction in nonfatal MI (odds ratio [OR] 0.83; 95% CI, 0.75–0.93) and a 15% reduction in events related to CHD (OR 0.85; 95% CI, 0.77–0.93) but no significant reductions in stroke or all-cause mortality.[62] Another meta-analysis of only ADVANCE, ACCORD, VADT, and UKPDS was directionally consistent with these findings, suggesting pooled RRRs of 10% (95% CI, 2%–17%) for CVD and 11% (95% CI, 4–19) for CHD but not in CV death or all-cause mortality. Severe hypoglycemia was increased 2-fold: RR 2.03 (95% CI, 1.46–2.81) in the pooled analysis.[63] Other analyses support the conclusions that tighter glycemic control can result in some, albeit small, reductions in CV events but not in overall mortality, and that for some individuals tighter control may results in more harm, whether due to hypoglycemia or other patient-specific factors.[64] The overall data at this point support individualization of glycemic targets to patient characteristics so the risks and benefits of treatment goals can be considered.

CALIBRATING TARGETS TO PATIENTS AND DISEASE

The extensive evidence for glucose lowering, reviewed previously, helps guide the treatment of patients with diabetes and specifically in the determination of glycemic treatment targets. The evidence is reasonably clear for microvascular disease—achieving near-normal glucose levels can prevent its development and progression. Even though data on major life-altering complications, such as visual or limb loss, or the need for dialysis are more limited, it is logical to presume that preventing the progression of more subtle endpoints will translate into long-term benefits for these outcomes. The DCCT, UKPDS, and Kumamoto study all provide rationale for glycemic targets associated with minimal risk of microvascular complications and form the basis for current treatment guidelines (**Tables 2** and **3**). Complications were essentially avoided in individuals

Table 2
Glycemic targets in tight control groups of various trials and the time after the trials began when significant complication reductions were reported

Glycemic Parameter	DCCT	Kumamato	UKPDS
Fasting glucose (mg/dL)	<120	<140	<108
2 h Postmeal (mg/dL)	<180	<200	—
HbA$_{1c}$ (%)	<7.0	<7.0	7.0[a]
Microvascular benefit (y)	6	6	10
Macrovascular benefit (y)	17	—	16.8

[a] HbA$_{1c}$ of 7% was not a target but was the median value achieved during the main study (nonmetformin) where there was evidence for microvascular disease reduction.

with HbA$_{1c}$ less than 7% in DCCT, less than 6.2% in UKPDS, and less than 6.5% in the Kumamoto study. In ADVANCE and VADT, nephropathy progression was reduced, with HbA$_{1c}$ less than 7% despite shorter time frames than other trials.

The evidence for macrovascular disease is extremely limited, with the suggestion of a benefit on nonfatal MI but not on other outcomes or overall mortality. There may, however, be benefits in select patient groups—younger, newly diagnosed patients, and those with minimal CVD at baseline. In ADVANCE, ACCORD, and VADT, there was evidence for benefit in those with shorter diabetes durations (<5 years), age less than 65, and absence of micro- or macrovascular disease at baseline.[60,61] Moreover, the follow-up studies of DCCT (in type 1) and UKPDS (in type 2) do suggest that any benefits of tight glycemic control on atherosclerosis-related endpoints are only observed over many years of treatment (see **Table 1**).

The costs of tight glycemic control are clear and consistent across studies and age groups: increased hypoglycemic events and weight gain, particularly with insulin. The increased mortality in ACCORD and lack of overall CV benefit in ACCORD, ADVANCE, and VADT coupled with adverse events make it difficult to recommend tight glycemic control for all patients.

What are the considerations for individualized diabetes treatment? Each patient presents a unique set of circumstances and for each a rational HbA$_{1c}$ target should be determined. This approach has been discussed extensively by Ismail-Beigi and

Table 3
Current diagnostic criteria for diabetes in nonpregnant adults and treatment targets set by various organizations

Glycemic Parameter	ADA Diagnostic Criteria for DM	ADA Guidelines	AACE Guidelines	IDF-Europe Guidelines Type 1	IDF-Europe Guidelines Type 2
Fasting glucose (mg/dL)	≥126	70–130	<110	91–120	<115
2 h Postmeal (mg/dL)	≥200[a]	<180	<140	136–160	<160
HbA$_{1c}$ (%)	≥6.5	<7.0	≤6.5	6.2–7.5	<7.0

Abbreviations: ADA, American Diabetes Association; AACE, American Association of Clinical Endocrinologists; DM, diabetes mellitus; IDF, International Diabetes Federation.
[a] After OGTT or random glucose + symptoms of diabetes.
Data from Refs.[67–70]

colleagues[65] and more recently in an American Diabetes Association (ADA)–European Association for the Study of Diabetes (EASD) position statement.[66] In each, the calibration of glycemic targets was encouraged to be based on a variety of patient- and disease-based considerations (**Fig. 10**). In general, keeping HbA$_{1c}$ as close to 7% as possible or slightly lower is an excellent start. For those who can, without significant additional expense or side effects, especially in younger and healthier individuals, approaching an HbA$_{1c}$ as close to 6% is reasonable. Conversely, older individuals, especially those with multiple comorbidities, should have more conservative targets, such as 7.5% to 8% or even higher. Many factors can modify targets: psychological well-being; ability to care for oneself; and safety risk, such as use of insulin in occupations where hypoglycemia could be life threatening (eg, driving).[65] Tight

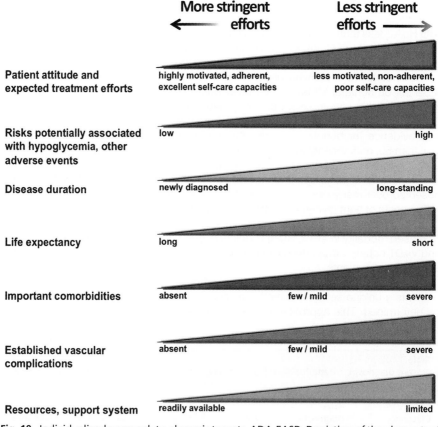

Fig. 10. Individualized approach to glycemic targets, ADA-EASD. Depiction of the elements of decision making used to determine appropriate efforts to achieve glycaemic targets. Greater concerns about a particular domain are represented by increasing height of the ramp. Thus, characteristics/predicaments toward the left justify more stringent efforts to lower HbA$_{1c}$, whereas those toward the right are compatible with less stringent efforts. Where possible, such decisions should be made in conjunction with the patient, reflecting his or her preferences, needs, and values. This scale is designed not to be applied rigidly but to be used as a broad construct to help guide clinical decisions. (*From* Inzucchi SE, Bergenstal RM, Buse JB, Diamant M, Ferrannini E, Nauck M, Peters AL, Tsapas A, Wender R, Matthews DR. Management of hyperglycemia in type 2 diabetes: A patient-centered approach. Diabetes Care 2012;35:1366; with permission.)

control may be reasonable in older patients on medications with minimal risk for hypoglycemia, little comorbidity, no CVD, and a good life expectancy with a high functional status. Alternatively, it may be harmful or impractical in younger patients with a history of severe hypoglycemia or advanced diabetes duration and complications; the frail; and those with limited life expectancy, limited social resources, and poor self-care ability or functional status.[65–67] These are some of several considerations that must be made in the context of shared decision making between physician and patient in developing a comprehensive treatment plan.

Finally, although glucose remains a central feature of diabetes mellitus and glucose lowering has been confirmed as a way to reduce the complications of diabetes, it has become clear that this alone is not the only factor that must be addressed in the treatment of diabetes.[67] Age, blood pressure, lipid levels, other risk factors, and the side effects of glucose-lowering therapies must be incorporated into individualized treatment strategies that aim to achieve maximal benefits in both complication reduction and quality of life, while minimizing harm.

REFERENCES

1. Joslin EP. The diabetic. Can Med Assoc J 1943;48:488–97.
2. Available at: http://www.nei.nih.gov/health/fact_sheet.asp. Accessed May 9, 2014.
3. Available at: http://kidney.niddk.nih.gov/KUDiseases/pubs/kdd/index.aspx. Accessed May 9, 2014.
4. Available at: http://www.ninds.nih.gov/disorders/peripheralneuropathy/detail_peripheralneuropathy.htm. Accessed May 9, 2014.
5. Nathan DM. Long-term complications of diabetes mellitus. N Engl J Med 1993; 328(23):1676–85.
6. Report of the Expert Committee on the Diagnosis and Classification of Diabetes Mellitus. Diabetes Care 1997;20:1183–97.
7. Tapp RJ, Zimmet PZ, Harper CA, et al. Diagnostic thresholds for diabetes: the association of retinopathy and albuminuria with glycemia. Diabetes Res Clin Pract 2006;73:315–21.
8. Klein R, Myers CE, Lee KE, et al. 15-Year cumulative incidence and associated risk factors for retinopathy in nondiabetic persons. Arch Ophthalmol 2010; 128(12):1568–75.
9. Klein R, Klein BE, Moss SE. Relation of glycemic control to diabetic microvascular complications in diabetes mellitus. Ann Intern Med 1996;124(1):90–6.
10. Klein R, Knudston MD, Lee KE, et al. The Wisconsin epidemiologic study of diabetic retinopathy XXII: the twenty-five-year progression of retinopathy in persons with type 1 diabetes. Ophthalmology 2008;115:1859–68.
11. Hillege HL, Janssen WM, Bak AA, et al, for The Prevend Study Group. Microalbuminuria is common, also in a nondiabetic, nonhypertensive population, and an independent predictor of cardiovascular risk factors and cardiovascular morbidity. J Intern Med 2001;249:519–26.
12. Dyck PJ, Kratz KM, Karnes JL, et al. The prevalence by staged severity of various types of diabetic neuropathy, retinopathy, and nephropathy in a population-based chohort: The Rochester diabetic neuropathy study. Neurology 1993;43:817–24.
13. Tesfaye S, Stevens LK, Stephenson JM, et al, The EURODIAB IDDM Study Group. Prevalence of diabetic peripheral neuropathy and its relation to glycaemic control and potential risk factors: the EURODIAB IDDM Complications Study. Diabetologia 1996;39:1377–84.

14. Engelgau MM, Thompson TJ, Herman WH, et al. Comparison of fasting and 2-hour glucose and HbA1c levels for diagnosing diabetes: diagnostic criteria and performance revisited. Diabetes Care 1997;20:785–91.

15. McCance DR, Hanson RL, Charles MA, et al. Comparison of tests for glycated hemoglobin and fasting and two hour plasma glucose concentrations as diagnostic methods for diabetes. BMJ 1994;308:1323–8.

16. Rajala U, Laakso M, Qiao Q, et al. Prevalence of retinopathy in people with diabetes, impaired glucose tolerance, and normal glucose tolerance. Diabetes Care 1998;21:1664–9.

17. Van Leiden HA, Dekker JM, Moll AC, et al. Blood pressure, lipids, and obesity are associated with retinopathy: the hoorn study. Diabetes Care 2002;25:1320–5.

18. Wong TY, Liew G, Tapp RJ, et al. Relationship between fasting glucose and retinopathy for diagnosis of diabetes: three population-based cross-sectional studies. Lancet 2008;371:736–43.

19. Brownlee M. Biochemistry and molecular cell biology of diabetic complications. Nature 2001;414:813–20.

20. Kannel WB, McGee DL. Diabetes and cardiovascular disease. JAMA 1979;241: 2035–8.

21. Stamler J, Vaccaro O, Neaton JD, et al, For The Multiple Risk Factor Intervention Trial Research Group. Diabetes, other risk factors, and 12-yr cardiovascular mortality for men screened in the multiple risk factor intervention trial. Diabetes Care 1993;16:434–44.

22. Gregg EW, Li Y, Wang J, et al. Changes in diabetes-related complications in the United States, 1990-2010. N Engl J Med 2014;370:1514–23.

23. Haffner SM, Lehto S, Ronnemaa T, et al. Mortality from coronary heart disease in subjects with type 2 diabetes and in nondiabetic subjects with and without prior myocardial infarction. N Engl J Med 1998;339:229–39.

24. Juutilainen A, Lehto S, Ronnemaa T, et al. Type 2 diabetes as a "coronary heart disease equivalent". Diabetes Care 2005;28:2901–7.

25. Saely CH, Drexel H. Is type 2 diabetes really a coronary heart disease risk equivalent? Vascul Pharmacol 2013;59:11–8.

26. Bulugahapitiya U, Siyambalapitiya S, Sithole J, et al. Is diabetes a coronary risk equivalent? Systematic review and meta-analysis. Diabet Med 2009;26:142–8.

27. Andersson DK, Svardsudd K. Long-term glycemic control relates to mortality in type II diabetes. Diabetes Care 1995;18(12):1534–43.

28. Eeg-Olofsson K, Cederholm J, Nilsson PM, et al. New Aspects of HbA1c as a risk factor for cardiovascular disease in type 2 diabetes: an observational study from the Swedish National Diabetes Register (NDR). J Intern Med 2010;268:471–82.

29. Eeg-Olofsson K, Cederholm J, Nilsson PM, et al. Glycemic control and cardiovascular disease in 7,454 patients with type 1 diabetes: an observational study from the Swedish National Diabetes Register (NDR). Diabetes Care 2010;33: 1640–6.

30. The Emerging Risk Factors Collaboration. Diabetes mellitus, fasting glucose concentration, and risk of vascular disease: a collaborative meta-analysis of 102 prospective studies. Lancet 2010;375:2215–22.

31. Khaw KT, Wareham N, Luben R, et al. Glycated hemoglobin, diabetes, and mortality in men in Norfolk cohort of European Prospective Investigation of Cancer and Nutrition (EPIC-Norfolk). BMJ 2001;322:1–6.

32. Khaw KT, Wareham N, Bingham S, et al. Association of hemoglobin A1c with cardiovascular disease and mortality in adults: the European Prospective Investigation into Cancer in Norfolk. Ann Intern Med 2004;141:413–20.

33. Rodriguez BL, Lau N, Burchfiel CM, et al. Glucose intolerance and 23-year risk of coronary heart disease and total mortality. the Honolulu Hear Program. Diabetes Care 1999;22:1262–5.
34. The DECODE Study Group, on behalf of the European Diabetes Epidemiology Group. Prediction of the risk of cardiovascular mortality using a score that includes glucose as a risk factor. The DECODE study. Diabetologia 2004;47:2118–28.
35. Balkau B, Shipley M, Jarrett RJ, et al. High blood glucose concentration is a risk factor for mortality in middle-aged nondiabetic men. 20-year follow-up in the Whitehall Study, the Paris prospective study, and the Helsinki policemen study. Diabetes Care 1998;21:360–7.
36. Jackson CA, Yudkin JS, Forrest RD. A comparison of the relationships of the glucose tolerance test and the glycated hemoglobin assay with diabetic vascular disease in the community. The Islington diabetes survey. Diabetes Res Clin Pract 1992;17:111–23.
37. Beks PJ, Mackaay AJ, de Neeling JN, et al. Peripheral arterial disease in relation to glycaemic level in an elderly Caucasian population: the Hoorn study. Diabetologia 1995;38:86–96.
38. Brownlee M. The pathobiology of diabetic complications: a unifying mechanism. Diabetes 2005;54:1615–25.
39. The Diabetes Control and Complications Trial Research Group. The effect of intensive treatment of diabetes on the development and progression of long-term complications in insulin-dependent diabetes mellitus. N Engl J Med 1993;329:977–86.
40. Nathan DM. The diabetes control and complications trial/epidemiology of diabetes interventions and complications study at 30 years: overview. Diabetes Care 2014;37:9–16.
41. Lachin JM, Genuth S, Nathan DM, et al, for The DCCT/EDIC Research Group. Effect of glycemic exposure on the risk of microvascular complications in the diabetes control and complications trial—revisited. Diabetes 2008;57:995–1001.
42. The Diabetes Control and Complications Trial/Epidemiology of Diabetes Interventions and Complications (DCCT/EDIC) Study Research Group. Intensive diabetes treatment and cardiovascular disease in patients with type 1 diabetes. N Engl J Med 2005;353:2643–53.
43. Larkin ME, Barnie A, Braffett BH, et al, The Diabetes Control and Complications Trial/Epidemiology of Diabetes Interventions and Complications (DCCT/EDIC) Study Research Group. Musculoskeletal complications in type 1 diabetes. Diabetes Care 2014;37:1863–9.
44. De Boer IH, for the DCCT/EDIC Research Group. Kidney disease and related findings in the diabetes control and complications trial/epidemiology of diabetes interventions and complications study. Diabetes Care 2014;37:24–30.
45. UK Prospective Diabetes Study (UKPDS) VIII. Study design, progress and performance. Diabetologia 1991;34:877–90.
46. UK Prospective Diabetes Study Group. Intensive blood-glucose control with sulphonylureas or insulin compared with conventional treatment and risk of complications in patients with type 2 diabetes (UKPDS 33). Lancet 1998;352:837–53.
47. UK Prospective Diabetes Study Group. Effect of intensive blood-glucose control with metformin on complications in overweight patients with type 2 diabetes (UKPDS 34). Lancet 1998;352:854–65.
48. Holman RR, Sanjoy PK, Bethel A, et al. 10-year follow up of intensive glucose control in type 2 diabetes. N Engl J Med 2008;359:1577–89.

49. Wright A, Burden AC, Paisey RB, et al, for The U.K. Prospective Diabetes Study Group. Sulfonylurea inadequacy: effect of addition of insulin over 6 years in patients with type 2 diabetes in the U. K. Prospective Diabetes Study (UKPDS 57). Diabetes Care 2002;25(2):330–6.

50. Stratton IM, Kohner EM, Aldington SJ, et al, for The UKPDS Group. UKPDS 50: risk factors for incidence and progression of retinopathy in type II diabetes over 6 years from diagnosis. Diabetologia 2001;44:156–63.

51. Stratton IM, Adler AI, Neil AW, et al, on behalf of the UK Prospective Diabetes Study Group. Association of glycemia with macrovascular and microvascular complications of type 2 diabetes (UKPDS 35): prospective observational study. BMJ 2000;321:405–12.

52. Ohkubo Y, Kishikawa H, Araki E, et al. Intensive insulin therapy prevents the progression of diabetic microvascular complications in Japanese patients with non-insulin-dependent diabetes mellitus: a randomized prospective 6-year study. Diabetes Res Clin Pract 1995;28:103–17.

53. Shichiri M, Kishikawa H, Ohkubo Y, et al. Long-term results from the Kumamoto study on optimal diabetes control in type 2 diabetic patients. Diabetes Care 2000;23(S2):B21–9.

54. The Action to Control Cardiovascular Risk in Diabetes Study Group. Effects of intensive glucose lowering in type 2 diabetes. N Engl J Med 2008;358: 2545–59.

55. The ADVANCE Collaborative Group. Intensive blood glucose control and vasculat outcomes in patients with type 2 diabetes. N Engl J Med 2008; 358:2560–72.

56. Zoungas S, Chalmers J, Neal L, et al. Follow-up of blood pressure lowering and glucose control in type 2 diabetes. NEJM 2014;371:1392–406.

57. Duckworth W, Abriara C, Moritz T, et al, for the VADT Investigators. Glucose control and vascular complications in veterans with type 2 diabetes. N Engl J Med 2009;360:129–39.

58. Riddle MC, Ambrosius WT, Brillon DJ, et al, for the Action to Control Cardio-vascular Risk in Diabetes (ACCORD) Investigators. Epidemiologic relation-ships between A1C and all-cause mortality during a median 3.4 year follow-up of glycemic treatment in the ACCORD trial. Diabetes Care 2010; 33(5):983–90.

59. Bonds DE, Miller ME, Bergenstall RM, et al. The association between symptom-atic, severe hypoglycaemia and mortality in type 2 diabetes: retrospective epidemiological analysis of the ACCORD study. BMJ 2010;340:b4909.

60. Reaven PD, Moritz TE, Schwenke DC, et al, for the Veterans Affairs Diabetes Trial. Intensive glucose-lowering therapy reduces cardiovascular disease events in veterans affairs diabetes trial participants with lower calcified coronary atherosclerosis. Diabetes 2009;58:2642–8.

61. Duckworth WC, Abraira C, Moritz TE, et al, for the Investigators of the VADT. The duration of diabetes affects the response to intensive glucose control in type 2 diabetes subjects: the VA Diabetes Trial. J Diabetes Complications 2001;25: 355–61.

62. Ray KK, Seshasai RK, Wijesuriya S, et al. Effect of intensive control of glucose on cardiovascular outcomes and death in patients with diabetes mellitus: a meta-analysis of randomized controlled trials. Lancet 2009;373:1765–72.

63. Kelly TN, Bazzano LA, Fonseca VA, et al. Systematic review: glucose control and cardiovascular disease in type 2 diabetes. Ann Intern Med 2009;151: 394–403.

64. Turnbull FM, Abraira C, Anderson RJ, et al. Intensive glucose control and macro-vascular outcomes in type 2 diabetes. Diabetologia 2009;52:2288–98.

65. Ismail-Beigi F, Moghissi E, Tiktin M, et al. Individualizing glycemic targets in type 2 diabetes mellitus: implications of recent clinical trials. Ann Intern Med 2011; 154:554–9.

66. Inzucchi SI, Bergenstal RM, Buse JB, et al. Management of hyperglycemia in type-2 diabetes: a patient-centered approach. Diabetes Care 2012;35:1364–79.

67. American Diabetes Association. Standards of medical care in diabetes—2014. Diabetes Care 2014;37(S1):S14–80.

68. American Association of Clinical Endocrinologists. American College of Endo-crinology Consensus Statement on Guidelines for Glycemic Control. Endocr Pract 2002;8(S1):5–11.

69. Available at: http://www.staff.ncl.ac.uk/philip.home/t1dgch3b.htm#AssessLevels. Accessed May 15, 2014.

70. Available at: http://www.idf.org/sites/default/files/IDF-Guideline-for-Type-2-Diabetes.pdf. Accessed May 15, 2014.

Lifestyle Intervention
Nutrition Therapy and Physical Activity

 CrossMark

Alison B. Evert, MS, RD, CDE[a],*, Michael C. Riddell, PhD[b]

KEYWORDS

- Medical nutrition therapy • Weight loss • Carbohydrate • Lifestyle intervention
- Physical activity • Exercise

KEY POINTS

- An individualized nutrition plan should be discussed with patients in a series of encounters with a registered dietitian starting at the time of diabetes diagnosis.
- Diabetes meal planning approaches should include instruction on a variety of topics including carbohydrate counting, healthy food choices, glycemic index, Mediterranean-style diet, low and high sodium foods, low-fat and low-carbohydrate diets.
- Early engagement in physical activity halts or slows the progression of type 2 diabetes development. Activities should include aerobic activities (at least 150 minutes per week) and resistance training 2-3 days per week.
- Accommodation to permit physical activity engagement for all patients with obesity and or diabetes should be performed.
- For patients attempting to lose weight, a mild to moderate daily energy deficit is needed (10-25% relative caloric restriction).

INTRODUCTION

Diabetes and obesity are major health concerns in the United States.[1–5] It is estimated that more than 3 out of every 4 adults with diabetes are overweight.[6] In a nationally representative sample of US adults, the prevalence of diabetes was found to increase with increasing weight classes.[7] The survey revealed that nearly one-fourth of adults with diabetes in this sample had poor glycemic control (defined as hemoglobin A1c [HbA1c] level >8.0%) and nearly half were considered obese.[7] Being obese with diabetes increases insulin resistance and negatively affects glucose tolerance, thereby making glycemic targets more difficult to achieve pharmacologically.

[a] Diabetes Education Programs, Diabetes Care Center, University of Washington Medical Center, 4245 Roosevelt Way Northeast, 3rd Floor, Seattle, WA 98105, USA; [b] Muscle Health Research Center, School of Kinesiology and Health Science, Bethune College, York University, 4700 Keele Street, 3rd Floor, Toronto, Ontario M3J1P3, Canada
* Corresponding author.
E-mail address: atevert@u.washington.edu

Med Clin N Am 99 (2015) 69–85
http://dx.doi.org/10.1016/j.mcna.2014.09.001   **medical.theclinics.com**
0025-7125/15/$ – see front matter © 2015 Elsevier Inc. All rights reserved.

Public health authorities and medical professionals have recommended weight loss as a therapeutic strategy for patients who are obese or who are overweight with co-morbid conditions such as diabetes for several years.[8] The 1998 Clinical Guidelines on the Identification, Evaluation, and Treatment of Overweight and Obesity in Adults state that, "the initial goal of weight loss therapy should be to reduce body weight by approximately 10% from baseline."[9] Recommended weight-loss strategies included a low-calorie diet to create a deficit of 500 to 1000 kcal/d, behavior therapy, and increased physical activity. More recently, lifestyle intervention strategies have been incorporated into clinically effective diabetes prevention trials around the world.[5,10,11] These strategies have also been found to be integral components of the treatment and management of type 2 diabetes, with documented improvements in weight, depression scores, quality of life, and various biochemical markers of health status.[12,13] Lifestyle intervention seems to be particularly beneficial early in the natural history of type 2 diabetes, before loss of beta cell function and mass becomes so extensive that multidrug pharmacotherapy is required to achieve optimal glycemic control.[14,15]

As type 2 diabetes progresses over the years with the continued loss of beta cell function and enduring insulin resistance, medications are often added to the treatment plan to achieve optimal glycemic control. From a lifestyle perspective, a reduced energy intake with an emphasis on nutrient-dense, fiber-rich foods (**Box 1**) along with regular physical activity should be priorities for all individuals living with type 2 diabetes.[2] However, people with diabetes, as well as their health care providers, are reluctant to initiate the use of medication for fear of weight gain. Referral to a registered dietitian (RD) for nutrition therapy has been shown to help mitigate this unwanted side effect of treatment.[16–20] In addition, successful lifestyle intervention typically reduces the reliance on pharmacologic agents to achieve glycemic targets.[12] Therefore, regardless of duration of diabetes in years, nutrition therapy remains a key treatment strategy.

Because of the importance of physical activity in enhancing weight loss and supporting weight maintenance, and the increasingly strong evidence that increased physical activity and fitness level can affect health independently of body mass index,[21] it is important to have interventions available that can lead to sustained changes in physical activity. The role of physical activity in treatment of type 2 diabetes is elaborated later in this article.

Box 1
Nutrient-dense foods

Nutrient density is a measure of the amount of nutrients a food contains compared with the number of calories. A food is more nutrient dense when the level of nutrients is high in relation to the number of calories the food contains.

Nutrient-dense food choices include the following:

- Grains, especially whole grains
- Fruits and vegetables: fresh, frozen, or canned with so-called lite sodium
- Fat-free or low-fat milk or dairylike products
- Lean protein sources or meat alternatives such as beans, lentils, and unsalted nuts
- Substitute unsaturated (liquid fats such as olive, canola, corn, safflower oil) for foods higher in saturated (solid fats) or *trans* fats as much as possible.

NONPHARMACOLOGIC TREATMENT OPTIONS: LIFESTYLE INTERVENTION: NUTRITION THERAPY

In a recent position statement for the management of hyperglycemia in type 2 diabetes the American Diabetes Association (ADA) and European Association for the Study of Diabetes endorse a patient-centered approach.[22] At diagnosis, before initiating pharmacotherapy, highly motivated patients with HbA1c already near target levels (eg, 7.5%) should be given the opportunity to participate in lifestyle change for a period of 3 to 6 months. Individuals with moderate hyperglycemia or in whom lifestyle changes are anticipated to be unsuccessful could be started on an antihyperglycemic agent (usually metformin) at diagnosis, which can later be modified or possibly discontinued if lifestyle changes are successful. Pharmacologic treatment options for type 2 diabetes are discussed in detail elsewhere in this issue.

Diabetes Nutrition Therapy: How Is It Provided?

People with diabetes should ideally be referred to an RD, and preferably one who is knowledgeable and skilled in providing diabetes medical nutrition therapy (MNT) soon after diagnosis.[23] Another option is participation in a comprehensive diabetes self-management education (DSME) program that includes instruction on nutrition.[23] Many insurance plans and Medicare cover MNT and DSME. These services require a referral or prescription from the health care provider and it is important to confirm coverage in advance of receiving service. Some insurance plans require preauthorization before diabetes self-management or nutrition consultation services are covered. Medicare typically covers up to 10 hours of initial DSME and 3 hours of MNT, and up to 2 hours of each type of service in subsequent years. However, national data in the United States indicate that only about a half of all persons with diabetes receive diabetes education and even fewer see an RD.[6] One study of more than 18,000 people with diabetes revealed that only 9.1% had at least 1 nutrition visit within a 9-year period.[24]

Diabetes Medical Nutrition Therapy: The Process

MNT is based on an assessment of lifestyle changes that would assist the person with diabetes in achieving and maintaining clinical goals[3] and has been shown to be effective in diabetes management.[2] The Academy of Nutrition and Dietetics Evidence-Based Nutrition Practice Guidelines recommend the following structure for the implementation of MNT for adults with diabetes[25]:

- A series of 3 to 4 encounters with RDs lasting from 45 to 90 minutes
  - The series of encounters should begin at diagnosis of diabetes or at first referral to an RD for MNT for diabetes and should be completed within 3 to 6 months.
- The RD should determine whether additional MNT encounters are needed.
- At least 1 follow-up encounter is recommended annually to reinforce lifestyle changes and to evaluate and monitor outcomes that indicate the need for changes in MNT or medications.
  - An RD should determine whether additional MNT encounters are needed.

The RD prioritizes nutrition therapy based on a thorough nutrition assessment of the individual. Once an assessment has been completed, the RD determines the nutrition diagnosis, which includes the presence of, risk of, or potential for developing a nutritional deficit that can be addressed by nutrition therapy. Nutrition interventions are specific actions to remedy the nutrition diagnosis and can include clinical and behavioral goals collaboratively agreed on with the person with diabetes, as well as specific nutrition intervention strategies. These strategies might include selecting a meal-planning strategy such as carbohydrate counting or the plate method, or education on topics such as how to read food labels, portion control, or tips for eating out. In addition, monitoring outcomes and providing ongoing support are also key components of MNT.

Individualization of the Eating Plan

The ADA 2013 position statement, *Nutrition Therapy: Recommendations for the Management of Adults with Diabetes* recommends the development of an individualized eating plan as needed to achieve treatment goals with ongoing support and encouragement to assist with health behavior change.[2] The eating plan should be based on the individual's personal and cultural preferences, literacy and numeracy, and readiness to change, because there is no single eating plan that meets the needs of all adults with diabetes. Food choices should not be limited unnecessarily but should be guided by scientific evidence and the need to delay or prevent complications of diabetes.

In the past a nutrition prescription included a specified calorie level and macronutrient percentage. However, despite efforts since 1994 to promote the individualization of the meal plan, the ADA diet continues to be prescribed. A recent systematic review found that there continues to be no ideal macronutrient distribution for the nutritional management of diabetes.[26] Research has also shown that a wide variety of diabetes meal-planning approaches and eating patterns can be clinically effective, with many including a reduced energy component.[2] Examples include carbohydrate counting, healthy food choices, glycemic index, as well as eating patterns such as the Mediterranean-style diet, Dietary Approach to Stop Hypertension, vegan or vegetarian, and low-fat and low-carbohydrate diets.

NONPHARMACOLOGIC TREATMENT OPTIONS: LIFESTYLE INTERVENTION: PHYSICAL ACTIVITY

Regular physical activity can help people with type 2 diabetes achieve a variety of goals,[27,28] including:

- Increased cardiorespiratory fitness and vigor
- Improved glycemic control
- Decreased insulin resistance
- An improved lipid profile
- Reduced blood pressure
- Maintenance of a healthy body mass after weight loss
- Less depression and anxiety
- Less sleep apnea
- Less medication use
- An overall improved quality of life

However, it is doubtful whether increased physical activity provides significant protection against premature mortality from heart disease and stroke in patients already diagnosed with type 2 diabetes.[12] Nonetheless, a healthful eating plan and regular exercise when implemented soon after diagnosis in a real-world health care setting improves markers of inflammation and the cardiovascular risk profile in patients with type 2 diabetes.[29] In adolescents with type 2 diabetes, regular physical activity is associated with lower HbA1c levels, lower body mass index, and higher HDL-cholesterol levels but not lower medication use.[30]

Definitions and Types of Activity

Physical activity is defined as any body movement caused by the contraction of skeletal muscle that substantially increases energy expenditure.[31] Physical activity comes in a variety of forms and may be performed during a person's occupation or as a leisure activity. It can also be performed at a range of intensities and this is typically expressed either in absolute terms (eg, metabolic equivalents, mL/kg/min, kcal/min), or in relative terms (eg, percent heart rate reserve, percent maximal oxygen consumption [Vo_{2max}], ratings of perceived exertion scale).

Exercise is a structured form of physical activity that can be prescribed as a therapeutic dose with a recommended type, intensity, and volume (ie, duration and frequency). Aerobic exercise, such as walking, bicycling, or jogging, is physical activity that involves continuous, rhythmic movements of large muscle groups lasting for at least 10 minutes at a time. Resistance exercise is physical activity involving brief repetitive exercises with weights, weight machines, resistance bands, or the person's own body weight to increase muscle strength (eg, pushups, sit-ups, and pull-ups). Flexibility exercise, such as lower back or hamstring stretching, is a form of activity that enhances the ability of joints to move through their full ranges of motion.

Recommendations on Type, Intensity, and Volume of Exercise

The American College of Sports Medicine and the ADA joint Position Stands recommendations suggest both aerobic and resistance-type exercise for people with prediabetes or type 2 diabetes.[32] A summary of recommendations is shown in **Table 1**. A goal of 150 minutes per week of accumulated moderate-intensity aerobic exercise is recommended for all patients with diabetes as long as this volume of exercise can be tolerated by the individual.[32] In general, aerobic exercise in the form of brisk walking on level ground, cycling, or recumbent cycling for those with joint pain with walking, are preferred activities for overweight/obese elderly patients with diabetes.[33]

Table 1
American College of Sports Medicine and the ADA recommendations for aerobic and resistance-type exercise for people with prediabetes or type 2 diabetes (PMID: 21115771)

Definitions, Examples and Frequency	Intensity	Examples
Aerobic exercise: rhythmic, repeated, and continuous movements of large muscle groups for at least 10 min at a time Performed daily or every other day Total amount = 150–175 min/wk (moderate to vigorous intensity)	Moderate: 50%–70% of person's maximum heart rate, or 40%–60% of heart rate reserve, or about 4–6 metabolic equivalents Vigorous: >70% of a person's maximum heart rate, or 60%–85% of heart rate reserve, or about 6–8 metabolic equivalents	Brisk walking (9–12 min per km [15–20 min per mile]), dancing, continuous swimming, biking, raking leaves, water aerobics Jogging, walking up an incline, aerobics, team sports (soccer, hockey, basketball), fast swimming, fast dancing
Resistance exercise: activities that use muscular strength to move against a weight or against a load[a] Performed 2–3 times per week	Start with 1 set of 10–15 repetitions at moderate weight Progress to 2 sets of 10–15 repetitions Progress to 3 sets of 8 repetitions at heavier weight	Exercise with weight machines Weight lifting Sit-ups, pull-ups (assisted), and pushups (modified if necessary)

[a] Initial instruction and periodic supervision by a qualified exercise professional are recommended.

More vigorous activities, such as walking up hills or jogging, can be encouraged for middle-aged and younger patients. In addition, resistance exercise performed 2 or 3 times per week provides additional benefits that complement those of aerobic training (eg, increased lean mass and strength, reduced body fat, increased resting metabolic rate).[34,35]

TREATMENT RESISTANCE AND COMPLICATIONS: NUTRITION THERAPY AND PHYSICAL ACTIVITY

It is essential that people with diabetes are actively involved with health professionals to collaboratively develop appropriate nutrition interventions and an individualized eating pattern that they can implement. Multiple encounters to provide education and counseling initially and on a continued basis are also essential.[36] Because of the progressive nature of type 2 diabetes, nutrition therapy recommendations often need to be adjusted over time based on changes in life circumstance, preferences, and disease course. Progression of diabetes complications may be modified by improving glycemic control, reducing blood pressure, and reducing fat intake.[2]

Because cardiovascular disease (CVD) is a common cause of death among individuals with and without diabetes, nutrition recommendations similar to those for the general population to manage CVD risk factors should be followed. The Dietary Guidelines for Americans 2010 recommendations include reducing saturated fats to less than 10% of calories, aiming for 300 mg of dietary cholesterol per day, and limiting *trans* fat as much as possible.[37] In people with type 2 diabetes, a Mediterranean-style, monounsaturated fatty acid–rich eating pattern may also benefit glycemic control and CVD risk factors and can, therefore, be recommended as an effective alternative to a lower-fat, higher-carbohydrate eating pattern.[2,14,38–40]

Evidence from 2 meta-analyses shows no clear benefits for individuals with diabetic neuropathy on renal parameters from protein-restricted diets.[41,42] Therefore reducing protein intake to less than the usual intake for people with diabetes and diabetic kidney disease (either microalbuminuria or macroalbuminuria) is not recommended because it does not alter glycemic measures, cardiovascular risk measures, or the course of glomerular filtration rate decline.[2]

Although regular physical activity is clearly beneficial for patients with diabetes, compliance with recommendations is often poor. Compared with physical activity advice only, supervised programs involving both aerobic and resistance exercise are associated with better improvements in glycemic control in people with type 2 diabetes.[43] Supervision helps with instruction, safety, motivation, and the capacity to overcome any physical barriers. Unsupervised exercise programs usually fail to improve glycemic control on their own, but can be associated with improved HbA1c levels if they are done with dietary intervention.[43] Exercise dropout remains a major limitation, with ~ 60% of patients failing to maintain both aerobic and resistance-type exercises after a lifestyle intervention.[44] However, motivational interviewing following a lifestyle intervention improves the maintenance of physical activity in people with type 2 diabetes.[45]

Although having diabetes increases the risk of having underlying CVD and other comorbidities, there is little evidence to suggest that moderate-intensity exercise triggers adverse cardiovascular events or worsens disease complications in people with diabetes.[46] Nonetheless, before beginning a program of vigorous physical activity, people with diabetes should be assessed for conditions that might increase risks associated with certain types of exercise or predispose them to injury.[33] Before establishing an exercise prescription, health care providers should pay attention to and talk to patients about the following relative contraindications for vigorous exercise[46]:

- Severe autonomic neuropathy (symptoms during exertion may include dizziness)
- Severe peripheral neuropathy (feet should be inspected regularly and proper footwear is required)
- Proliferative retinopathy (should be treated before starting resistance exercise or vigorous aerobic exercise)
- CVD (symptoms may or may not include dyspnea, or chest discomfort)
- Musculoskeletal issues (back, hip, and/or knee problems)

Initial physical assessment before initiating a new program of vigorous exercise should include a resting electrocardiogram and possibly a stress test for individuals with possible CVD.[27] Patients with severe autonomic neuropathy, severe peripheral neuropathy, preproliferative or proliferative retinopathy, and unstable angina should be stabilized and exercise only at a low intensity for brief periods (eg, 10–15 minutes of walking) under appropriate supervision. This type of activity may be best done in a cardiac rehabilitation setting.[47,48] Patients with severe peripheral neuropathy should be instructed to inspect their feet daily, especially on days in which they are physically active, and to wear appropriate footwear.[33] Patients with movement disorders, pain, or any physical limitations should be supervised by a qualified exercise professional.

The risk of hypoglycemia during exercise is of concern for all patients with diabetes who are taking insulin or insulin secretagogues (sulfonylureas and meglitinides). Reductions in insulin administration or oral secretagogues may be needed once the new exercise pattern is established. Patients should be encouraged to monitor their blood glucose levels regularly and to treat hypoglycemia accordingly. As a general rule, patients should indicate in their log books the level of blood glucose just before initiating an exercise session (eg, walking, physically demanding chores) and following every 30 to 45 minutes of sustained activity. Hypoglycemia can be prevented and/or treated by the consumption of 15 to 30 g of fast-acting carbohydrate before exercise or when hypoglycemia develops. If hypoglycemia develops regularly with increased activity levels, perhaps because of a change in routine, then a reduction in exogenous insulin (or oral hypoglycemic agent) should be considered. Patients taking insulin can reduce mealtime insulin by 25% to 50% at the meal before exercise if the activity follows after a meal.[49] Reductions in basal insulin should also be made if the activity is particularly prolonged or regular (every day).

Education on the treatment of mild hypoglycemia includes the assessment of the individual's ability to recognize foods that contain carbohydrate and how these foods affect blood glucose. Based on the 2013 ADA/Endocrine Society Scientific Statement, as a starting point the treatment of hypoglycemia should include carrying carbohydrate foods such as glucose tablets, as well as education on how to use them[50]:

- Take 15 g of glucose or half a cup of fruit juice
- Wait 15 minutes
- Remeasure blood glucose level
- Repeat if hypoglycemia persists

People with diabetes may be more susceptible to adverse events associated with hot environments, perhaps because of reduced capacity to dissipate heat.[51] Thus, elderly patients in particular and those with autonomic neuropathy, cardiac disease, or pulmonary disease should take care to avoid heat-related illness. Precautions may include exercising indoors in cool environments or outdoors in the early or later hours of the day during hot or sunny days.

EVALUATION OF OUTCOME: NUTRITION THERAPY AND PHYSICAL ACTIVITY

Diabetes nutrition therapy has been found to be an effective component of a comprehensive group education program or an individualized session.[23] Evidence from meta-analyses, randomized controlled trials, and observational studies shows that nutrition therapy improves metabolic outcomes such as HbA1c, lipids, and blood pressure in people with diabetes.[13,14,16,36,52] Individualized education sessions or group education programs including nutrition therapy have shown HbA1c reductions of 0.5% to 2% for type 2 diabetes.[2–4,16,17,53,54]

The evaluation of exercise interventions can be performed by conducting an initial assessment of exercise fitness and body composition. Maximal exercise testing on a motorized treadmill or cycle ergometer can be useful for exercise prescription and postintervention assessment. This is best done before an intervention, because the appropriate exercise intensity can be prescribed and assessed more accurately when the maximum heart rate or Vo_{2max} is determined from exercise testing by a qualified clinical exercise physiologist or equivalent health care expert. Estimating target heart rate or work rate from age-predicted calculations is simpler but is prone to measurement error and medication interactions with the cardiovascular system. Exercise testing can also be useful for risk stratification, given that lower aerobic capacity and the presence of ischemic changes on electrocardiogram are each associated with higher risks of cardiovascular and overall morbidity and mortality in diabetes[55,56] and in prediabetes.[57] Exercise testing may also help detect coronary disease and allow the aerobic exercise prescription to be below the ischemic threshold. Several other assessments should be considered both as a baseline and as outcome follow-up[58]:

- An assessment of fall risk (eg, the Timed Up and Go Test, Functional Reach Test, Berg Balance Scale, Dynamic Gait Index)
- Baseline physical activity level (pedometer/accelerometer)
- Body composition (bioelectrical impedance, waist circumference)
- Muscle strength (manual muscle testing, handgrip dynamometer, or repetition maximal testing of certain muscle groups)

LONG-TERM RECOMMENDATIONS: CLINICAL PRIORITIES: NUTRITION THERAPY AND PHYSICAL ACTIVITY

The ADA 2013 nutrition therapy recommendations provide a summary of priority topics for persons with diabetes[2]:

- Portion control with emphasis on choosing nutrient-dense, high-fiber foods, whenever possible, instead of processed foods with added sodium, fat, and sugars.
- Carbohydrate-containing foods and beverages are the greatest determinant of the postmeal blood glucose excursions in people with diabetes, along with the capacity to secrete endogenous insulin. Therefore it is important for individuals with diabetes to know what foods contain carbohydrates (starchy vegetables, whole grains, fruit, milk and milk products, vegetables, and sugar) and how the various forms of carbohydrate influence their glycemia.

- For individuals trying to lose weight, a mild to moderate daily energy deficit is needed (10%–25% relative caloric restriction). Modest weight loss (of >6 kg or ~7.0%–8.5% loss of initial body weight) may provide clinical benefits such as improved glycemia, blood pressure, and/or lipid levels in some individuals with diabetes, especially those early in the disease process. Intensive lifestyle interventions (counseling about nutrition therapy, physical activity, and behavior change) with ongoing support are recommended to achieve and sustain a modest energy deficit until a goal weight is achieved.
- Limitation of any caloric sweetener, including high-fructose corn syrup and sucrose, reduces risk of worsening the cardiometabolic risk profile and weight gain.[2] The term free fructose refers to the consumption of fructose that is naturally occurring in foods such as fruit, and does not include the fructose that is found in the form of the disaccharide sucrose or the fructose in high-fructose corn syrup.[2] It seems that free fructose is not more harmful than other forms of sugar unless it is consumed in excessive amounts (>12% of the total caloric intake).[59,60]
- The selection of lean protein sources and meat alternatives and the substitution of foods high in unsaturated fat (liquid oils) should be preferred rather than those high in trans or saturated fats. Fat quality seems to be more in important than quantity.
- Micronutrients, vitamins, herbal products, and supplements are not recommended for management of diabetes because of a lack of evidence at this time. However, without well-designed clinical trials to prove efficacy, the benefit of pharmacologic doses of micronutrients and supplements is unknown, and findings from small clinical and animal studies is frequently extrapolated to clinical practice.[61]
- Use of nonnutritive sweeteners (NNS), also commonly referred to as artificial sweeteners, continues to be an area of much debate and misinformation. The US Food and Drug Administration has reviewed several types of hypocaloric sweeteners (eg, aspartame, sucralose, saccharin, and sugar alcohols) for safety and has approved them for consumption by the general public, including people with diabetes.[62] **Table 2** shows the acceptable daily intake of popular nonnutritive sweeteners (based on a 70-kg [150-lb] adult). Research supports that nonnutritive sweeteners do not produce a glycemic effect; however, foods containing

Table 2
Acceptable daily intake of popular nonnutritive sweeteners (based on 70-kg [150-lb] adult)

Type of Sweetener	Acceptable Daily Intake[a] (mg/kg Body Weight)	Amount of Diet Soda/Day (355-mL [12-ounce] can)	Amount of Artificial Sweetener (Packets)
Aspartame	50	17	97
Saccharin	5	2	9
Sucralose	5	5	68
Acesulfame K	15	26	20
Stevia	0–4	[b]	30

[a] The US Food and Drug Administration sets an acceptable daily intake (ADI) for each sweetener, which is the maximum amount considered safe to consume each day during a person's lifetime. The ADI is set at about 100 times less than the smallest amount that might cause health concerns, based on studies done in laboratory animals.
[b] Product information not available; sodas containing Stevia are not widely available.

NNSs may affect glycemia based on other ingredients in the product.[63] In a recently published meta-analysis that included 15 randomized controlled trials, the use of NNSs and other low-calorie sweeteners (LCSs) such as sugar alcohols was associated with lower body weight, BMI, and waist circumference when substituted for calorically dense alternatives. The meta-analysis also included 9 cohort studies that reported that the use of NNSs and LCSs were associated with less weight gain but a slightly greater BMI.[64]

- The recommendation for the general population to limit sodium intake to less 2300 mg/d is also appropriate for individuals with diabetes. Lower levels should only be considered on an individual basis for people with diabetes and hypertension.
- Moderate alcohol consumption (1 drink/d or less for adult women and 2 drinks/d or less for adult men) has minimal acute or long-term effects on blood glucose and may have beneficial effects on cardiovascular risk. To reduce the risk of hypoglycemia for individuals using insulin or insulin secretagogues, alcohol should be consumed with food.

Key strategies for individuals requiring medications or insulin include:

- Eating moderate amounts of carbohydrate at meals (and snacks, if desired)
- Not skipping meals
- If on a multiple-daily injection plan or an insulin pump, take mealtime insulin before eating
- If on a premixed or fixed insulin plan, meals need to be eaten at similar times every day and contain similar amounts of carbohydrate that match set doses of insulin

According to the ADA/American College of Sports Medicine position statement[32] and the guide to prescribing physical activity for patients with diabetes by Colberg[65]:

- At least 2.5 h/wk of moderate to vigorous physical activity should be undertaken as part of lifestyle changes to prevent type 2 diabetes onset in high-risk adults.
- Persons with type 2 diabetes should undertake at least 150 min/wk of moderate to vigorous aerobic exercise spread over at least 3 days during the week, with no more than 2 consecutive days between bouts of aerobic activity.
- In addition to aerobic training, persons with type 2 diabetes should undertake moderate to vigorous resistance training at least 2 to 3 d/wk.
- Supervised and combined aerobic and resistance training may confer additional health benefits, although milder forms of physical activity (such as yoga) have shown mixed results.
- Persons with type 2 diabetes are encouraged to increase their total daily unstructured physical activity.
- Flexibility training may be included but should not be undertaken in place of other recommended types of physical activity.
- Although hyperglycemia can be worsened by exercise in type 1 diabetic individuals who are insulin deficient and ketotic (caused by missed or insufficient insulin), few persons with type 2 diabetes develop such a profound degree of insulin deficiency. As such, individuals with type 2 diabetes may engage in physical activity, using caution when exercising with blood glucose levels exceeding 300 mg/dL (16.7 mmol/L) without ketosis, provided they are feeling well and are adequately hydrated.
- Known CVD is not an absolute contraindication to exercise. Individuals with angina classified as moderate or high risk should likely begin exercise in a supervised cardiac rehabilitation program.

- Patients with intermittent claudication are advised to walk at a speed that induces claudication pain within 3 to 5 minutes. Walking should be stopped when claudication pain is rated as moderate and the patient should rest until the claudication pain has resolved. At that point, the patient should resume walking until moderate claudication pain is induced again. The walking exercise program should begin with exercise and rest cycles of at least 30 minutes and should progress to 60 minutes.[66]
- Individuals with peripheral neuropathy and without acute ulceration may participate in moderate weight-bearing exercise. Comprehensive foot care including daily inspection of feet and use of proper footwear (correct sizing and with custom-made foot beds with some cushioning, if feasible) is recommended for prevention and early detection of sores or ulcers. In general, shoes should:
  ○ Fit well
  ○ Be made out of breathable material
  ○ Have a firm heel
  ○ Have hook and loop type fasteners or shoelaces
  ○ Have good shock absorption
  ○ Not be bent or twisted
  ○ Have no seams in the toe box
  ○ Stabilize overpronation or oversupination
- Moderate walking likely does not increase risk of foot ulcers or reulceration in patients with peripheral neuropathy.
- Individuals with cardiac autonomic neuropathy should be screened and receive physician approval and possibly an exercise stress test before exercise initiation. Exercise intensity is best prescribed using the heart rate reserve method with direct measurement of maximal heart rate.
- In individuals with proliferative or preproliferative retinopathy or macular degeneration, careful screening and physician approval are recommended before initiating an exercise program. Activities that greatly increase intraocular pressure, such as high-intensity aerobic or resistance training (with large increases in systolic blood pressure) and head-down activities, are not advised with uncontrolled proliferative disease, nor are jumping or jarring activities, all of which increase hemorrhage risk.
- Individuals with nephropathy often have exercise intolerance. However, exercise training improves cardiovascular risk profile, muscle mass, physical function, and quality of life in individuals with kidney disease[67] and may even be undertaken during dialysis sessions. Animal models suggest that regular exercise delays the progression of diabetic nephropathy[68,69] although good evidence for this in humans is currently lacking. The presence of microalbuminuria per se does not necessitate exercise restrictions.
- Patients with knee pain from osteoarthritis and obesity should be encouraged to participate in modified exercise programs to help with weight loss and improvements in pain, physical function, mental health, and quality of life.[70] Walking, if tolerated, should be encouraged, as should resistance exercise as long as the affected joints are not overly stressed. Other exercise modes, such as recumbent cycling and aquatic exercises, may also help limit knee pain.
- Efforts to promote physical activity should focus on developing self-efficacy and fostering social support from family, friends, and health care providers. Encouraging mild or moderate physical activity may be most beneficial to adoption and maintenance of regular physical activity participation. Lifestyle interventions may have some efficacy in promoting physical activity behavior.

Box 2
The 5 As

Assess: establish current physical activity level and readiness for change (consider the frequency, intensity, duration, and type of activity)

- Not active, not thinking about physical activity
- Not active, ready for physical activity
- Active and ready to maintain or progress

Advise: strongly encourage all patients to get more active by reviewing the health risks of inactivity and the benefits of physical activity. Advise on the appropriate amount and type of physical activity.

Agree: collaboratively develop goals and a personalized action plan. Provide individually relevant exercise prescriptions, time frames, and monitoring of strategies to meet the goals.

Assist: identify personal barriers and strategies to overcome barriers. Identify connections and resources for exercise and physical activity in the community.

Arrange: specify plan for follow-up at diabetes-focused visits with telephone calls or email reminders. Review physical activity level at subsequent visits and provide advice to achieve the next level of activity.

Adapted from Glynn TJ, Manley MW. How to help your patients stop smoking: a National Cancer Institute manual for physicians. Bethesda (MD): National Cancer Institute; 1989. NIH publication no. 89-3064.

To help facilitate changes in physical activity and eating habits, diabetes health care professionals can incorporate the use of the so-called 5 As (assess, advise, agree, assist, and arrange). This approach does not require a lot of training and offers a simple framework that can be integrated with other education and counseling resources. The 5 As concept was introduced by the National Cancer Institute as a guide to help physicians counsel their patients about smoking cessation.[71] This framework has since been expanded to address broader issues of health behavior change and to give care providers the flexibility of addressing important lifestyle topics in a manner ranging from simple to in-depth (depending on time, training, and resources). **Box 2** provides an example of how to use the 5 As for development of a physical activity prescription[71,72]:

FUTURE CONSIDERATIONS/SUMMARY

Lifestyle intervention for the treatment of type 2 diabetes should focus on a reduced energy intake with modification of food choices (increased whole grains, fiber, vegetables, and fruit; reduced total and saturated fat, sugar, and refined grains) and increased physical activity (150 min/wk of aerobic exercise plus strength training 2–3 times per week). In order to be successful another critical component of lifestyle intervention is the use of behavior modification, such as motivational interviewing, self-monitoring, and individualized goal setting, to support long-term results.

REFERENCES

1. Centers for Disease Control and Prevention. National diabetes fact sheet, United States. 2014. Available at: http://www.cdc.gov/diabetes/pubs/statsreport14.htm. Accessed May 23, 2014.

Lifestyle Intervention   **81**

2. Evert AB, Boucher JL, Cypress M, et al. Nutrition therapy recommendations for the management of adults with diabetes. Diabetes Care 2013;36:3821–42.

3. Franz MJ, Powers MA, Leontos C, et al. The evidence for medical nutrition therapy for type 1 and type 2 diabetes in adults. J Am Diet Assoc 2010;110:1852–89.

4. Academy of Nutrition and Dietetics. Diabetes type 1 and 2 for adults evidence-based nutrition practice guidelines. 2008. Available at: http://www.adaevidencelibrary.com/topic.cfm?cat=3253. Accessed May 23, 2014.

5. Diabetes Prevention Program Research Group (DPP). Reduction in the incidence of type 2 diabetes with lifestyle intervention or metformin. N Engl J Med 2011;346:393–403.

6. Ali MK, Bullard KM, Saaddine JB, et al. Achievement of goals in US diabetes care. 1999–2010. N Engl J Med 2013;368:1613–24.

7. Nguyen NT, Nguyen XM, Lane J, et al. Relationship between obesity and diabetes in a US adult population: findings from the National Health and Nutrition Examination Survey, 1999-2006. Obes Surg 2011;21:351–5.

8. Clinical guidelines on the identification, evaluation, and treatment of overweight and obesity in adults–the evidence report. National Institutes of Health. Obes Res 1998;6:51S–209S.

9. National Heart, Lung, and Blood Institute; Clinical Guidelines on the Identification, Evaluation, and Treatment of Overweight and Obesity in Adults. The Evidence Report NHLBI Obesity Education Initiative Expert Panel on the Identification, Evaluation, and Treatment of Obesity in Adults (US). Bethesda (MD):1998 Sep. Report No 98-4083.

10. Lindstrom J, Ilanne-Parikka P, Peltonen M, et al, Finnish Diabetes Prevention Study Group. Sustained reduction in the incidence of type 2 diabetes by lifestyle intervention: follow-up of the Finnish Diabetes Prevention Study. Lancet 2006; 368:1673–9.

11. Li G, Zhang P, Wang J, et al. The long-term effect of lifestyle interventions to prevent diabetes in the China Da Qing Diabetes Prevention Study: a 20-year follow-up study. Lancet 2008;371:1783–9.

12. Look AHEAD Research Group. Cardio-vascular effects of intensive lifestyle intervention in type 2 diabetes. N Engl J Med 2013;369:145–54.

13. Look AHEAD Research Group. Impact of intensive lifestyle intervention on depression and health-related quality of life in type 2 diabetes: the Look AHEAD Trial. Diabetes Care 2014;37:1544–53.

14. Esposito K, Maiorino MI, Ciotola M, et al. Effects of a Mediterranean-style diet on the need for antihyperglycemic drug therapy in patients with newly diagnosed type 2 diabetes: a randomized trial. Ann Intern Med 2009;151:306–14.

15. Feldstein AC, Nichols GA, Smith DH, et al. Weight change in diabetes and glycemic and blood pressure control. Diabetes Care 2008;31:1960–5.

16. Andrews RC, Cooper AR, Montgomery AA, et al. Diet or diet plus physical activity versus usual care in patients with newly diagnosed type 2 diabetes: the early ACTID randomized controlled trial. Lancet 2011;378:129–39.

17. Coppell KJ, Kataoka M, Williams SM, et al. Nutritional intervention in patients with type 2 diabetes who are hyperglycaemic despite optimized drug treatment—Lifestyle Over and Above Drugs in Diabetes (LOADD) study: randomized controlled trial. BMJ 2010;341:c3337.

18. Battista MC, Labonté M, Ménard J, et al. Dietitian-coached management in combination with annual endocrinologist follow up improves global metabolic and cardiovascular health in diabetic participants after 24 months. Appl Physiol Nutr Metab 2012;37:610–20.

19. Banister NA, Jastrow ST, Hodges V, et al. Diabetes self-management training program in a community clinic improves patient outcomes at modest cost. J Am Diet Assoc 2004;104:807–10.

20. Barratt R, Frost G, Millward DJ, et al. A randomized controlled trial investigating the effect of an intensive lifestyle intervention v. standard care in adults with type 2 diabetes immediately after initiating insulin therapy. Br J Nutr 2008;99: 1025–31.

21. Lee DC, Sui X, Church TS, et al. Changes in fitness and fatness on the development of cardiovascular disease risk factors hypertension, metabolic syndrome, and hypercholesterolemia. J Am Coll Cardiol 2012;59:665–72.

22. Inzucchi SE, Bergenstal RM, Buse JB, et al, American Diabetes Association (ADA), European Association for the Study of Diabetes (EASD). Management of hyperglycemia in type 2 diabetes: a patient-centered approach. Position statement of the American Diabetes Association (ADA) and the European Association for the Study of Diabetes (EASD). Diabetes Care 2012;35:1364–79.

23. American Diabetes Association. Standards of medical care in diabetes–2014. Diabetes Care 2014;37(Suppl 1):S14–90.

24. Robbins JM, Thatcher GE, Webb DA, et al. Nutritionist visits, diabetes classes, and hospitalization rates and charges: the Urban Diabetes Study. Diabetes Care 2008;31:655–60.

25. Lacey K, Pritchett E. Nutrition care process and model: ADA adopts road map to quality care and outcomes management. J Am Diet Assoc 2003;103: 1061–72.

26. Wheeler ML, Dunbar SA, Jaacks LM, et al. Macronutrients, food groups and eating patterns in the management of diabetes: a systematic review of the literature, 2010. Diabetes Care 2012;35:434–45.

27. Canadian Diabetes Association Clinical Practice Guidelines Expert Committee, Sigal RJ, Armstrong MJ, et al. Physical activity and diabetes. Can J Diabetes 2013;7(Suppl 1):S40–4.

28. Steinberg H, Jacovino C, Kitabchi AE. Look inside look ahead: why the glass is more than half-full. Curr Diab Rep 2014;7:500.

29. Thompson D, Walhin JP, Batterham AM, et al. Effect of diet or diet plus physical activity versus usual care on inflammatory markers in patients with newly diagnosed type 2 diabetes: the Early ACTivity In Diabetes (ACTID) randomized, controlled trial. J Am Heart Assoc 2014;3:e000828.

30. Herbst A, Kapellen T, Schober E, et al, for the DPV-Science-Initiative. Impact of regular physical activity on blood glucose control and cardiovascular risk factors in adolescents with type 2 diabetes mellitus - a multicenter study of 578 patients from 225 centres. Pediatr Diabetes 2014. http://dx.doi.org/10.1111/pedi.12144.

31. Balducci S, Sacchetti M, Haxhi J, et al. Physical exercise as therapy for type 2 diabetes mellitus. Diabetes Metab Res Rev 2014;30(Suppl 1):13–23.

32. Colberg SR, Sigal RJ, Fernhall B, et al, American College of Sports Medicine, American Diabetes Association. Exercise and type 2 diabetes: the American College of Sports Medicine and the American Diabetes Association: joint position statement executive summary. Diabetes Care 2010;33:2692–6.

33. Colberg SR, Sigal RJ. Prescribing exercise for individuals with type 2 diabetes: recommendations and precautions. Phys Sportsmed 2014;39:13–26.

34. Church TS, Blair SN, Cocreham S, et al. Effects of aerobic and resistance training on hemoglobin A1c levels in patients with type 2 diabetes: a randomized controlled trial. JAMA 2010;304(20):2253–62.

35. Sigal RJ, Kenny GP, Boulé NG, et al. Effects of aerobic training, resistance training, or both on glycemic control in type 2 diabetes: a randomized trial. Ann Intern Med 2007;147(6):357–69.
36. Pastors JG, Franz MJ. Effectiveness of medical nutrition therapy in diabetes. In: Franz MJ, Evert AB, editors. American Diabetes Association guide to nutrition therapy for diabetes. Alexandria (VA): American Diabetes Association; 2012. p. 1–18.
37. US Department of Health and Human Services and US Department of Agriculture. Dietary guidelines for Americans, 2010. [Internet]. Available at: www.health.gov/dietaryguidelines/. Accessed 12 July 7, 2014.
38. Schwingshackl L, Strasser B, Hoffmann G. Effects of monounsaturated fatty acids on glycaemic control in patients with abnormal glucose metabolism: a systematic review and meta-analysis. Ann Nutr Metab 2011;58:290–6.
39. Itsiopoulos C, Brazionis L, Kaimakamis M, et al. Can the Mediterranean diet lower HbA1c in type 2 diabetes? Results from a randomized cross-over study. Nutr Metab Cardiovasc Dis 2011;21:740–7.
40. Brehm BJ, Lattin BL, Summer SS, et al. One-year comparison of a high-monounsaturated fat diet with a high-carbohydrate diet in type 2 diabetes. Diabetes Care 2009;32:215–20.
41. Pan Y, Guo LL, Jin HM. Low-protein diet for diabetic nephropathy: a meta-analysis of randomized controlled trials. Am J Clin Nutr 2008;88:660–6.
42. Robertson L, Waugh N, Robertson A. Protein restriction for diabetic renal disease. Cochrane Database Syst Rev 2007;(4):CD002181.
43. Umpierre D, Ribeiro PA, Kramer CK, et al. Physical activity advice only or structured exercise training and association with HbA1c levels in type 2 diabetes: a systematic review and meta-analysis. JAMA 2011;305:1790–9.
44. Tulloch H, Sweet SN, Fortier M, et al. Exercise facilitators and barriers from adoption to maintenance in the diabetes aerobic and resistance exercise trial. Can J Diabetes 2013;37:367–74.
45. Armstrong MJ, Campbell TS, Lewin AM, et al. Motivational interviewing-based exercise counselling promotes maintenance of physical activity in people with type 2 diabetes. Can J Diabetes 2013;37(Suppl 4):S3.
46. Riddell MC, Burr J. Evidence-based risk assessment and recommendations for physical activity clearance: diabetes mellitus and related comorbidities. Appl Physiol Nutr Metab 2011;36(Suppl 1):S154–89.
47. Colberg SR, Vinik AI. Exercising with peripheral or autonomic neuropathy: what health care providers and diabetic patients need to know. Phys Sportsmed 2014;42(1):15–23.
48. Armstrong MJ, Martin BJ, Arena R, et al. Patients with diabetes in cardiac rehabilitation: attendance and exercise capacity. Med Sci Sports Exerc 2014;46(5):845–50.
49. Rabasa-Lhoret R, Bourque J, Ducros F, et al. Guidelines for premeal insulin dose reduction for postprandial exercise of different intensities and durations in type 1 diabetic subjects treated intensively with a basal-bolus insulin regimen (ultralente-lispro). Diabetes Care 2001;24:625–30.
50. Seaquist ER, Anderson J, Childs B, et al. Hypoglycemia and diabetes: a report of a workgroup of the American Diabetes Association and the Endocrine Society. Diabetes Care 2013;36:1384–95.
51. Yardley JE, Stapleton JM, Sigal RJ, et al. Do heat events pose a greater health risk for individuals with type 2 diabetes? Diabetes Technol Ther 2013;15:520–9.

52. Pi-Sunyer X, Blackburn G, Brancati FL, et al. Reduction in weight and cardiovascular disease risk factors in individuals with type 2 diabetes: on-year results of the Look AHEAD trial. Diabetes Care 2007;30:1374–83.

53. Metz JA, Stern JS, Kris-Etherton P, et al. A randomized trial of improved weight loss with a prepared meal plan in overweight and obese patients: impact on cardiovascular risk reduction. Arch Intern Med 2000;160:2150–8.

54. Nield L, Moore HJ, Hooper L, et al. Dietary advice for treatment of type 2 diabetes mellitus in adults. Cochrane Database Syst Rev 2007;(3):CD004097.

55. Church TS, LaMonte MJ, Barlow CE, et al. Cardiorespiratory fitness and body mass index as predictors of cardiovascular disease mortality among men with diabetes. Arch Intern Med 2005;16:2114–20.

56. Lyerly GW, Sui X, Lavie CJ, et al. The association between cardiorespiratory fitness and risk of all-cause mortality among women with impaired fasting glucose or undiagnosed diabetes mellitus. Mayo Clin Proc 2009;84:780–6.

57. McAuley PA, Artero EG, Sui X, et al. Fitness, fatness, and survival in adults with pre-diabetes. Diabetes Care 2014;37:529–36.

58. Hansen D, Peeters S, Zwaenepoel B, et al. Exercise assessment and prescription in patients with type 2 diabetes in the private and home care setting: clinical recommendations from AXXON (Belgian Physical Therapy Association). Phys Ther 2013;93:597–610.

59. Sievenpiper JL, Carleton AJ, Chatha S, et al. Heterogeneous effects of fructose on blood lipids in individuals with type 2 diabetes: systematic review and meta-analysis of experimental trials in humans. Diabetes Care 2009;32:1930–7.

60. Livesey G, Taylor R. Fructose consumption and consequences for glycation, plasma triacylglycerol, and body weight: meta-analyses and meta-regression models of intervention studies. Am J Clin Nutr 2008;88:1419–37.

61. Nuemiller JJ. Micronutrients and diabetes. In: Franz MJ, Evert AB, editors. American Diabetes Association guide to nutrition therapy for diabetes. Alexandria (VA): American Diabetes Association; 2012. p. 41–68.

62. US Department of Agriculture. Nutritive and nonnutritive sweetener resources [Internet]. National Agricultural Library, Food and Nutrition Information Center. 2013. Available at: http://fnic.nal.usda.gov/food-composition/nutritive-and-nonnutritive-sweetener-resources. Accessed May 23, 2014.

63. Gardner C, Wylie-Rosett J, Gidding SS, et al, American Heart Association Nutrition Committee of the Council on Nutrition, Physical Activity and Metabolism, Council on Arteriosclerosis, Thrombosis and Vascular Biology, Council on Cardiovascular Disease in the Young, American Diabetes Association. Nonnutritive sweeteners: current use and health perspectives: a scientific statement from the American Heart Association and the American Diabetes Association. Diabetes Care 2012;35:1798–808.

64. Miller PE, Perez V. Low-calorie sweeteners and body weight and composition: a meta-analysis of randomized controlled trials and prospective cohort studies. Am J Clin Nutr 2014;100:765–77.

65. Colberg SR. Exercise and diabetes. A clinician's guide to prescribing physical activity. Alexandria (VA): American Diabetes Association; 2013.

66. Brunelle CL, Mulgrew JA. Exercise for intermittent claudication. Phys Ther 2011;91:997–1002.

67. Smith AC, Burton JO. Exercise in kidney disease and diabetes: time for action. J Ren Care 2012;38(Suppl 1):52–8.

68. Tufescu A, Kanazawa M, Ishida A, et al. Combination of exercise and losartan enhances renoprotective and peripheral effects in spontaneously type 2 diabetes mellitus rats with nephropathy. J Hypertens 2008;26:312–21.
69. Ghosh S, Khazaei M, Moien-Afshari F, et al. Moderate exercise attenuates caspase-3 activity, oxidative stress, and inhibits progression of diabetic renal disease in db/db mice. Am J Physiol Renal Physiol 2009;296:F700–8.
70. Foy CG, Lewis CE, Hairston KG, et al, Look AHEAD Research Group. Intensive lifestyle intervention improves physical function among obese adults with knee pain: findings from the Look AHEAD trial. Obesity (Silver Spring) 2011;19:83–93.
71. Glynn TJ, Manley MW. How to help your patients stop smoking: a National Cancer Institute manual for physicians. Bethesda (MD): National Cancer Institute; 1989. NIH publication no. 89–3064.
72. Estabrooks PA, Glasgow RE, Dzewaltowski DA. Physical activity promotion through primary care. JAMA 2003;289:2913–6.

Oral Antihyperglycemic Treatment Options for Type 2 Diabetes Mellitus

Stephen A. Brietzke, MD

KEYWORDS

- Metformin • Sulfonylureas • Thiazolidinediones
- Sodium-glucose transporter-2 inhibitors (SGLT2 inhibitors) • Colesevelam
- Bromocriptine • Type 2 diabetes mellitus

KEY POINTS

- Metformin is the best available combination of low-cost, low-risk, high-efficacy oral therapy for type 2 diabetes mellitus.
- The lowest-cost oral add-on drug to metformin is a sulfonylurea.
- A sodium-glucose transporter type 2 inhibitor, an alpha-glucosidase inhibitor, or a thiazolidinedione, is a reasonable second or tertiary add-on option.
- Alpha-glucosidase inhibitors, colesevelam, and bromocriptine mesylate are niche drugs and may have value in cardiovascular risk reduction, but more information from clinical trials and/or meta-analyses is needed.

INTRODUCTION

The worldwide epidemic of type 2 diabetes mellitus (T2DM) has made diagnosing, counseling, and prescribing for newly diagnosed patients an almost reflex process for many primary care physicians. Patients overwhelmingly prefer initial therapy to be with an oral medication, rather than an injectable (ie, insulin) and, as patient advocates, their treating physicians comply with this request. The past 20 years have transformed oral treatment options for T2DM from a single option (sulfonylureas [SUs]) to at least 9 different classes of drugs, enabling rational, individually customized combination therapy. Incretin analogues and dipeptidyl peptidase-4 (DPP-4) inhibitors are covered in detail elsewhere in this issue. This article reviews the mechanism of action, efficacy, major untoward effects, and impact of other oral therapies on T2DM and associated health risks; most notably, cardiovascular disease.

The likelihood of success for prescribed oral therapy can be estimated from simple observations and measurements at the point of care. **Box 1** emphasizes the

Division of Endocrinology, Diabetes, and Metabolism, Department of Medicine, University of Missouri-Columbia, DC043 UMHC, 1 Hospital Drive, Columbia, MO 65212, USA
E-mail address: brietzkes@health.missouri.edu

Med Clin N Am 99 (2015) 87–106
http://dx.doi.org/10.1016/j.mcna.2014.08.012
0025-7125/15/$ – see front matter © 2015 Elsevier Inc. All rights reserved.
medical.theclinics.com

Box 1
Predictors of response to oral antihyperglycemic drugs (consider initial therapy with insulin if multiple points are negative)

- Newly diagnosed T2DM
- Obesity (body mass index >30 kg/m^2)
- Absence of symptomatic diabetes mellitus (eg, rapid weight loss, severe polyuria, severe polydipsia)
- Hemoglobin A1c (HbA1c) less than 10%
- Fasting serum glucose less than 250 mg/dL
- Absence of nonfasting ketonuria

---

characteristics of patients likely to respond well to oral therapy for T2DM; patients who lack multiples of these characteristics are best served by an initial prescription for insulin therapy (covered in a separate article by Meah and Juneja in this issue).

Rules of thumb estimating the impact of drug monotherapy, and subsequent add-on drugs, are highlighted in **Box 2**. Available drug therapies, by class, are overviewed individually, with regard to mechanism of action, efficacy, adverse effects, and influence on cardiovascular disease and neoplasia.

METFORMIN

Metformin was first available in the United States in 1995, and was long delayed because of fear of fatal lactic acidosis, which had led to market withdrawal of another biguanide drug, phenformin, in 1970. Practitioners have learned to use the drug cautiously or not at all in patients thought to be at increased risk for lactic acidosis, including the elderly, patients with congestive heart failure (CHF), and patients with chronic kidney disease. However, it has become the number 1 most prescribed oral antihyperglycemic agent in the world, while also becoming one of the lowest-cost and lowest-risk agents available. As metformin approaches its 20th anniversary in the United States, its track record of low cost, low risk, and low frequency of troublesome side effects justifies its place as the first choice when oral therapies for T2DM are prescribed for patients. Many of the original cautions and presumed contraindications for prescribing should be relearned.

Metformin's primary action is suppression of hepatic glucose generation, and the exact molecular action is still not understood. Enhanced activity of AMP kinase (AMPK) may be either caused by a direct agonist effect on AMPK, or by suppression of hepatic mitochondrial oxidation, resulting in a higher AMP/ATP ratio, and thence secondary activation of AMPK.[1,2] An apparent insulin-sensitizing effect of metformin on muscle glucose uptake may simply be escape from the glucose toxicity phenomenon, caused by reduced endogenous glucose production.

Box 2
Anticipated efficacy of initial and add-on oral antihyperglycemic drugs

- Initial drug: ΔHbA1c = -1.5% to -2.0%
- First add-on: ΔHbA1c = -1% to -1.5%
- Second add-on: ΔHbA1c = -0.5% to -1%

Efficacy of metformin, either as a stand-alone or in combination with SU, was established in the United Kingdom Prospective Diabetes Study (UKPDS). After 3 years' usage in the UKPDS study, 79% of 207 obese patients originally randomized to metformin only were still taking the drug; only 10% required addition of another agent because of inadequate response to monotherapy. Mean hemoglobin A1c (HbA1c) at the 3-year point in the study was 7.1% for metformin only, versus 7.8% for the obese control group.[3] In a US trial, DeFronzo and Goodman[4] randomized 289 patients to metformin versus placebo, attaining a mean on-treatment HbA1c level of 7.1% versus 8.6%, in a 29-week trial.

In the UKPDS, users of metformin had significantly reduced rates of microvascular diabetic complications. A subsequent 10-year follow-up study of UKPDS patients showed risk reduction for cardiovascular disease events favoring metformin users, with relative risks versus nonusers of 0.79 for any diabetes-related end point, 0.70 for diabetes-related death, 0.73 for all-cause mortality, and 0.67 for myocardial infarction (MI).[5] Metformin plus insulin was not allowed in the UKPDS study protocol, but Hemingsen and colleagues[6] conducted a meta-analysis of 23 clinical trials totaling 2117 patients, which compared outcomes of metformin plus insulin versus insulin-only treatment regimens. The quality of evidence from these trials was generally poor, but identified significantly lower HbA1c (-0.5%), less weight gain (by 1 kg), and reduced insulin dose (by 5 units/d) in the metformin plus insulin groups, with a greater risk of hypoglycemia (odds ratio, 2.83) and no conclusive difference in cardiovascular or all-cause mortality.

There is evidence that metformin may reduce cancer risk, possibly by ameliorating hyperinsulinemia's activation of the proneoplastic enzyme, mammalian target of rapamycin (mTOR).[7] In a 10-year follow-up study of patients with T2DM, new cancer incidence was 7.3% in users, versus 11.6% in nonusers.[8] Breast cancer incidence was significantly lower in women with T2DM who used metformin, as opposed to women who did not (odds ratio, 0.44).[9] In another study of patients with diagnosed breast cancer, complete response to neoadjuvant chemotherapy occurred in 24% of metformin-treated patients with T2DM, versus 8% of non–metformin-treated patients with T2DM, and in 16% of nondiabetic individuals.[10] A hospital-based study of pancreatic adenocarcinoma identified an odds ratio of 0.38 for metformin users. Metformin use may reduce both the incidence[11] and the prognosis of prostate cancer.[12]

The most common adverse effects limiting use of metformin are gastrointestinal, most commonly diarrhea/fecal urgency and nausea. These adverse effects are reported by up to 30% of users within the first 1 to 2 weeks of usage, but resolve in all but 5% to 10%. The adverse effects are severe enough to preclude use in approximately 5% of users[13]; in the UKPDS, 11% of patients randomized to metformin were unable to tolerate therapy.[3] Common interventions to improve tolerance of metformin include taking the medication with meals (rather than on an empty stomach), starting the medication at a low dose (500 mg, with the evening meal), and advancing the dose gradually week by week, and using an extended-release preparation. There is anecdotal evidence that these interventions help some patients, but this has not been validated by evidence from clinical trials. Metformin impairs intestinal absorption of vitamin B_{12}, and in one study vitamin B_{12} levels were 19% lower in the metformin versus the placebo group at the end of the 52-month study period. Vitamin B_{12} deficiency (serum level <150 pmol/L) occurred in 9.9% of the metformin group, versus 2.7% of the placebo group; low vitamin B_{12} (serum level 150–220 pmol/L) was found in 18.2% of the metformin group, and in 7% of the placebo group.[14] Periodic measurement of serum B_{12} levels is warranted, in the authors opinion.

Fear of lactic acidosis was a major concern when metformin first became available in the United States.[15] The estimated frequency of lactic acidosis is not in excess of 3 cases per 100,000 patients treated[16]; furthermore, a recent Cochrane Review of 347 clinical trials and observational studies concluded that, compared with other treatments for T2DM, metformin was not associated with any risk for lactic acidosis.[17] A comprehensive review by Scheen and Paquot[18] identified reduced risk for all-cause mortality in metformin users versus other T2DM treatment regimens, in the settings of stable coronary heart disease (relative risk, 0.72–0.76), following acute coronary syndrome (relative risk, 0.4–0.8), and in CHF (relative risk, 0.65–0.87). In a systematic review of observational studies numbering more than 34,000 patients with CHF, Eurich and colleagues[19] found metformin use to be associated with reduced (not increased) risk for mortality (relative risk vs nonusers, 0.80), and even when left ventricular ejection fraction was severely reduced the relative risk for mortality was not significantly different than for nonusers (0.91). Among patients with CHF and chronic kidney disease, metformin use was also associated with reduced mortality risk (relative risk, 0.81 for metformin users vs nonusers). The following recommendations for metformin use based on renal function have been offered independently by several critical reviews: no dose adjustment for estimated glomerular filtration rate (eGFR) greater than or equal to 45 mL/min/1.73 m^2; limit dose to 50% of maximum recommended for eGFR greater than or equal to 30 to less than 45 mL/min/1.73 m^2; and discontinue metformin only for eGFR less than 30 mL/min/1.73 m^2.[16,20,21] Based on the Eurich and colleagues[19] systematic review, and based on US Food and Drug Administration (FDA) change in prescribing information for metformin in 2010, CHF independent of eGFR less than 30 mL/min/1.73 m^2 should no longer be considered a contraindication to metformin use.[19]

INSULIN SECRETOGOGUES
Sulfonylureas

Until the introduction of metformin in 1995, SUs were the only oral antihyperglycemic class available in the United States. The SU class might now be considered the "Rodney Dangerfield" of oral therapies for T2DM. Like the late comedian, whose signature line bemoaned that "he got no respect at all," the SU class has been disrespected over the years for possibly increasing cardiovascular risk, and possibly accelerating pancreatic islet cell burnout. Despite the concerns, SUs remain widely prescribed, because of familiarity, relative lack of nonglycemic adverse effects, very low cost, and generally good efficacy in controlling glycemia, at least in the early phases of T2DM. The SUs prevalently used in the United States are the second-generation SUs glyburide and glipizide, and the third-generation SU, glimepiride.

The mechanism of action common to all the SU drugs involves binding to the pancreatic islet cell sulfonylurea receptor 1 (SUR1), which results in closure of the cell membrane ATP-sensitive potassium channel (K^+_{ATP}), thereby causing membrane depolarization, influx of calcium ions, and subsequent release of insulin from storage vesicles.[22,23] A Cochrane Review of clinical trial and observation study data totaling more than 22,000 patients, and including both first-generation and second-generation SUs, identified a mean 1.01% reduction in HbA1c with SU monotherapy.[24] Initiation of SU monotherapy in previously treatment-naive individuals with T2DM can be expected to produce a 1% to 2% reduction in HbA1c,[25] averaging about 1.5%.[26,27]

Based on the UKPDS trial results, slightly more than half of patients newly diagnosed with T2DM can be expected to attain a goal HbA1c less than 7% on SU monotherapy. In the UKPDS, only 24% of patients treated by intent to a goal HbA1c level of less than 7.0% were achieving that goal with SU alone after 9 years; 50% were failing to reach goal by 3 years.[28] With regard to purported accelerated burnout of islet cells with SU therapy, some investigators have pointed out that the rate of monotherapy failure for metformin in UKPDS was similar to that for SU, suggesting that progressive loss of islet cell function is simply part of the natural history of T2DM.[29,30] In the ADOPT (A Diabetes Outcome Progression Trial) trial, monotherapy failure after 5 years of treatment was 34% for glyburide, 21% for metformin, and 15% for rosiglitazone.[31] Based on available dose-response curves, many experienced clinicians recommend a maximum clinical dose of an SU drug of approximately half the US FDA-approved maximal dose.[25,32] In one dose-response trial of glimepiride, the mean reduction in HbA1c was 1.9% at the maximal dose, 8 mg daily, and 1.8% at 4 mg daily.[33] Some investigators have suggested a tachyphylaxis response to high-dose SU, with downregulation of SUR1 binding and signaling transduction.[34]

Efficacy of SU as add-on therapy to metformin, and thiazolidinedione (TZD) has been established, with efficacy of ΔHbA1c −0.47% to −1.3%,[27] and −1.76% to −2.68%,[35] respectively. In these studies of combination oral therapy including SU, adverse events except for hypoglycemia were similar: SU-plus groups experienced hypoglycemia about twice as often as the comparator groups (relative risk, 2.41).[27]

The most frequent serious adverse effect of SUs is hypoglycemia, occurring at a frequency of 1.7% of glimepiride users and 5% of glyburide users within the first month of therapy in one study.[25] In a German study, glyburide was responsible 6 times as often as was glimepiride for severe hypoglycemic events requiring professional care, despite many more active prescriptions in use for glimepiride.[36] Because risk for hypoglycemia is greater in persons with chronic kidney disease, all of the SUs are considered contraindicated at serum creatinine greater than 1.8 mg/dL (eGFR <30 mL/min/1.73 m^2); at any degree of impaired renal function, glipizide or glimepiride is preferred to glyburide, because of its longer half-life and inherently greater risk for hypoglycemia. Weight gain is also a frequent, possibly ubiquitous occurrence in SU-treated patients; over a 6-year period in the United Kingdom Prospective Diabetes Study, patients randomized to treatment with an SU gained a mean of 5.3 kg.[37] In the UKPDS, the prevalent SUs were chlorpropamide and glyburide; there is evidence that glimepiride may be associated with less weight gain over time than other drugs of the SU class.[25,26] Glyburide, glipizide, and glimepiride are all rated as class C in pregnancy, and glyburide has been studied and established as noninferior to insulin therapy in gestational diabetes, with no evidence of adverse fetal or maternal outcomes.[38,39]

The cardiovascular safety question that has dogged the SU class remains unresolved 43 years after the University Group Diabetes Project (UGDP) study reported a disproportionate number of acute MIs in patients receiving tolbutamide, a first-generation SU.[40] The UKPDS study partly assuaged concerns, with a nonsignificant decreased number of cardiovascular events during the original trial,[41] and a reduced rate (vs the non–SU-using usual care group) during the 10-year follow-up study, including risk ratios of 0.87 for all-cause mortality and 0.85 for MI, versus usual care.[5] However, a large retrospective cohort study of patients attending US Veterans Administration care facilities compared 98,665 veterans who received SU monotherapy with 155,025 receiving metformin monotherapy. After adjustment for confounding factors, a hazard ratio of 1.26 for glyburide versus metformin (95% confidence interval [CI], 1.16–1.37), and 1.15 for glipizide versus metformin (CI, 1.06–1.26) was identified in this study for the composite end point of acute MI, stroke, or death.[42]

It is possible that some of the disparity in cardiovascular outcomes with SU drugs can be explained by different pharmacologic properties of individual SUs. Although the various SU agents have similar agonist effects on the pancreatic islet SUR1 receptor, they differ in the degree of agonist activity on myocardial and coronary vascular SUR2 receptors.[43,44] Glipizide and glimepiride have low agonist effects on the

SUR2 receptor, whereas glyburide has significant agonist effect on SUR2. Opening of the myocardial $K^+{}_{ATP}$ is important in the ischemic preconditioning phenomena, which can limit infarct size following the acute ischemic insult. Closure of this channel by activation of the SUR2 receptor is thought to interfere with ischemic preconditioning, thereby potentially extending infarct size and adversely affecting prognosis.[45] There is experimental and observational evidence to support a concept that glyburide is uniquely hazardous among the 3 SUs in common use in the United States with regard to coronary disease outcomes. In a study conducted in Taiwan, Lee and Chou[46] noted differential response to glimepiride and glyburide in both nondiabetic and diabetic patients undergoing coronary angioplasty, with lower ischemic burden scores in patients receiving glimepiride as opposed to glyburide. In a prospective study of 1310 patients admitted for acute MI over a 1-month period to French hospitals in 2005, SU use at the time of admission was not associated with an in-hospital increased risk for complications or mortality. On the contrary, SU use before admission was associated with lower mortality (3.9%) than was use of other oral agents (mortality 6.4%), insulin (mortality 9.4%), or no T2DM drug therapy (mortality 8.4%). However, the shorter-acting and more pancreatic islet–specific ATP channel agonists gliclazide and glimepiride were associated with lower in-hospital mortality (2.7%) than was the longer-acting, non–organ-specific K^+ ATP channel agonist glyburide (in-hospital mortality, 7.9%).[47]

There is controversy as to whether or not SUs are associated with increased risk for common cancers, with data from several studies summarized in **Table 1**. Taken in the aggregate, findings from these studies lead to a conclusion that, although SUs may not definitely increase the risk for malignancies, there is no evidence that they reduce cancer risk.

Based on low toxicity, low cost, and extensive worldwide experience, SU drugs are still deserving of a role as add-on therapy for patients failing to achieve treatment goals on regimens of 1 or 2 drugs that include metformin. Glyburide is associated with both a greater risk of hypoglycemia and greater association with complications arising from acute coronary presentations. It therefore seems prudent to preferentially use glipizide or glimepiride. It is unclear whether glyburide offers any justification for continued use, given the concerns with disproportionate risk,[51,52] except in pregnancy and in countries in which glyburide is the only available SU.

Glinides

Two drugs of the glinide class, repaglinide and nateglinide, are available for use. Like SUs, these drugs work as agonists of the SUR1 receptor, but have extremely short

Table 1			
Relative risk of incident cancer with sulfonylureas (vs nonusers)			
Study	**Cancer Type**	**Number of Patients**	**Relative Risk**
Singh et al,[48] 2013	Hepatocellular	334,307	1.61 (95% CI, 1.16–2.24)
Chang et al,[49] 2012	Any	40,970	1.08 (95% CI, 1.01–1.15)
Thakkar et al,[50] 2013	Any (meta-analysis)	315,517	1.55 (cohort studies) (95% CI, 1.48–1.63) 1.02 (case-control studies) (95% CI, 0.93–1.13) 1.17 (RCTs) (95% CI, 0.95–1.45)
Soranna et al,[7] 2012	Any (meta-analysis)	35,642	0.97 (95% CI, 0.82–1.14)

Abbreviation: RCTs, randomized controlled trials.

durations of action. They are best considered as non-SU SUs," and use is best reserved for persons responsive to SU but susceptible to fasting hypoglycemia, or for persons with true SU allergy.[53,54]

THIAZOLIDINEDIONES

If SUs are the "Rodney Dangerfield," it seems fair to label TZDs as the "Warren G. Harding" of antihyperglycemic drugs, because Harding was a US President elected largely on the basis that he looked like a president, and many TZD effects look as if they should be ideal treatment of T2DM. Rosiglitazone and pioglitazone bind to peroxisome proliferator activating receptor gamma (PPARγ) receptors to form heterodimers with retinoid-X receptors, which then bind to various response elements of the genome, resulting in transactivation of gene products enhancing insulin action, and transrepression of nuclear signal pathways generally unfavorable to insulin action (notably, nuclear factor kappa B [NF-kB]).[55,56] In adipose tissue, PPARγ activation blocks release of free fatty acids (FFAs), reduces tumor necrosis factor alpha (TNF-α), and increases adiponectin. TZDs promote expansion of the subcutaneous adipose compartment, and contraction of the visceral adipose compartment.[57] The lipid steal hypothesis suggests that increased uptake of FFAs by adipose tissue allows FFAs to escape from muscle, liver, and islet cells, resulting in improved insulin action and increased insulin secretion.[55,56]

Clinical efficacy trials of the TZD drugs have all shown significant improvement in HbA1c, as monotherapy versus placebo, or as add-on therapy to metformin, SU, and insulin regimens. Monotherapy trials of pioglitazone 15 to 45 mg produced ΔHbA1c versus placebo of up to −1.6%, at the study end points.[58] Compared with placebo as add-on therapy to metformin, pioglitazone produced ΔHbA1c up to −1.4%; as add-on therapy to SU, it produced ΔHbA1c up to −1.6%; and as add-on to insulin, it produced ΔHbA1c up to −1.0%.[58,59] Monotherapy trials of rosiglitazone 2 to 8 mg daily likewise produced ΔHbA1c of up to −1.5% versus placebo.[58] Compared with placebo as add-on therapy to metformin, SU, and insulin, rosiglitazone 2 to 8 mg daily produced ΔHbA1c up to −2.3%, −1.0%, and −1.3%, respectively.[58,59]

TZDs have shown nonglycemic pleiotropic effects on numerous surrogate markers of atherosclerotic cardiovascular disease, including reduced carotid artery intimal media thickness on carotid ultrasonography. Because of the numerous salutary effects of TZDs on markers of inflammation, thrombosis, and endothelial health (summarized in **Box 3**), the use of these agents attracted widespread interest among both researchers and clinicians interested in preventing microvascular and atherosclerotic complications of T2DM.[60-65]

Pioglitazone has shown some utility in the treatment of nonalcoholic fatty liver disease (NAFLD), which is frequently associated with T2DM, and is clinically heralded by variable transaminitis and hepatomegaly. NAFLD is now recognized as a cause of formerly cryptogenic cirrhosis. Use of both rosiglitazone and pioglitazone have been associated with net reduction in hepatic fat; in some studies, pioglitazone seems to reduce hepatic fibrosis in patients with severe NAFLD.[70]

The favorable pleiotropic effects of TZDs on multiple cardiovascular risk factors contrasts with a general lack of disease outcomes improvements. By contrast, the evidence is confluent that these drugs cause or aggravate edema and CHF. Overall, when used as monotherapy, a TZD is associated with edema in 2% to 5% of users; if combined with another oral agent, the risk increases to 6% to 8%; and, if combined with insulin, the risk is about 15%.[71] Relative risk for CHF from 17,579 patients in 3 rosiglitazone and 2 pioglitazone trials ranges from 1.41 to 7.0 versus a comparator

---

Box 3
Pleiotropic effects of TZDs

Antiinflammatory effects
- ↓hsCRP
- ↓TNF-α
- ↓IL-6
- ↓Vascular adhesion molecules

Antithrombotic effects
- ↓PAI-1
- ↓MMP-9

Lipid composition effects
- ↑HDLc
- ↓TG
- ↑LDL particle size (large fluffy LDLc)

Salutary vascular effects
- ↑eNOS
- ↓Smooth muscle proliferation
- ↓Systolic blood pressure
- ↓Restenosis after coronary angioplasty[66]

Abbreviations: eNOS, endothelial nitric oxide synthase; HDLc, high-density lipoprotein cholesterol; hsCRP, highly sensitive C-reactive protein; IL-6, interleukin 6; LDL, low-density lipoprotein; LDLc, low-density lipoprotein cholesterol; MMP-9, matrix metallopeptidase 9; PAI-1, plasminogen activator inhibitor-1; TG, triglycerides.
   Data from Refs.[67–69]

---

group[71]; a meta-analysis of 7 trials totaling 20,191 participants established a relative risk for CHF of 1.72 (95% CI, 1.21–2.42) for TZD users, versus comparator groups.[72] Estimation of cardiovascular disease risk beyond edema and CHF comes from multiple clinical trials of TZDs. The diabetes reduction assessment with ramipril and rosiglitazone Medication (DREAM) trial of rosiglitazone versus placebo, in 5269 subjects with impaired glucose tolerance, showed reduced incident T2DM, but no reduction in the pooled cardiovascular outcomes of MI, stroke, and cardiovascular death. Incident CHF was greater in the rosiglitazone group, occurring in 0.5%, versus 0.1% in the placebo group.[73] The ADOPT trial, comparing magnitude and durability of response of glycemia in T2DM with rosiglitazone, metformin, or glyburide as oral monotherapy, identified rosiglitazone as the most durable response with regard to HbA1c, but it had no advantage with regard to incident cardiovascular events.[31] The RECORD (Rosiglitazone Evaluated for Cardiovascular Outcomes in Oral Agent Combination Therapy for Type 2 Diabetes) trial of 4447 patients T2DM compared rosiglitazone plus either metformin or SU, versus the combination of metformin and SU, specifically for cardiovascular outcomes. Analysis of RECORD trail data identified an increased risk of CHF among rosiglitazone users (hazard ratio 2.1 [95% CI, 1.35–3.27], vs non-users), but no significant advantage with regard to microvascular disease, or cardiovascular event-related hospitalization or death.[74] A meta-analysis by Nissen, which drew heavily from unpublished clinical trials registry data, identified odds ratios of

1.43 (95% CI, 1.03–1.98; P = .03) for MI, and 1.64 (95% CI, 0.98–2.74; P = .06) for cardiovascular death for rosiglitazone use versus comparator groups in the pooled trial data.[75] With subsequent reviews reaching similar conclusions, albeit at lower magnitude of risk, rosiglitazone virtually disappeared from clinical use.

The PROspective pioglitAzone clinical trial in macroVascular events (PROActive) trial, which compared pioglitazone versus placebo as add-on therapy to existing treatment of T2DM, was specifically designed to measure rate of incident cardiovascular disease events and cardiovascular mortality in a high-risk group of patients with prior cardiovascular disease events, but there was no difference in the primary outcomes in the pioglitazone versus placebo groups.[76] Head-to-head comparison seems to favor pioglitazone rather than rosiglitazone, with regard to cardiovascular outcomes, based on data from a meta-analysis of 4 case-control and 12 retrospective cohort studies, in which relative risk for MI was 1.16 (95% CI, 1.07–1.24; P<.001) and relative risk of death was 1.14 (95% CI, 1.09–1.20; P<.001), for rosiglitazone versus pioglitazone.[77] Caution in accepting that conclusion has been urged based on methodologic flaws in many of the studies.[71] Pioglitazone, but not rosiglitazone, has been associated with an increased risk for bladder cancer; a meta-analysis by Bosetti and colleagues[78] identified a relative risk of 1.42 (95% CI, 1.17–1.72) for pioglitazone use beyond 2 years, versus never-users. No other cancer risk has thus far been linked with either rosiglitazone or pioglitazone.

TZD drugs seem to have an adverse effect on bone health. Among 666 participants with T2DM in the Health, Aging, and Body Composition observational study, self-reported TZD use in women (but not in men) was associated with annualized bone loss of −1.23% at the lumbar spine, and −0.65% at the hip by dual-energy x-ray absorptiometry (DEXA), compared with nonusers.[79] Other investigators have identified increased risk of fracture in TZD users; these studies are summarized in **Table 2**. In summary, literature to date establishes that TZD use is associated with bone loss, which translates into a roughly 50% increased risk of fracture, over time.

The increase and decrease in popularity of the TZD class represents a new age of awareness in which glycemic efficacy is no longer the sole determinant leading to drug approval, marketing, and prescribing. Henceforth, cardiovascular safety will be as important as blood glucose normalization. The TZD experience is a reminder that favorable effects on surrogate markers of disease do not necessarily translate to clinical outcomes.

SODIUM-GLUCOSE TRANSPORTER TYPE 2 INHIBITORS

The concept of sodium-glucose transporter type 2 (SGLT2) inhibitors has been described as "turning symptoms into therapy"[85] for T2DM. In the proximal renal

Table 2
Relative risk of TZD use for incident fractures (vs nonusers)

Study	Number of Subjects	Relative Risk of Fracture (TZD vs Non-TZD)
Aubert et al,[80] 2010	69,047	1.39 (95% CI, 1.32–1.46)
Meier et al,[81] 2008	66,696	2.43 (95% CI, 1.49–3.45)
Dormuth et al,[82] 2009	84,000	1.28 (95% CI, 1.10–1.48)
Kahn et al,[83] 2008	1840 (ADOPT trial)	1.81 (rosiglitazone vs metformin) (95% CI, 1.17–2.80) 2.13 (rosiglitazone vs glyburide) (95% CI, 1.30–3.51)
Loke et al,[84] 2009	45,394	1.45 (95% CI, 1.18–1.79)

tubule, the SGLT2 is the predominant transport system, normally reclaiming about 144 g of filtered glucose from glomerular filtrate per 24 hours. The avidity of SGLT2-mediated glucose transport in the kidney is such that normally serum glucose must exceed 180 mg/dL for the volume of filtered glucose to exceed transport capacity and produce glucosuria. Inhibition of SGLT2 causes glycosuria at a lower level of filtered (and hence, serum) glucose and thus lowers serum glucose through increased selective glycosuria.[86]

Canagliflozin and dapagliflozin are the first two SGLT2 inhibitor drugs available in the United States. They are indicated for treatment of T2DM, based on monotherapy trials versus placebo, and as add-on therapy for patients failing to reach HbA1c treatment goals with metformin monotherapy. Monotherapy with canagliflozin produced ΔHbA1c of −0.77% to −1.03%, along with body weight change of −2.5 to −3.4 kg at doses of 100 mg and 300 mg daily, respectively, versus placebo.[87] Canagliflozin proved equal to glimepiride as add-on therapy for subjects inadequately controlled on metformin, in the CANagliflozin treatment and trial analysis-sulfonylurea (CANTATA-SU) trial, with ΔHbA1c −0.93% (vs baseline value) in the canagliflozin add-on group, and ΔHbA1c −0.81% in the glimepiride group, although on average weight changed by −3.7 kg in the canagliflozin groups and by +0.7 kg in the glimepiride group.[88] Hypoglycemia was more frequent in the glimepiride plus metformin group, whereas genital mycotic infections were more frequent in the canagliflozin plus metformin groups. Another trial examining canagliflozin versus sitagliptin as tertiary therapy for patients failing metformin plus SU slightly favored canagliflozin, with ΔHbA1c −1.03% in the canagliflozin plus SU plus metformin group, and ΔHbA1c −0.67% in the sitagliptin plus SU plus metformin group; weight changed −2.3 kg in the canagliflozin-plus group and by +0.3 kg in the sitagliptin-plus group.[89] Dapagliflozin has been studied versus placebo, as add-on therapy to metformin in inadequately controlled T2DM, with ΔHbA1c of −0.67% to −0.84% for dapagliflozin doses ranging from 2.5 to 10 mg daily, versus ΔHbA1c of +0.3% in the placebo plus metformin group. Body weight changed by −2.2 to −3.0 kg with canagliflozin plus metformin, and by −0.9 kg for placebo plus metformin, with similar frequency of adverse events.[90]

Vasilakou and colleagues[91] conducted a meta-analysis of all clinical trial data, to estimate the overall efficacy of the SGLT2 drug class, and found an overall ΔHbA1c of −0.79% in patients treated with SGLT2 monotherapy, and ΔHbA1c of −0.61% with SGLT2 as add-on therapy. Other associations with SGLT2 therapy included mean −1.8 kg weight loss, −4.5 mm Hg systolic blood pressure, and up to a 5-fold increased rate of genital mycotic infections, versus comparator groups. These investigators, and others, have been critical of missing data in trials and strong possibility of overestimation of benefit, caused by the last observation carried forward when subjects dropped out or were lost to follow-up in the trials.[91,92] It is hoped that an ongoing cardiovascular safety trial will establish long-term safety for canagliflozin[93]; dapagliflozin will be monitored closely not only for cardiovascular safety but for incident breast and bladder cancer, which was noted to have occurred more frequently in dapagliflozin users in the meta-analysis.[91] For now, SGLT2s can be viewed as equivalent to other available agents as add-on therapy to metformin, albeit at high financial cost and with increased risk for genital mycotic infections. Small but significant weight loss of up to 5 kg in the first year of therapy is expected, and risk of hypoglycemia is low. Long-term safety (benefit or noninferiority with regard to other drug classes) with regard to cardiovascular disease events and neoplasia has not yet been established.[94] Based on relative absence of long-term safety information, and high financial cost of treatment, it seems prudent to recommend SGLT2 inhibitors as third-line therapy for T2DM at the present time.

ALPHA-GLUCOSIDASE INHIBITORS

An orally administered inhibitor of intestinal alpha-glucosidases, acarbose is poorly absorbed (<1%) by the gut, and reduces peak postprandial glycemia by delaying absorption of ingested disaccharides and complex carbohydrates.[95] It has minimal effect on fasting glucose, and, when added to metformin in patients with baseline HbA1c greater than 7.0%, reduces HbA1c by approximately 0.7%.[96] Based on its mechanism of action, it has little potential for drug-induced hypoglycemia, unless used in combination with exogenously administered insulin or insulin secretogogue (SU or glinides).

Acarbose was approved by the FDA for treatment of T2DM in 1996. One clinical trial compared acarbose only with SU only, and with SU plus acarbose, and found that ΔHbA1c was −0.54% for acarbose only, −0.93% for SU only, and −1.32% for acarbose plus SU.[97] Another trial compared acarbose or placebo as add-on therapy to diet only, metformin, glyburide, or insulin; at the 1-year study termination, ΔHbA1c was −0.9% for acarbose plus diet, −0.8% for acarbose plus metformin, −0.9% for acarbose plus glyburide, and −0.4% for acarbose plus insulin.[98] Adverse effects associated with acarbose were limited to flatulence, diarrhea, and abdominal cramping.

Efficacy of acarbose in the delay of onset or prevention of T2DM, and on incident cardiovascular disease events and hypertension, was established by The Study to Prevent Non–insulin-dependent Diabetes Mellitus (STOP-NIDDM) trial. This randomized, placebo-controlled study compared acarbose 100 mg 3 times a day with meals, versus placebo, on rates of incident T2DM in 1429 at-risk subjects, selected from impaired glucose tolerance on standard oral glucose tolerance testing; over a mean period of follow-up of 3.3 years, incident T2DM occurred in 32% of acarbose-treated subjects, versus 42% of placebo-treated subjects (absolute risk reduction, 10%; number needed to treat, 10).[99] Furthermore, an absolute risk reduction for new cardiovascular events of 2.5% favoring acarbose (cardiovascular disease incidence, 2.2%) versus placebo (cardiovascular disease incidence, 4.6%), and a 5.3% absolute risk reduction (adjusted by multivariate analysis) for new-onset hypertension favoring acarbose (new hypertension in 24% in 3.3 years) versus placebo (new hypertension in 33.7% in 3.3 years) were also noted in this trial.[100] No serious adverse events were reported in either study group; gastrointestinal symptoms were far more frequent in the acarbose group than in the placebo group.

Aside from flatulence and loose stool, adverse effects of acarbose are minimal. Malabsorption of iron is possible. Acarbose reduces bioavailability of metformin, and, if used in combination with metformin, markedly increases the likelihood of gastrointestinal adverse effects.[95] Contraindications to use of acarbose include severe irritable bowel syndrome, severe renal disease, and severe hepatic disease.[101]

COLESEVELAM

Bile acids are involved in glucose homeostasis signal pathways as activators of the farnesoid X receptor alpha, which is a regulator of gluconeogenesis and glucagon synthesis; bile acids may also induce glucagon-like peptide-1 production.[102] The glycemic efficacy of a bile acid sequestrant, colesevelam, was first formally tested in a randomized, placebo-controlled fashion in the glucose lowering effect of WelChol study (GLOWS) (GLP-1) trial, which showed a ΔHbA1c of −0.5% versus placebo, and also showed decreased low-density lipoprotein cholesterol (LDLc) level of −9.6% (vs baseline value), compared with +2.1% (vs baseline value) in the placebo group. Gastrointestinal symptoms, primarily constipation, were 3 times more frequent in the colesevelam group than in the placebo group.[103]

The efficacy of colesevelam as add-on therapy for T2DM was subsequently tested in clinical trials in patients receiving monotherapy with SUs, metformin, combined oral therapies (excluding DPP-4 inhibitors), and insulin. In a 26-week clinical trial of 316 subjects at multiple centers in the United States and Mexico, patients treated with metformin or metformin plus combinations of SU, glinides, TZDs, and/or alpha-glucosidase inhibitors, were randomized to colesevelam 3.75 g per day, or placebo. At study conclusion, the colesevelam group's HbA1c level was 0.54% lower than the placebo group's; LDLc, and highly sensitive C-reactive protein (hsCRP) were also lower in the colesevelam group.[104] A 26-week multicenter trial, also including US and Mexican sites, of 461 subjects with T2DM with baseline HbA1c of 8.2%, randomized patients treated with SU or with SU plus metformin, TZD, and/or alpha-glucosidase inhibitor to receive either colesevelam 3.75 g daily or placebo. At the study's conclusion, HbA1c was 0.54% lower in the colesevelam than in the comparator groups, and LDLc level was also significantly lower.[105] A 16-week clinical trial added colesevelam or placebo to patients with mean HbA1c of 8.3% treated with insulin-based therapies, either as insulin alone or in combination with oral therapies that included metformin, SUs, or glinides, and/or a TZD. In this study of 287 randomized patients, HbA1c changed by −0.41%, and LDLc by −12.3% in the colesevelam group, whereas HbA1c changed by +0.09% and LDLc by +0.5% in the placebo group.[106]

A 2012 Cochrane Review of the available clinical trial data for colesevelam concluded that the overall strength of evidence supported adjunctive use of colesevelam, but that further research to establish long-term risks and benefits would be necessary before widespread or early use of colesevelam for glycemic control could be strongly encouraged.[107] Among other concerns, the mechanism by which colesevelam effects improved glycemia has not been elucidated. Radiolabeled tracer study of mixed meal feedings has suggested that the major action of colesevelam is to increase splanchnic sequestration of meal-derived glucose,[108] which is consistent with the clinical data from the Zieve and colleagues[103] trial, in which postprandial glycemia was significantly reduced in the colesevelam group compared with the placebo group.[103] At the present time, perhaps the best niche for colesevelam in the treatment arsenal of oral antihyperglycemic therapies is in patients adjudged to have unsatisfactory glycemic control, as well as unsatisfactory LDLc, on other well-tolerated antihyperglycemic and lipid-lowering (specifically, statin) drug therapies.[102,109,110]

BROMOCRIPTINE MESYLATE

Approved by FDA in 2010 for the indication of treatment of T2DM, the mechanism of action of bromocriptine mesylate (also known as bromocriptine-QR [quick release]) is largely inferred from animal studies. The drug is ingested within 2 hours of waking in the morning, with breakfast, and is rapidly cleared by first-pass action of cytochrome P450 34A (CYP34A) in the liver, with less than 10% of the ingested dose reaching the systemic circulation. It is thought to increase dopamine in the hypothalamus, thereby reducing sympathetic nervous activity, hepatic glucose production, and lipolysis, with resultant improvement in insulin sensitivity.[111]

Bromocriptine mesylate has been studied as monotherapy versus placebo, and as add-on therapy to SU, with ΔHbA1c of −0.5% to −0.7%, and also with lower FFAs and triglycerides, versus placebo.[112,113] Vinik and colleagues[114] showed similar efficacy of bromocriptine added to failing monotherapy or combined therapies with various combinations of metformin, SU, and TZDs, finding ΔHbA1c of −0.47% in the bromocriptine group, versus +0.26% in the placebo group, at 24 weeks.

A 52-week safety trial compared bromocriptine mesylate versus placebo, in randomized fashion, in 3095 subjects treated with various monotherapies, oral combinations, or insulin alone or in combination with oral therapies, for the purpose of comparing incidence of serious adverse events in the two groups[115] Composite major adverse cardiovascular events, including MI, stroke, coronary revascularization, or hospitalization for unstable angina or CHF, occurred in 1.8% of the bromocriptine group and in 3.2% of the placebo group; a risk reduction of 40% (hazard ratio, 0.61; 95% CI, 0.38–0.97; P = .02).[116] Reasons for the apparent risk reduction are thought to be related to reduced sympathetic nervous system activation or to reduced circulating inflammatory markers such as hsCRP, and TNF-α, although to date such markers have not been measured in studies.[117,118] The lack of long-term efficacy data (ie, studies longer than 24 weeks), the high financial cost of bromocriptine mesylate, and a high frequency of significant adverse effects (nausea in 26%, asthenia/malaise in 15%) have led some authorities to recommend against widespread use of this therapy.[118,119] As further experience accumulates, the magnitude of benefit may allow a more optimistic benefit versus risk estimation for select patients.

SUMMARY

Table 3 provides an overview of the oral antihyperglycemic drugs reviewed in this article. A 2011 meta-analysis by Bennett and colleagues[120] found low or insufficient quality of evidence favoring an initial choice of metformin, SUs, glinides, TZDs, or

Table 3
Oral antihyperglycemic drug: suggested dosing, action, expected efficacy, and cost

Class/Drug	Suggested Dosing	Mechanism of Action	Expected ΔHbA1c (%)	Cost/ Month (US$)
Biguanide				
Metformin	500–2000 mg/d	↓Gluconeogenesis	−1 to −2	4 (generic)
Sulfonylureas				
Glipizide	2.5–10 mg/d	↑Insulin release	−1 to −2	4 (generic)
Glimepiride	1–4 mg/d			4 (generic)
Glinides				
Repaglinide	0.5–2 mg TID with meals	—	—	200 (generic)
Nateglinide	60–120 mg TID with meals	—	—	120
TZDs				
Rosiglitazone	2–4 mg/d	↓FFA release	−1 to −2	130
Pioglitazone	15–30 mg/d	↑Insulin sensitivity		45 (generic)
SGLT2s				
Canagliflozin	100–300 mg/d	↑Glycosuria	−1 to −1.5	290
Dapagliflozin	5–10 mg/d			290
Alpha-glucosidase Inhibitors				
Acarbose	25–100 mg TID with meals	↓Carbohydrate absorption	−0.5 to −1	45 (generic)
Bile Acid Sequestrants				
Colesevelam	3750 mg/d	Unclear	−0.5 to −1	335
Bromocriptine mesylate	1.6–4.8 mg/d	↑CNS dopamine	−0.5	120

Abbreviations: CNS, central nervous system; TID, 3 times a day.
Dose and price information from Anonymous. Drugs for type 2 diabetes. Treat Guidel Med Lett 2014;12(139):17–24.

DPP-4 inhibitors (alpha-glucosidase inhibitors, bromocriptine mesylate, and SGLT2 inhibitors were not included in this meta-analysis) with regard to the outcomes measures of all-cause mortality, cardiovascular events and mortality, and incidence of microvascular disease (retinopathy, nephropathy, and neuropathy) in previously healthy individuals with newly diagnosed T2DM. Likewise, the Bennett and colleagues[120] meta-analysis judged these drugs to be of roughly equal efficacy with regard to reduction of HbA1c (1%–1.6%) from the pretreatment baseline. The ADOPT clinical trial of 3 different and, at the time, popular, oral monotherapies for T2DM provides support for the consensus recommendation of metformin as first-line therapy. The ADOPT trial showed slightly superior HbA1c reduction for rosiglitazone compared with metformin, which was in turn superior to glyburide. However, significant adverse events, including edema, weight gain, and fractures, were more common in the rosiglitazone-treated patients.[31,83] The implication of this trial is that the combination of low cost, low risk, minimal adverse effects, and efficacy of metformin justifies use of this agent as the cornerstone of oral drug treatment of T2DM. Judicious use of metformin in groups formerly thought to be at high risk for lactic acidosis (ie, those with CHF, chronic kidney disease [eGFR >30 mL/min/1.73 m^2], and the elderly) may be associated with mortality benefit rather than increased risk. Secondary and tertiary add-on drug therapy should be individualized based on cost, personal preferences, and overall treatment goals, taking into account the wishes and priorities of the patient.

REFERENCES

1. Miller RA, Birnbaum MJ. An energetic tale of AMPK-independent effects of metformin. J Clin Invest 2010;120:2267–70.
2. Andujar-Plata P, Pi-Sunyer X, Laferrere B. Metformin effects revisited. Diabetes Res Clin Pract 2012;95:1–9.
3. United Kingdom Prospective Diabetes Study Group. United Kingdom Prospective Diabetes Study (UKPDS) 13: relative efficacy of randomly allocated diet, sulphonylurea, insulin, or metformin in patients with newly diagnosed non-insulin dependent diabetes followed for three years. BMJ 1995;310:83–8.
4. DeFronzo RA, Goodman AM. Efficacy of metformin in patients with non-insulin-dependent diabetes mellitus. Multicenter Metformin Study Group. N Engl J Med 1995;333:541–9.
5. Holman RR, Paul SK, Bethel MA, et al. 10-year follow-up of intensive glucose control in type 2 diabetes. N Engl J Med 2008;359:1577–89.
6. Hemmingsen B, Christensen LL, Wetterslev J, et al. Comparison of metformin and insulin versus insulin alone for type 2 diabetes: systematic review of randomized clinical trials with meta-analyses and trial sequential analyses. BMJ 2012;344:e1771.
7. Soranna D, Scotti L, Zambon A, et al. Cancer risk associated with use of metformin and sulfonylurea in type 2 diabetes: a meta-analysis. Oncologist 2012;17:813–22.
8. Libby G, Donnelly LA, Donnan PT, et al. New users of metformin are at low risk of incident cancer: a cohort study among people with type 2 diabetes. Diabetes Care 2009;32:1620–5.
9. Bodmer M, Meier C, Krahenbuhl S, et al. Long-term metformin use is associated with decreased risk of breast cancer. Diabetes Care 2010;33:1304–8.
10. Jiralerspong S, Palla SL, Giordano SH, et al. 2009 Metformin and pathologic complete responses to neoadjuvant chemotherapy in diabetic patients with breast cancer. J Clin Oncol 2009;27:3297–302.

11. Li D, Yeung SC, Hassan MM, et al. Antidiabetic therapies affect risk of pancreatic cancer. Gastroenterology 2009;137:482–8.
12. Wright JL, Stanford JL. Metformin use and prostate cancer in Caucasian men: results from a population-based case–control study. Cancer Causes Control 2009;20:1617–22.
13. Bouchoucha M, Uzza B, Cohen R. Metformin and digestive disorders. Diabetes Metab 2010;37:90–6.
14. de Jager J, Kooy A, Lehert P, et al. Long term treatment with metformin in patients with type 2 diabetes and risk of vitamin B-12 deficiency: randomised placebo controlled trial. BMJ 2010;340:c2181.
15. Anonymous. Metformin for non-insulin-dependent diabetes mellitus. Med Lett Drugs Ther 1995;37:41–2.
16. Lipska KJ, Bailey CJ, Inzucchi SE. Use of metformin in the setting of mild-to-moderate renal insufficiency. Diabetes Care 2011;34:1431–7.
17. Salpeter SR, Greyber E, Pasternak GA, et al. Risk of fatal and nonfatal lactic acidosis with metformin use in type 2 diabetes. Cochrane Database Syst Rev 2010;(4):CD002967.
18. Scheen AJ, Paquot N. Metformin revisited: a critical review of the benefit-risk balance in at-risk patients with type 2 diabetes. Diabetes Metab 2013;39: 179–90.
19. Eurich DT, Majumdar SR, McAlister FA, et al. Improved clinical outcomes associated with metformin in patients with diabetes and heart failure. Diabetes Care 2005;28:2345–51.
20. Nye HJ, Herrington WG. Metformin: the safest hypoglycaemic agent in chronic kidney disease? Nephron Clin Pract 2011;118:c380–3.
21. Rocha A, Almeda M, Santos J, et al. Metformin in patients with chronic kidney disease: strengths and weaknesses. J Nephrol 2013;26:55–60.
22. Seino S. Cell signaling in insulin secretion: the molecular targets of ATP, cAMP and sulfonylurea. Diabetologia 2012;55:2096–108.
23. Ashcroft FM. ATP-sensitive potassium channelopathies: focus on insulin secretion. J Clin Invest 2005;115:2047–58.
24. Hemmingsen B, Schroll JB, Lund SS, et al. Sulphonylurea monotherapy for patients with type 2 diabetes mellitus (review). Cochrane Database Syst Rev 2013;(4):CD009008.
25. Bell DS. Practical considerations and guidelines for dosing sulfonylureas as monotherapy or combination therapy. Clin Ther 2004;26:1715–27.
26. Davis SN. The role of glimepiride in the effective management of type 2 diabetes. J Diabetes Complications 2004;18:367–76.
27. Hirst JA, Farmer AJ, Dyar A, et al. Estimating the effect of sulfonylurea on HbA1c in diabetes: a systematic review and meta-analysis. Diabetologia 2013;56: 973–84.
28. Turner RC, Cull CA, Frighi V, et al. Glycemic control with diet, sulfonylurea, metformin, or insulin in patients with type 2 diabetes mellitus: progressive requirement for multiple therapies (UKPDS 49). UK Prospective Diabetes Study (UKPDS) Group. JAMA 1999;281:2005–12.
29. Del Prato S, Pulizzi N. The place of sulfonylureas in the therapy for type 2 diabetes mellitus. Metabolism 2006;55(Suppl 1):S20–7.
30. Holman RR. Long-term efficacy of sulfonylureas: a United Kingdom Prospective Diabetes Study perspective. Metabolism 2006;55(Suppl 1):S2–5.
31. Kahn SE, Haffner SM, Helse MA, et al. Glycemic durability of rosiglitazone, metformin, or glyburide monotherapy. N Engl J Med 2006;355:2427–43.

32. Rambiritch V, Naidoo P, Butkow N. Dose-response relationships of sulfonylureas: will doubling the dose double the response? South Med J 2007;100:1132–6.

33. Goldberg RB, Holvey SM, Schneider J. A dose-response study of glimepiride in patients with NIDDM who have previously received sulfonylurea agents. The Glimepiride Protocol #201 Study Group. Diabetes Care 1996;19:849–56.

34. Melander A. Kinetics-effect relations of insulin-releasing drugs in patients with type 2 diabetes—brief overview. Diabetes 2004;53(Suppl 3):S151–5.

35. Horton ES, Whitehouse F, Ghazzi MN, et al. Troglitazone in combination with sulfonylurea restores glycemic control in patients with type 2 diabetes. The Troglitazone Study Group. Diabetes Care 1998;21:1462–9.

36. Holstein A, Plaschke A, Egberts EH. Lower incidence of severe hypoglycemia in patients with type 2 diabetes treated with glimepiride versus glibenclamide. Diabetes Metab Res Rev 2001;17:467–73.

37. United Kingdom Prospective Diabetes Study Group. United Kingdom Prospective Diabetes Study 24: a 6-year, randomized, controlled trial comparing sulfonylurea, insulin, and metformin therapy in patients with newly diagnosed type 2 diabetes that could not be controlled with diet therapy. Ann Intern Med 1998;128:165–75.

38. Caritis SN, Hebert MF. A pharmacologic approach to the use of glyburide in pregnancy. Obstet Gynecol 2013;121:1309–12.

39. Dhulkotia JS, Ola B, Fraser R, et al. Oral hypoglycemic agents versus insulin in management of gestational diabetes: a systematic review and meta-analysis. Am J Obstet Gynecol 2010;203:457.e1–9.

40. Goldner MG, Knatterud GL, Prout TE. Effects of hypoglycemic agents on vascular complications in patients with adult-onset diabetes. 3. Clinical implications of UGDP results. JAMA 1971;218:1400–10.

41. UK Prospective Diabetes Study (UKPDS) Group. Intensive blood-glucose control with sulphonylureas or insulin compared with conventional treatment and risk of complications in patients with type 2 diabetes (UKPDS 33). Lancet 1998;352:837–53.

42. Roumie CL, Hung AM, Greevy RA, et al. Comparative effectiveness of sulfonylurea and metformin monotherapy on cardiovascular events in type 2 diabetes mellitus. Ann Intern Med 2012;157:612–5.

43. Quast U, Stephan D, Bieger S, et al. The impact of ATP-sensitive K^+ channel subtype selectivity of insulin secretagogues for the coronary vasculature and the myocardium. Diabetes 2004;53(Suppl 3):S156–64.

44. Nagashima K, Takahashi A, Ikeda H, et al. Sulfonylurea and non-sulfonylurea hypoglycemic agents: pharmacological properties and tissue selectivity. Diabetes Res Clin Pract 2004;66(Suppl 1):S75–8.

45. Thisted H, Johnsen SP, Rungby J. Sulfonylureas and the risk of myocardial infarction. Metabolism 2006;55(Suppl 1):S16–9.

46. Lee TM, Chou TF. Impairment of myocardial protection in type 2 diabetic patients. J Clin Endocrinol Metab 2003;88:531–7.

47. Zeller M, Danchin N, Simon D, et al. Impact of type of preadmission sulfonylureas on mortality and cardiovascular outcomes in diabetic patients with acute myocardial infarction. J Clin Endocrinol Metab 2010;95:4993–5002.

48. Singh S, Singh PP, Singh AG, et al. Anti-diabetic medications and the risk of hepatocellular cancer: a systematic review and meta-analysis. Am J Gastroenterol 2013;108:881–91.

49. Chang CH, Lin JW, Wu LC, et al. Oral insulin secretogogues, insulin, and cancer risk in type 2 diabetes mellitus. J Clin Endocrinol Metab 2012;97:E1170–5.

50. Thakkar B, Aronis KN, Vamvini MT, et al. Metformin and sulfonylureas in relation to cancer risk in type 2 diabetes patients: a meta-analysis using primary data of published studies. Metabolism 2013;62:922–34.
51. Riddle MC. Editorial: sulfonylureas differ in effects on ischemic preconditioning—is it time to retire glyburide? J Clin Endocrinol Metab 2003;88:528–30.
52. Riddle MC. Editorial: more reasons to say goodbye to glyburide. J Clin Endocrinol Metab 2010;95:4867–70.
53. Anonymous. Repaglinide for type 2 diabetes. Med Lett Drugs Ther 1998;40:55–6.
54. Anonymous. Nateglinide for type 2 diabetes. Med Lett Drugs Ther 2001;43:29–31.
55. Cariou B, Charbonnel B, Staels B. Thiazolidinediones and PPARγ agonists: time for a reassessment. Trends Endocrinol Metab 2012;23:205–15.
56. Decker M, Hofflich H, Elias AN. Thiazolidinediones and the preservation of β-cell function, cellular proliferation and apoptosis. Diabetes Obes Metab 2008;10:617–25.
57. Ovalle F, Ovalle-Berumen JF. Thiazolidinediones: a review of their benefits and risks. South Med J 2002;95:1188–94.
58. Diamant M, Heine RJ. Thiazolidinediones in type 2 diabetes mellitus: current clinical evidence. Drugs 2003;63:1373–405.
59. Derosa G, Maffioli P. Thiazolidinediones plus metformin association on body weight in patients with type 2 diabetes. Diabetes Res Clin Pract 2011;91:265–70.
60. Viberti G. Thiazolidinediones—benefits on microvascular complications of type 2 diabetes. J Diabetes Complications 2005;19:168–77.
61. Riera-Guardia N, Rothenbacher D. The effect of thiazolidinediones on adiponectin serum level: a meta-analysis. Diabetes Obes Metab 2008;10:367–75.
62. Quinn CE, Hamilton PK, Lockhart CJ, et al. Thiazolidinediones: effects on insulin resistance and the cardiovascular system. Br J Pharmacol 2008;153:636–45.
63. Lebovitz HE. Rationale for and role of thiazolidinediones in type 2 diabetes mellitus. Am J Cardiol 2002;90(Suppl):34G–41G.
64. Kendall DM. Thiazolidinediones—the case for early use. Diabetes Care 2006;29:154–7.
65. Ceriello A. Thiazolidinediones as anti-inflammatory and anti-atherogenic agents. Diabetes Metab Res Rev 2008;24:14–26.
66. Choi D, Kim SK, Choi SH, et al. Preventative effects of rosiglitazone on restenosis after coronary stent implantation in patients with type 2 diabetes. Diabetes Care 2004;27:2654–60.
67. Gilling L, Suwattee P, DeSouza C, et al. Effects of thiazolidinediones on cardiovascular risk factors. Am J Cardiovasc Drugs 2002;2:149–56.
68. Wyne KL. The metabolic syndrome: evolving evidence that thiazolidinediones provide rational therapy. Diabetes Obes Metab 2006;8:365–80.
69. Parulkar AA, Pendergrass ML, Granda-Ayala R, et al. Nonhypoglycemic effects of thiazolidinediones. Ann Intern Med 2001;134:61–71.
70. Yki-Jarvinen H. Thiazolidinediones and the liver in humans. Curr Opin Lipidol 2009;20:477–83.
71. Khanderia U, Pop-Busui R, Eagle KA. Thiazolidinediones in type 2 diabetes: a cardiology perspective. Ann Pharmacother 2008;42:1466–74.
72. Lago RM, Singh PP, Nesto RW. Congestive heart failure and cardiovascular death in patients with prediabetes and type 2 diabetes given thiazolidinediones: a meta-analysis of randomized clinical trials. Lancet 2007;370:1129–36.

73. DREAM Trial Investigators. Effect of rosiglitazone on the frequency of diabetes in patients with impaired glucose tolerance or impaired fasting glucose: a randomized controlled trial. Lancet 2006;368:1096–105.

74. Home PD, Pocock SJ, Beck-Nielsen H, et al. Rosiglitazone Evaluated for Cardiovascular Outcomes in Oral Agent Combination Therapy for Type 2 Diabetes (RECORD): a multicenter, randomized, open-label trial. Lancet 2009;373: 2125–35.

75. Nissen SE, Wolski K. Effect of rosiglitazone on the risk of myocardial infarction and death from cardiovascular causes. N Engl J Med 2007;356: 2457–71.

76. Dormandy JA, Charbonnel B, Eckland DJ, et al. Secondary prevention of macrovascular events in patients with type 2 diabetes in the PROactive study (Prospective Pioglitazone Clinical Trial in Macrovascular Events): a randomized controlled trial. Lancet 2005;266:1279–89.

77. Loke YK, Kwok CS, Singh S. Comparative cardiovascular effects of thiazolidinediones: systematic review and meta-analysis of observational studies. BMJ 2011;342:d1309.

78. Bosetti C, Rosato V, Buniato D, et al. Cancer risk for patients using thiazolidinediones for type 2 diabetes: a meta-analysis. Oncologist 2013;18:148–56.

79. Schwartz AV, Sellmeyer DE, Vittinghoff E, et al. Thiazolidinedione use and bone loss in older diabetic adults. J Clin Endocrinol Metab 2006;91:3349–54.

80. Aubert RE, Herrera V, Chen W, et al. Rosiglitazone and pioglitazone increase fracture risk in women and men with type 2 diabetes. Diabetes Obes Metab 2010;12:716–21.

81. Meier C, Kraenzlin ME, Bodmer M, et al. Use of thiazolidinediones and fracture risk. Arch Intern Med 2008;168:820–5.

82. Dormuth CR, Carney G, Carleton B, et al. Thiazolidinediones and fractures in men and women. Arch Intern Med 2009;169:1395–402.

83. Kahn SE, Zinman B, Lachin JM, et al. Rosiglitazone-associated fractures in type 2 diabetes. An analysis from A Diabetes Outcome Progression Trial (ADOPT). Diabetes Care 2008;31:845–51.

84. Loke YK, Singh S, Furberg CD. Long-term use of thiazolidinediones and fractures in type 2 diabetes: a meta-analysis. CMAJ 2009;180:32–9.

85. Diamant M, Morsink LM. SGLT2 inhibitors for diabetes: turning symptoms into therapy. Lancet 2013;382:917–8.

86. Nair S, Wilding JP. Sodium glucose cotransporter 2 inhibitors as a new treatment for diabetes mellitus. J Clin Endocrinol Metab 2010;95:34–42.

87. Stenlof K, Cefalu WT, Kim KA, et al. Efficacy and safety of canagliflozin monotherapy in subjects with type 2 diabetes mellitus inadequately controlled with diet and exercise. Diabetes Obes Metab 2013;15:372–82.

88. Cefalu WT, Leiter LA, Yoon KH, et al. Efficacy and safety of canagliflozin versus glimepiride in patients with type 2 diabetes inadequately controlled with metformin (CANTATA-SU): 52 week results from a randomised, double-blind, phase 3 non-inferiority trial. Lancet 2013;382:941–50.

89. Schernthaner G, Gross JL, Rosenstock J, et al. Canagliflozin compared with sitagliptin for patients with type 2 diabetes who do not have adequate glycemic control with metformin plus sulfonylurea-a 52-week randomized trial. Diabetes Care 2013;36:2508–15.

90. Bailey CF, Gross JL, Pieters A, et al. Effect of dapagliflozin in patients with type 2 diabetes who have inadequate glycaemic control with metformin: a randomised, double-blind, placebo-controlled trial. Lancet 2010;375:2223–33.

91. Vasilakou D, Karagiannis T, Athanasiadou E, et al. Sodium–glucose cotransporter 2 inhibitors for type 2 diabetes: a systematic review and meta-analysis. Ann Intern Med 2013;159:262–74.
92. Stack CB, Localio R, Griswold ME, et al. Handling of rescue and missing data affects synthesis and interpretation of evidence: the sodium–glucose cotransporter 2 inhibitor example. Ann Intern Med 2013;159:285–8.
93. Neal B, Perkovic V, de Zeeuw D, et al. Rationale, design, and baseline characteristics of the Canagliflozin Cardiovascular Assessment Study (CANVAS)—a randomized placebo-controlled trial. Am Heart J 2013;166:217–23.
94. Anonymous. Canagliflozin for type 2 diabetes. Med Lett Drugs Ther 2013;55:37–9.
95. Anonymous. Acarbose for diabetes mellitus. Med Lett Drugs Ther 1996;38:9–10.
96. Gross JL, Kramer CK, Leitao CB, et al. Effect of antihyperglycemic agents added to metformin and sulfonylurea on glycemic control and weight gain in type 2 diabetes: a network meta-analysis. Ann Intern Med 2011;154:672–9.
97. Coniff RF, Shapiro JA, Robbins D, et al. Reduction of glycosylated hemoglobin and postprandial hyperglycemia by acarbose in patients with NIDDM. A placebo-controlled dose-comparison study. Diabetes Care 1995;18:817–24.
98. Chiasson JL, Josse RG, Hunt JA, et al. The efficacy of acarbose in the treatment of patients with non-insulin-dependent diabetes mellitus. Ann Intern Med 1994;121:928–35.
99. Chiasson JL, Josse RG, Gomis R, et al. Acarbose for prevention of type 2 diabetes mellitus: the STOP-NIDDM randomized trial. Lancet 2002;359:2072–7.
100. Chiasson JL, Josse RG, Gomis R, et al. Acarbose treatment and the risk of cardiovascular disease and hypertension in patients with impaired glucose tolerance: the STOP-NIDDM Trial. JAMA 2003;290:486–94.
101. Cheng AY, Fantus IG. Oral antihyperglycemic therapy for type 2 diabetes mellitus. CMAJ 2005;172:213–26.
102. Reasner CA. Reducing cardiovascular complications of type 2 diabetes by targeting multiple risk factors. J Cardiovasc Pharmacol 2008;52:136–44.
103. Zieve FJ, Kalin MF, Schwartz SL, et al. Results of the Glucose-Lowering Effect of WelChol Study (GLOWS): a randomized, double-blind, placebo-controlled pilot study evaluating the effect of colesevelam hydrochloride on glycemic control in subjects with type 2 diabetes. Clin Ther 2007;29:74–83.
104. Bays HE, Goldberg RB, Truitt KE, et al. Colesevelam hydrochloride therapy in patients with type 2 diabetes mellitus treated with metformin. Glucose and lipid effects. Arch Intern Med 2008;168:1975–83.
105. Fonseca VA, Rosenstock J, Wang AC, et al. Colesevelam HCl improves glycemic control and reduces LDL cholesterol in patients with inadequately controlled type 2 diabetes on sulfonylurea-based therapy. Diabetes Care 2008;31:1479–84.
106. Goldberg RB, Fonseca VA, Truitt KE, et al. Efficacy and safety of colesevelam in patients with type 2 diabetes mellitus and inadequate glycemic control receiving insulin-based therapy. Arch Intern Med 2008;168:1531–40.
107. Ooi CP, Loke SC. Colesevelam for type 2 diabetes mellitus. Cochrane Database Syst Rev 2012;(12):CD009361. http://dx.doi.org/10.1002/14651858.CD009361.pub2.
108. Smushkin G, Sathananthan M, Piccinini F, et al. The effect of a bile acid sequestrant on glucose metabolism in subjects with type 2 diabetes. Diabetes 2013;62:1094–101.

109. Aggarwal S, Loomba RS, Arora RR. Efficacy of colesevelam on lowering glycemia and lipids. J Cardiovasc Pharmacol 2012;59:198–205.

110. Goldfine AB. Modulating LDL cholesterol and glucose in patients with type 2 diabetes mellitus: targeting the bile acid pathway. Curr Opin Cardiol 2008;23: 502–11.

111. DeFronzo RA. Bromocriptine: a sympatholytic, D2-dopamine agonist for the treatment of type 2 diabetes. Diabetes Care 2011;34:789–94.

112. Cincotta AH, Meier AH, Cincotta M Jr. Bromocriptine improves glycaemic control and serum lipid profile in obese type 2 diabetic subjects: a new approach in the treatment of diabetes. Expert Opin Investig Drugs 1999;8:1683–707.

113. Kerr JL, Timpe EM, Petkewicz KA. Bromocriptine mesylate for glycemic management in type 2 diabetes mellitus. Ann Pharmacother 2010;44:1777–86.

114. Vinik AI, Cincotta AH, Scranton RE, et al. Effect of bromocriptine-QR on glycemic control in subjects with uncontrolled hyperglycemia on one or two oral anti-diabetes agents. Endocr Pract 2012;18:931–43.

115. Gaziano JM, Cincotta AH, O'Connor CM, et al. Randomized clinical trial of quick-release bromocriptine among patients with type 2 diabetes on overall safety and cardiovascular outcomes. Diabetes Care 2010;33:1503–8.

116. Gaziano JM, Cincotta AH, Vinik A, et al. Effect of bromocriptine-QR (a quick-release formulation of bromocriptine mesylate) on major adverse cardiovascular events in type 2 diabetes subjects. J Am Heart Assoc 2012;1:e002279. http://dx.doi.org/10.1161/JAHA.112.002279.

117. Bell DS. Why does quick-release bromocriptine decrease cardiac events? Diabetes Obes Metab 2011;13:880–4.

118. Garber AJ, Blonde L, Bloomgarden ZT, et al. The role of bromocriptine-QR in the management of type 2 diabetes expert panel recommendations. Endocr Pract 2013;19:100–6.

119. Anonymous. Bromocriptine (Cycloset) for type 2 diabetes. Med Lett Drugs Ther 2010;52:97–9.

120. Bennett WL, Maruthur NM, Singh S, et al. Comparative effectiveness and safety of medications for type 2 diabetes: an update including new drugs and 2-drug combinations. Ann Intern Med 2011;154:602–13.

Incretin-Based Therapies

Joshua J. Neumiller, PharmD, CDE

KEYWORDS

- Dipeptidyl peptidase 4 • DPP-4 inhibitors • GLP-1 receptor agonists
- Glucagon-like peptide 1 • Incretin effect • Incretin mimetics • Pharmacotherapy

KEY POINTS

- Incretin hormones (glucagon-like peptide 1 [GLP-1] and gastric inhibitory peptide) play a key role in glucose homeostasis.
- Two classes of incretin-based therapies are currently available: GLP-1 receptor agonists and dipeptidyl peptidase 4 (DPP-4) inhibitors.
- Potential key benefits of GLP-1 receptor agonist therapy include a low risk of hypoglycemia and a potential for weight loss with treatment.
- GLP-1 receptor agonists have variable effects on glycemia, with short-acting agents having a greater effect on postprandial glucose and longer-acting agents having a relatively greater effect on fasting glucose levels.
- Potential key benefits of DPP-4 inhibitor therapy include a low risk of hypoglycemia, a relatively mild side-effect profile, and simple daily oral administration.
- Incretin-based therapies have been associated with rare adverse events such as pancreatitis and acute renal failure, and patients should be selected and monitored accordingly.

INTRODUCTION

Hormonal regulation of glucose metabolism extends well beyond the physiologic effects of insulin and glucagon. Incretin hormones, namely glucagon-like peptide 1 (GLP-1) and gastric inhibitory peptide (GIP), have been recognized for some time as playing a key role in glucose homeostasis.[1] As a result, incretin-based therapies have emerged as valuable pharmacologic agents in the treatment of diabetes mellitus (DM). This article discusses the incretin effect, and reviews currently available incretin-based therapies and their potential role in the treatment of DM.

Disclosure Statement: J.J. Neumiller receives institutional research grant support from Amylin, AstraZeneca, Johnson & Johnson, Merck, and Novo Nordisk. J.J. Neumiller serves as a consultant to Janssen Pharmaceuticals and Sanofi and serves on the speaker's bureau for Janssen Pharmaceuticals. No financial support was received for writing this article.
Department of Pharmacotherapy, College of Pharmacy, Washington State University, PO Box 1495, Spokane, WA 99210-1495, USA
E-mail address: jneumiller@wsu.edu

Med Clin N Am 99 (2015) 107–129
http://dx.doi.org/10.1016/j.mcna.2014.08.013
0025-7125/15/$ – see front matter © 2015 Elsevier Inc. All rights reserved.

medical.theclinics.com

The Incretin Effect

The term incretin effect (INtestinal seCRETion of INsulin) is used to describe the finding that oral glucose induces a more pronounced insulin response in comparison with intravenous glucose administration.[2] This observation supports the notion that signals originating from the gut are instrumental in the stimulation of prandial insulin release. The first incretin hormone identified in the 1970s was gastric inhibitory peptide (GIP). On study, GIP was shown to stimulate insulin secretion from pancreatic β cells.[3,4] Glucagon-like peptide 1 (GLP-1) was later identified in the 1980s as another principal incretin hormone.[5] The effects of incretin hormones are believed to be responsible for up to 60% of postprandial insulin release,[6] which has been shown to be impaired in persons with type 2 diabetes mellitus (T2DM).[7] In light of the important contribution of the incretin effect to prandial insulin release, augmentation of this system is an important pharmacologic approach to glycemic management.

Glucagon-like peptide 1

GLP-1 is secreted following oral nutrient intake from intestinal L cells located in the ileum and colon. The glucoregulatory effects of GLP-1 derive from several mechanisms. GLP-1 induces glucose-dependent insulin secretion from pancreatic β cells,[8,9] decreases plasma glucagon concentrations,[9] and delays gastric emptying.[10] The delayed gastric emptying induced by GLP-1 helps decrease postprandial hyperglycemia but also induces a feeling of fullness, thus reducing appetite and food intake. GLP-1 is additionally believed to induce satiety via a direct effect on the central nervous system.[11] Results from preclinical data suggest that GLP-1 may also have beneficial effects on β-cell function and survival. Animal studies have shown GLP-1 to stimulate the proliferation and differentiation of pancreatic β cells and to inhibit β-cell apoptosis.[12,13] These and other effects of GLP-1 are mediated via activation of the GLP-1 receptor (GLP-1R). GLP-1R is known to be expressed in pancreatic β cells and the kidney, liver, myocardium, adipocytes, intestine, and hypothalamus.[14,15] Evidence additionally suggests that activation of GLP-1Rs may be cardioprotective, as demonstrated in animal models of ischemia/reperfusion injury.[16] **Fig. 1** illustrates the select direct and indirect effects of GLP-1 in peripheral tissues.[1]

Glucose-dependent insulinotropic polypeptide

GIP is produced and secreted in response to a meal from K cells of the small intestine.[17] While GLP-1-based treatments have been a focus of drug development for the management of T2DM, GIP-based therapies have been slow to develop, largely because of previous findings showing that the insulinotropic effects of GIP are blunted in persons with T2DM[18,19]; however, the insulinotropic effects of GIP were shown to be restored in T2DM patients following a 4-week normalization of hyperglycemia with insulin treatment.[20] In contrast to GLP-1, GIP stimulates glucagon release from pancreatic α cells,[21] stimulates lipogenesis, inhibits lipolysis in adipocytes, and enhances fatty acid uptake.[17] Because of these counterproductive effects the clinical advancement of GIP receptor agonists has proved to be more challenging, although they are still being studied.[22] GIP receptor antagonists are additionally being studied for the treatment of T2DM as a means to inhibit adverse GIP-mediated effects on levels of lipids and free fatty acids.[17]

PHARMACOLOGIC TREATMENT OPTIONS: INCRETIN-BASED THERAPIES

As mentioned previously, the incretin effect plays a major role in glucose homeostasis. Although native GLP-1 has been targeted as a therapeutic agent because

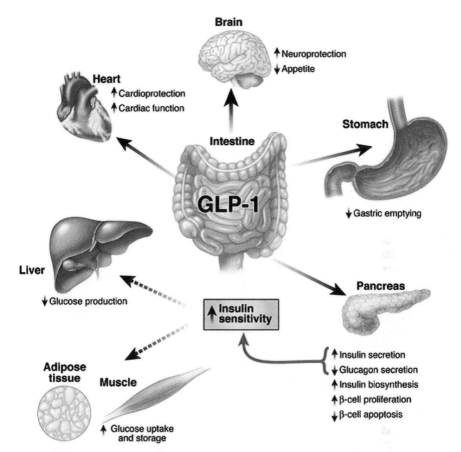

Fig. 1. Actions of glucagon-like peptide 1 (GLP-1) in peripheral tissues. Most of the effects of GLP-1 are mediated by direct interaction with GLP-1 receptor agonists on specific tissues. However, the actions of GLP-1 in liver, fat, and muscle most likely occur through indirect mechanisms. (*From* Baggio LL, Drucker DJ. Biology of incretins: GLP-1 and GIP. Gastroenterology 2007;132:2131–57; with permission.)

of its favorable effects on glycemia, its clinical utility in the ambulatory care setting is hindered owing to its extremely short half-life.[11] Both native GLP-1 and GIP are quickly cleared following release caused by renal clearance and rapid metabolism by the enzyme dipeptidyl peptidase-4 (DPP-4).[23] Owing to the short half-life of incretin hormones, 2 predominant therapeutic strategies have been developed and marketed to address the impaired incretin response (**Fig. 2**):

1. GLP-1 receptor agonists (RAs) resistant to degradation by DPP-4
2. DPP-4 inhibitors

Although both strategies are used to augment the incretin effect, there are key differences in clinical outcomes achieved with these 2 medication classes. **Table 1** provides a general clinical comparison of GLP-1 RAs and DPP-4 inhibitors for the treatment of T2DM.[24,25]

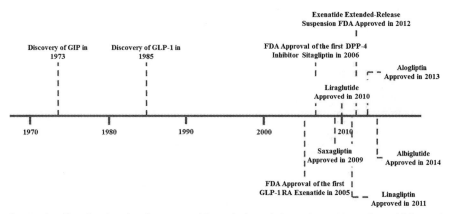

Fig. 2. Timeline for the development of incretin-based therapies. DPP-4, dipeptidyl peptidase 4; FDA, Food and Drug Administration; GIP, gastric inhibitory peptide; GLP-1, glucagon-like peptide 1; GLP-1RA, GLP-1 receptor agonist.

GLP-1 Receptor Agonists

GLP-1 RAs are continuing to grow in popularity for the treatment of T2DM because of their beneficial effects on glycemia and weight. At present, 4 GLP-1 RAs have received approval by the US Food and Drug Administration (FDA):

- Exenatide (Byetta)
- Liraglutide (Victoza)
- Exenatide extended-release suspension (Bydureon)
- Albiglutide (Tanzeum).

Table 2 outlines select clinical properties of these 4 agents.[25–48]

In addition to the glycemic effects of GLP-1 RAs, a host of extraglycemic effects have been noted with GLP-1 RA use, and are under active study (**Fig. 3**).[49] There are several important considerations when choosing a GLP-1 RA for a given patient.

Table 1
Select clinical properties of GLP-1 receptor agonists and DPP-4 inhibitors

	GLP-1 Receptor Agonists	DPP-4 Inhibitors
Slowing of gastric emptying?	Yes[a]	No
Effect on postprandial hyperglycemia?	Yes	Yes
Effect on weight	Weight loss	Weight neutral
Common side effects	Nausea, vomiting, diarrhea	Headache, sinusitis, rhinorrhea
Route of administration	Subcutaneous injection	Oral
Associated with hypoglycemia when used as monotherapy?	No	No

[a] Short-acting GLP-1 receptor agonist.
Adapted from Campbell RK. Clarifying the role of incretin-based therapies in the treatment of type 2 diabetes mellitus. Clin Ther 2011;33(5):511–27; and Meier JJ. GLP-1 receptor agonists for individualized treatment of type 2 diabetes mellitus. Nat Rev Endocrinol 2012;8:728–42.

Table 2
Comparison and contrast of currently available GLP-1 receptor agonists

	Exenatide	Liraglutide	Exenatide ER	Albiglutide
Administration frequency	Twice daily[26]	Once daily[27]	Once weekly[28]	Once weekly[29]
GLP-1 receptor agonist type[25]	Short-acting	Long-acting	Long-acting	Long-acting
Effect on gastric emptying rate[25]	Deceleration	No Effect	No Effect	No Effect
Effect on fasting blood glucose levels[25]	Modest reduction	Strong reduction	Strong reduction	Strong reduction
Effect on postprandial blood glucose levels[25]	Strong reduction	Modest reduction	Modest reduction	Modest reduction
Average hemoglobin A_{1C} lowering (%)[a]	0.5–1.0[30–33]	0.83–1.36[34–37]	1.5–2.0[38–42]	0.76–1.04[43–48]
Average weight change (kg)[a]	−0.3 to −3.1[30–33]	−2.6 to +0.8[34–37]	−2.3 to −4.7[38–42]	+0.3 to −0.21[43–48]

[a] Placebo-subtracted change from baseline for exenatide, liraglutide, and albiglutide, and absolute change from baseline for exenatide extended-release (ER). Baseline characteristics of study groups and concomitant medications varied from study to study.

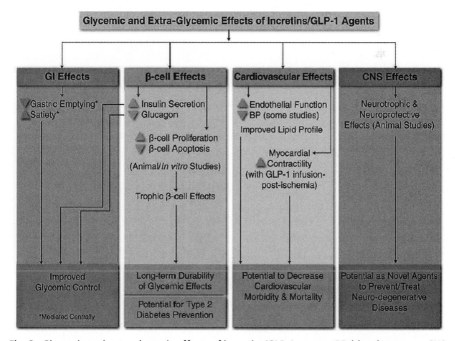

Fig. 3. Glycemic and extraglycemic effects of incretins/GLP-1 agents. BP, blood pressure; CNS, central nervous system; GI, gastrointestinal. (*From* Mudaliar S, Henry RR. Incretin therapies: effects beyond glycemic control. Eur J Intern Med 2009;20:S319–28; with permission.)

Certainly factors such as convenience (frequency of administration) and tolerability are important. Also of critical importance is determining the individualized glycemic needs of the individual. As noted in **Table 2**, currently available GLP-1 RAs have variable effects on fasting and postprandial blood glucose, with short-acting GLP-1 RAs having a greater effect on postprandial glucose and, conversely, long-acting agents having a greater effect on fasting glucose levels.[25] These differences may lead the clinician to choose a short-acting GLP-1 RA (such as exenatide) in a patient with predominant postprandial hyperglycemia.

Exenatide

Exenatide was the first GLP-1 RA approved by the FDA for the treatment of T2DM.[26] Compared with other longer-acting GLP-1 RAs, exenatide has a more robust effect on postprandial blood glucose excursions (for those meals in which it is administered prior).[39] Select key clinical information for exenatide is provided in **Box 1**.[26]

Nausea is the most common dose-limiting adverse event associated with exenatide therapy, with approximately 48% of participants receiving exenatide at the 10-μg twice-daily dose reporting nausea during clinical trials.[30–33] Accordingly, exenatide therapy should be initiated with caution in individuals with gastrointestinal disease. The following are select contraindications and warnings/precautions noted with exenatide.[26]

Contraindications

- A history of severe hypersensitivity to exenatide or any product components.

Warnings/precautions

- Pancreatitis
  The association between incretin-based medications and pancreatitis is controversial.[50] Overall, the incidence of acute pancreatitis in persons with T2DM is

---

Box 1
Exenatide (Byetta): key clinical information

Dosing	• 5 μg twice daily initially
	• Increase to 10 μg twice daily after 1 month based on clinical response
	• Inject within 60 minutes before the 2 main meals of the day
Renal dose adjustment	• Not recommended with CrCl <30 mL/min
How supplied	• 5-μg prefilled pen (60 doses)
	• 10-μg prefilled pen (60 doses)
Common side effects	• Nausea
	• Vomiting
	• Diarrhea
	• Headache
Key drug interactions	• May affect absorption of orally administered medications
	• Postmarketing reports of increased international normalized ratio (INR) when given in combination with warfarin

Adapted from Byetta (exenatide) [package insert]. Princeton, NJ: Bristol-Myers-Squibb Company; 2013.

higher in comparison with those without diabetes, and potential confounding factors such as alcohol use and hypertriglyceridemia are often unreported in postmarketing case reports.[51] Six cases of acute pancreatitis were noted during clinical trials (1.7 cases per 1000 patient-years) compared with 1 case reported among participants receiving placebo (3.0 cases per 1000 patient-years).[50]

- Hypoglycemia
  Whereas GLP-1 RAs are associated with a minimal risk of hypoglycemia when used as monotherapy, they can contribute to hypoglycemia when used in combination with medications associated with hypoglycemia, such as insulin secretagogues and insulin. When adding exenatide to such agents, a dose reduction of insulin secretagogue or insulin to minimize the risk of treatment-emergent hypoglycemia may be considered according to the individual needs and characteristics of the patient.
- Renal impairment
  Exenatide use has been associated with reports of altered renal function, including acute renal failure and acute renal insufficiency.[52] It is thought that acute changes in renal function primarily occur from dehydration in patients experiencing nausea and vomiting with treatment.

Liraglutide

Liraglutide is approved for once-daily subcutaneous administration for the treatment of T2DM. Select clinical information is provided in **Box 2**.[27] Liraglutide has been studied head-to-head versus exenatide as add-on therapy for persons with T2DM inadequately controlled on metformin and a sulfonylurea.[53] Once-daily liraglutide compared favorably with twice-daily exenatide, with similar effects on weight and hemoglobin A_{1C} observed with both agents (**Box 3**).[53]

The nausea associated with liraglutide therapy was reported most commonly during the initial 4 weeks of therapy in clinical trials, with nausea symptoms improving over time with continued use.[34–37] The following are contraindications and warnings/precautions for consideration with liraglutide.[27]

Box 2	
Liraglutide (Victoza): key clinical information	
Dosing	• 0.6 mg once daily initially without regard to meals
	• Increase to 1.2 mg once daily after 1 week
	• Increase to 1.8 mg once daily after 1 week if the 1.2-mg dose does not result in acceptable glycemic control
Renal dose adjustment	• Use with caution: no specific renal dose adjustments are provided by the manufacturer
How supplied	• Prefilled, multidose pen that delivers doses of 0.6 mg, 1.2 mg, or 1.8 mg
Common side effects	• Headache
	• Nausea
	• Diarrhea
Key drug interactions	• May affect absorption of orally administered medications
Adapted from Victoza (liraglutide) [package insert]. Plainsboro, NJ: Novo Nordisk, Inc; 2013.	

Box 3
Findings from head-to-head study of liraglutide and exenatide

Treatment	Hemoglobin A_{1C} Change (%)	Body Weight Change (kg)
Liraglutide 1.8 mg once daily	−1.12[a]	−3.2
Exenatide 10 μg twice daily	−0.79	−2.9

[a] $P<.0001$.

Adapted from Buse JB, Rosenstock J, Sesti G, et al. Liraglutide once a day versus exenatide twice a day for type 2 diabetes: a 26-week randomised, parallel-group, multinational, open-label trial (LEAD-6). Lancet 2009;374(9683):39–47.

Contraindications

- A history of serious hypersensitivity to liraglutide or any product components.
- Personal or family history of medullary thyroid carcinoma or in patients with multiple endocrine neoplasia syndrome type 2.

Warnings/precautions

- Thyroid C-cell tumors in animals
  An additional concern noted in the prescribing information is a warning of dose-dependent and treatment-duration–dependent thyroid C-cell tumors observed during preclinical studies with liraglutide. In rodent models, liraglutide was associated with an increased risk of thyroid C-cell focal hyperplasia and C-cell tumors at clinically relevant doses. The true meaning of these findings with regard to human use is currently unknown. According to the prescribing information for liraglutide, clinical trials have generated 4 reported cases of thyroid C-cell hyperplasia among liraglutide-treated patients, compared with 1 case in a patient treated with a comparator product. These cases equate to 1.3 versus 0.6 cases per 1000 patient-years, respectively. Data from long-term studies did not demonstrate differences in mean calcitonin levels (a surrogate marker for C-cell hyperplasia) between subjects treated with liraglutide and those in comparator groups during 2 years of follow-up.[54]
- Pancreatitis
  Like exenatide, the labeling for liraglutide includes a warning of pancreatitis. Seven cases of pancreatitis were reported during the phase 3 clinical trial program for liraglutide, compared with 1 case observed within the comparator groups. **Box 4** summarizes key recommendations provided as part of the REMS (Risk Evaluation and Mitigation Strategy) for liraglutide.[55]
- Hypoglycemia
  Similarly to exenatide, caution should be exercised when adding liraglutide in a patient receiving a sulfonylurea or insulin, and a decrease in the dose of sulfonylurea or insulin may be warranted to avoid hypoglycemic events.[27]
- Renal impairment
  Cases of renal impairment, typically associated with nausea, vomiting, and diarrhea, have been noted with liraglutide therapy. Caution should be used when initiating therapy or titrating up the dose of liraglutide in persons with renal impairment.[27]

Exenatide extended-release suspension

Exenatide extended-release (ER) was approved in 2012 for the treatment of T2DM. Exenatide ER uses microsphere technology to achieve its protracted duration of action.[56] Following subcutaneous injection, the biodegradable polymeric

---

Box 4
FDA recommendations to reduce the risk of pancreatitis in patients using liraglutide

- Patients using liraglutide should be counseled about the symptoms of pancreatitis, such as severe abdominal pain that may radiate to the back, possibly with nausea and vomiting
- If patients experience symptoms of pancreatitis, they should contact their health care provider immediately
- Patients must be provided a Medication Guide that provides information about pancreatitis that includes the following:
  - Conditions that may place patients at greater risk for pancreatitis, such as a prior history of pancreatitis, gallstones, excessive use of alcohol, or very high levels of triglycerides
  - Symptoms of pancreatitis and what to do if these symptoms occur
- If health care professionals suspect a patient has pancreatitis, liraglutide should be stopped immediately and the patient should undergo testing to confirm a diagnosis of pancreatitis and, if confirmed, liraglutide should not be resumed
- Liraglutide should be used cautiously in those with a history of pancreatitis

Adapted from US Food and Drug Administration. NDA 22-341 Victoza (liraglutide [rDNA origin] injection) risk evaluation and mitigation strategy (REMS). Available at: http://www.fda.gov/downloads/Drugs/DrugSafety/PostmarketDrugSafetyInformationforPatientsandProviders/UCM202063.pdf. Accessed June 1, 2014.

---

microspheres containing exenatide begin to absorb water, causing the microspheres to swell and degrade over time.[56] Select key clinical features of this product are provided in **Box 5**.[28]

Comparative efficacy data are available from a 30-week study comparing the effect of exenatide ER (n = 148) with exenatide 10 μg twice daily (n = 147).[38] Participants in the exenatide ER group experienced a greater reduction in hemoglobin A_{1C} when compared with those receiving exenatide twice daily. The once-weekly formulation additionally achieved a greater mean reduction in fasting glucose levels ($P<.0001$). In regard to postprandial glucose reductions, however, a more robust postprandial lowering effect with twice-daily exenatide at the meals in which it was administered was demonstrated (**Table 3**).[38]

Injection-site pruritus was seen in 26% of individuals receiving exenatide ER in comparison with 2% of persons on twice-daily exenatide.[38] Symptoms of pruritus are typically described as mild, and generally resolve with continued use of the medication. A warning/precaution is listed in the labeling, however, related to serious injection-site reactions with or without the presence of subcutaneous nodule formation.[28] Contraindications and warnings/precautions noted for exenatide ER are as follows.[28]

Contraindications
- A history of serious hypersensitivity to exenatide or any product components.
- Personal or family history of medullary thyroid carcinoma or in patients with multiple endocrine neoplasia syndrome type 2.

Warnings/precautions Warnings/precautions for exenatide ER are similar to those listed for liraglutide, and include:

- Thyroid C-cell tumors in animals
- Pancreatitis

Box 5
Exenatide ER (Bydureon): key clinical information

Dosing	• 2 mg once weekly without regard to meals
	• Administer immediately after the dose is prepared
Renal dose adjustment	• Not recommended with CrCl <30 mL/min
How supplied	• Single-dose 2-mg pen
	• Single-dose 2-mg vial for reconstitution
Common side effects	• Nausea
	• Diarrhea
	• Headache
	• Vomiting
	• Constipation
	• Injection-site pruritus
	• Injection-site nodules
	• Dyspepsia
Key drug interactions	• May affect absorption of orally administered medications
	• Postmarketing reports of increased INR when given in combination with warfarin

Adapted from Bydureon (exenatide extended-release for injectable suspension) [package inert]. Wilmington, DE: AstraZeneca Pharmaceuticals LP; 2014.

- Hypoglycemia
- Renal impairment
- Injection-site reactions

Albiglutide

Albiglutide is the newest FDA-approved once-weekly GLP-1 RA. The protracted duration of action of albiglutide is achieved by fusion of recombinant GLP-1 to human

Table 3
Comparison of exenatide ER with exenatide twice daily (30-week data)

	Exenatide ER Suspension	Exenatide Twice Daily
A$_{1c}$ reduction (%)	1.9[a]	1.5
FPG reduction (mg/dL)	41[b]	25
PPG reduction (mg/dL)	96	124[c]
Achievement of A$_{1c}$ <7%	77%[d]	61%
Change in body weight (kg)	−3.7	−3.6

Abbreviations: A$_{1c}$, hemoglobin A$_{1c}$; FPG, fasting plasma glucose; PPG, postprandial glucose.
  [a] $P = .0023$.
  [b] $P<.0001$.
  [c] $P = .0124$.
  [d] $P = .0039$ versus comparator.
Adapted from Drucker DJ, Buse JB, Taylor K, et al. Exenatide once weekly versus twice daily for the treatment of type 2 diabetes: a randomized, open-label, non-inferiority study. Lancet 2008;372(9645):1240–50.

albumin.[57] A summary of select clinical information for albiglutide is presented in **Box 6**.[29]

Albiglutide was studied head-to-head versus liraglutide in a 32-week study.[58] Participants enrolled had inadequate glycemic control despite treatment with oral antihyperglycemic agents, and were randomized to receive albiglutide 30 mg once weekly titrated up to 50 mg weekly (n = 404), or liraglutide 0.6 mg once daily titrated up to 1.8 mg (n = 408).[58] The mean change in hemoglobin A_{1C} achieved at week 32 in the 2 groups were −0.78% and −0.99%, respectively. In this study, the mean change in hemoglobin A_{1C} from baseline was significant for albiglutide ($P<.001$), but albiglutide had less of an effect on hemoglobin A_{1C} in this noninferiority trial when compared with liraglutide over 32 weeks (difference of 0.21% in favor of liraglutide), and albiglutide was thus unable to demonstrate noninferiority when studied against liraglutide.[58]

Contraindications and warnings/precautions listed for albiglutide include the following.[29]

Contraindications
- A history of serious hypersensitivity to albiglutide or any product components.
- Personal or family history of medullary thyroid carcinoma or in patients with multiple endocrine neoplasia syndrome type 2.

Warnings/precautions Warnings/precautions are similar to those previously discussed for other GLP-1 RAs, and include:

- Pancreatitis
- Hypoglycemia
- Renal impairment

Dipeptidyl Peptidase 4 Inhibitors

DPP-4 inhibitors are orally administered medications that prevent the inactivation of incretin hormones, in turn increasing the pool of active hormones that can carry out

---

Box 6
Albiglutide (Tanzeum): key clinical information

Dosing	• 30 mg once weekly without regard to meals initially
	• Increase to 50 mg once weekly in patients requiring additional glycemic control
	• If a dose is missed, administer within 3 days of missed dose
Renal dose adjustment	• No dose adjustment required
How supplied	• 30-mg single-dose pen
	• 50-mg single-dose pen
Common side effects	• Upper respiratory tract infection
	• Diarrhea
	• Nausea
	• Injection-site reactions
Key drug interactions	• May affect absorption of orally administered medications

Adapted from Tanzeum (albiglutide) [package insert]. Wilmington, DE: GlaxoSmithKline, LLC; 2014.

their glucoregulatory functions.[59] DPP-4 inhibitors possess actions similar to those seen with GLP-1 RAs, including glucose-dependent stimulation of insulin secretion, inhibition of glucagon secretion, and even preservation of β-cell mass via inhibition of apoptosis and increased proliferation.[60] DPP-4 inhibitor therapy is not associated with weight loss, however, which is attributed to a negligible effect of these agents on gastric emptying (as shown in **Table 1**).[24,25] DPP-4 inhibitors are generally well tolerated, with a low risk of contributing to hypoglycemia because of their glucose-dependent mechanism of action. Similarly to GLP-1 RAs, DPP-4 inhibitors are being studied for their potential vascular protective effects.[61] There are currently 4 DPP-4 inhibitors approved for use in the United States:

- Sitagliptin (Januvia)
- Saxagliptin (Onglyza)
- Linagliptin (Tradjenta)
- Alogliptin (Nesina)

Table 4 outlines select clinical properties of the 4 currently available DPP-4 inhibitors.[62–79]

Sitagliptin

Sitagliptin, the first DPP-4 inhibitor approved by the FDA, has been studied and used clinically in combination with numerous other antidiabetic therapies, and has emerged as a widely used oral antidiabetic medication (**Box 7**).[62] In line with DPP-4 inhibitors inducing insulin secretion in a glucose-dependent manner, the overall incidence of hypoglycemia in subjects receiving sitagliptin was similar to that of placebo controls. Caution is advised, however, if using sitagliptin in combination with insulin secretagogue medications, owing to an increased risk of hypoglycemia when used together.[66–69] Key contraindications, warnings, and precautions for sitagliptin are as follows.[62]

Contraindications

- A history of a serious hypersensitivity reaction to sitagliptin.

Warnings/precautions

- Pancreatitis

  The prescribing information for sitagliptin includes information regarding post-marketing reports of acute pancreatitis.[62] The FDA cited 88 cases of acute pancreatitis reported between October 2006 and February 2009, 2 of which were cases of hemorrhagic or necrotizing pancreatitis.[81] A large retrospective

Table 4
Comparison and contrast of currently available DPP-4 inhibitors

	Sitagliptin	Saxagliptin	Linagliptin	Alogliptin
Administration frequency	Once daily[62]	Once daily[63]	Once daily[64]	Once daily[65]
Average hemoglobin A_{1C} lowering (%)[a]	0.65–0.79[66–69]	0.36–0.82[70–72]	0.50–0.69[73–76]	0.47–0.85[77–80]
Average weight change (kg)[a]	+0.3 to +1.2[66,68,69]	−0.51 to +1.3[70–72]	+0.33 to +1.1[75,76]	+0.14 to +0.51[78,79]

[a] Placebo-subtracted change from baseline; baseline characteristics of study groups and concomitant medications varied from study to study.

Box 7	
Sitagliptin: key clinical information	
Dosing	• 100 mg once daily without regard to meals
Renal dose adjustment	• Decrease to 50 mg once daily if CrCl $\geq$30 mL/min to <50 mL/min
	• Decrease to 25 mg once daily if CrCl <30 mL/min
How supplied	• 100-mg tablets
	• 50-mg tablets
	• 25-mg tablets
Common side effects	• Upper respiratory tract infection
	• Nasopharyngitis
	• Headache
Key drug interactions	• No major drug interactions

Adapted from Januvia (sitagliptin) [package insert]. Whitehouse Station, NJ: Merck & Co., Inc; 2014.

study, however, determined the relative risk of pancreatitis in persons receiving sitagliptin to be 1.0 (95% confidence interval [CI] 0.5–2.0) compared with matched controls receiving metformin or glyburide.[82] Accordingly, the association between sitagliptin (and DPP-4 inhibitor use in general) and pancreatitis is controversial; however, the manufacturer warns against using DPP-4 inhibitors in individuals with a history of pancreatitis.

• Renal failure
Postmarketing reports of acute renal failure, sometimes requiring dialysis, have been reported. Dosage adjustment of sitagliptin is recommended based on renal function, and assessment of renal function is recommended before initiating and during treatment.

• Hypoglycemia
The risk of hypoglycemia may be increased when sitagliptin is used with an insulin secretagogue or insulin.

• Serious allergic reactions
Reports of serious allergic and hypersensitivity reactions such as angioedema, exfoliative skin conditions, and anaphylaxis have been reported.

Saxagliptin
Key clinical information for saxagliptin is summarized in **Box 8**.[63] A differentiating factor for saxagliptin in comparison with other DPP-4 inhibitors is that it is a substrate of CYP3A4/5, and a dose reduction is recommended when given in combination with a strong CYP3A4/5 inhibitor such as ketoconazole.[63] Similarly to sitagliptin, a higher risk of hypoglycemia was observed when saxagliptin was used in combination with an insulin secretagogue. The contraindications, warnings, and precautions for saxagliptin are similar to those noted for other agents in this class.[63]

Contraindications
• A history of a serious hypersensitivity reaction to saxagliptin.

Box 8	
Saxagliptin: key clinical information	
Dosing	• 2.5 to 5 mg once daily without regard to meals
Renal dose adjustment	• Limit to 2.5 mg once daily if CrCl ≤50 mL/min
How supplied	• 5-mg tablets
	• 2.5-mg tablets
Common side effects	• Upper respiratory tract infection
	• Urinary tract infection
	• Headache
Key drug interactions	• Strong CYP3A4/5 inhibitors (eg, ketoconazole) increases saxagliptin concentrations: limit saxagliptin dose to 2.5 mg once daily

Adapted from Onglyza (saxagliptin) [package insert]. Princeton, NJ: Bristol-Myers Squibb Company; 2013.

Warnings/precautions
- Pancreatitis
  Overall, the incidence of pancreatitis during clinical trials was 0.2% in the 3422 patients who received saxagliptin, compared with 0.2% in 1066 controls.[83]
- Hypoglycemia
- Serious allergic reactions

Linagliptin

In comparison with other currently available DPP-4 inhibitors, linagliptin has a long half-life (131 hours) owing to its extensive binding to plasma proteins.[84] Linagliptin is primarily eliminated hepatically (~85%), with an estimated 5% of a given dose undergoing renal elimination (**Box 9**).[64,84] A study of linagliptin use in patients with renal compromise concluded that dose adjustment is not required in various degrees of renal impairment,[85] a unique trait in comparison with other currently available DPP-4 inhibitors, which all require renal dose adjustment.

The following are contraindications, warnings, and precautions noted in the labeling for linagliptin.[64]

Contraindications
- A history of a serious hypersensitivity reaction to linagliptin.

Warnings/precautions
- Pancreatitis
  Eight of 4687 participants (4311 patient-years of exposure) who received linagliptin experienced pancreatitis while receiving treatment, compared with no cases in the 1183 participants (433 patient years of exposure) receiving placebo.
- Hypoglycemia
- Serious allergic reactions

Alogliptin

Alogliptin is the newest DPP-4 inhibitor marketed for the treatment of T2DM. Alogliptin monotherapy is generally well tolerated, with a generally mild overall side-effect profile.[65] Key clinical information on alogliptin, including the most common side effects

Box 9 Linagliptin: key clinical information	
Dosing	• 5 mg once daily without regard to meals
Renal dose adjustment	• No renal dose adjustment required
How supplied	• 5-mg tablets
Common side effects	• Nasopharyngitis
Key drug interactions	• Linagliptin efficacy may be reduced when given in combination with strong P-glycoprotein or CYP3A4 inducers

Adapted from Tradjenta (linagliptin) [package insert]. Ridgefield, CT: Boehringer Ingelheim Pharmaceuticals, Inc; 2014.

noted in clinical trials, is summarized in **Box 10**.[65] The contraindications, warnings, and precautions listed for alogliptin are similar to those discussed previously.[65]

Contraindications
- A history of a serious hypersensitivity reaction to alogliptin.

Warnings/precautions
- Pancreatitis
- Hypersensitivity
- Hepatic effects
  Postmarketing reports of hepatic failure for which causality could not be excluded have been noted in persons receiving alogliptin therapy. The manufacturer recommends prompt discontinuation of treatment for patients in whom liver injury is detected or suspected.
- Hypoglycemia

Box 10 Alogliptin: key clinical information	
Dosing	• 25 mg once daily without regard to meals
Renal dose adjustment	• Decrease to 12.5 mg once daily if CrCl ≥30 mL/min to <60 mL/min
	• Decrease to 6.25 mg once daily if CrCl <30 mL/min
How supplied	• 25-mg tablets
	• 12.5-mg tablets
	• 6.25-mg tablets
Common side effects	• Nasopharyngitis
	• Headache
	• Upper respiratory tract infection
Key drug interactions	• No major drug interactions

Adapted from Nesina (alogliptin) [package insert]. Deerfield, IL: Takeda Pharmaceuticals American, Inc; 2013.

CARDIOVASCULAR SAFETY

Given concerns of cardiovascular (CV) safety of drugs for the treatment of DM in recent years,[86–88] the Endocrinologic and Metabolic Drugs Advisory Committee of the FDA redefined the approval criteria for all new medications for the treatment of DM, requiring sponsors to demonstrate that products do not convey an unacceptable CV risk.[89] The potential effect of GLP-1 on CV function is an additional area of growing interest, with evidence suggesting that GLP-1 receptors are widely expressed on cardiomyocytes and in the peripheral vasculature.[25]

Findings from a large CV outcomes study with saxagliptin (SAVOR-TIMI 53) were recently published.[90] This trial, enrolling more than 16,000 participants with T2DM, compared the use of saxagliptin and placebo on rates of a composite primary end point of CV death, myocardial infarction, or ischemic stroke. Although saxagliptin was not shown to increase the risk of the primary end point (hazard ratio [HR] 1.00; 95% CI 0.89–1.12; $P = .99$ for superiority), more participants in the saxagliptin group were hospitalized for heart failure (3.5% vs 2.8%; HR 1.27, 95% CI 1.07–1.51, $P = .007$), thus raising potential concern about DPP-4 inhibitor use and occurrence

Table 5
Select cardiovascular outcome trials (CVOTs) recently completed or in progress with incretin-based therapies

Agent	Trial Name (ClinicalTrials.gov Identifier)	Primary Outcome Measures	Trial Status
Exenatide	EXSCEL (NCT01144338)	Time to first confirmed cardiovascular (CV) event: Composite defined as CV-related death, nonfatal myocardial infarction (MI), or nonfatal stroke	In progress
Liraglutide	LEADER (NCT01179048)	Time to first confirmed CV event: Composite defined as CV-related death, nonfatal MI, or nonfatal stroke	In progress
Sitagliptin	TECOS (NCT00790205)	Time to first confirmed CV event: Composite defined as CV-related death, nonfatal MI, nonfatal stroke, or unstable angina requiring hospitalization	In progress
Saxagliptin	SAVOR-TIMI 53 (NCT01107886)	Composite of CV-related death, nonfatal MI, or nonfatal ischemic stroke	Completed
Linagliptin	CARMELINA (NCT01897532)	Time to first confirmed CV event: Composite defined as CV-related death, nonfatal MI, nonfatal stroke, or unstable angina requiring hospitalization	In progress
Alogliptin	EXAMINE (NCT00968708)	Percentage of participants with primary major adverse cardiac events: Composite defined as CV-related death, nonfatal MI, or nonfatal stroke	Completed

Adapted from ClinicalTrials.gov. Available at: http://clinicaltrials.gov. Accessed July 28, 2014.

of heart failure. In response to these findings, a meta-analysis of randomized clinical trials of DPP-4 inhibitors was conducted, showing the overall risk of acute heart failure to be higher in patients treated with DPP-4 inhibitors when compared with those treated with placebo or an active comparator (odds ratio 1.19; 95% CI 1.03–1.37; $P = .015$).[91]

Questions regarding CV safety likewise exist for GLP-1 RAs. Although preliminary CV safety analyses of data with liraglutide and exenatide suggest a trend toward a reduction in CV events,[54] studies with long-acting GLP-1 RAs have consistently shown an increase in heart rate with the use of these agents.[41,92] The mechanism by which long-acting GLP-1 RAs increase heart rate is not currently known, nor is whether this finding conveys any increase in the risk of CV events.

While these and other findings have raised questions about incretin-based therapies and CV risk or benefit, ongoing CV outcome studies will provide additional information concerning the impact of incretin-based treatments on CV safety. **Table 5** provides a summary of CV outcome trials, recently completed and in progress, with the agents discussed herein.[93]

SUMMARY

Incretin-based therapies are steadily gaining clinical popularity, with many more products in the developmental pipeline. Current treatment recommendations incorporate GLP-1 RAs and DPP-4 inhibitors as important agents for consideration in the treatment of T2DM owing to their low hypoglycemia risk, ability to address postprandial hyperglycemia (DPP-4 inhibitors and short-acting GLP-1 RAs), and potential for weight reduction (GLP-1 RAs).[94,95] These properties may likewise prove advantageous in older adults in whom hypoglycemia is particularly undesirable, although older adults may be more prone to the nausea and vomiting associated with GLP-1 RA therapy.[96] Other safety issues for incretin-based therapies, such as pancreatitis, C-cell hyperplasia, and renal failure, should be considered when choosing an appropriate patient to receive such therapies. Ongoing CV outcome studies will further inform the health care community regarding the CV safety of incretin-based therapies. The availability of both short-acting and long-acting GLP-1 RAs currently allows practitioners to consider individualized blood glucose trends and therapeutic needs when choosing an optimal agent.

REFERENCES

1. Baggio LL, Drucker DJ. Biology of incretins: GLP-1 and GIP. Gastroenterology 2007;132:2131–57.
2. Elrick H, Stimmler L, Hlad CJ, et al. Plasma insulin response to oral and intravenous glucose administration. J Clin Endocrinol Metab 1964;24:1076–82.
3. Creutzfeldt W. The incretin concept today. Diabetologia 1979;16(2):75–85.
4. Dupre J, Ross SA, Watson D, et al. Stimulation of insulin secretion by gastric inhibitory polypeptide in man. J Clin Endocrinol Metab 1973;37(5):826–8.
5. Bell GI, Santerre RF, Mullenbach GT. Hamster preproglucagon contains the sequence of glucagon and two related peptides. Nature 1983;302(5910):716–8.
6. Nauck MA, Homberger E, Siegel EG, et al. Incretin effects of increasing glucose loads in man calculated from venous insulin and C-peptide responses. J Clin Endocrinol Metab 1986;63(2):492–8.
7. Nauck M, Stockmann F, Ebert R, et al. Reduced incretin effect in type 2 (non-insulin-dependent) diabetes. Diabetologia 1986;29(1):46–52.

8. Holst JJ, Orskov C, Nielsen OV, et al. Truncated glucagon-like peptide 1, an insulin-releasing hormone from the distal gut. FEBS Lett 1987;211(2):169–74.

9. Kreymann B, Williams G, Ghatei MA, et al. Glucagon-like peptide-1 7-36: a physiological incretin in man. Lancet 1987;2(8571):1300–4.

10. Wettergren A, Schjoldager B, Mortensen PE, et al. Truncated GLP-1 (proglucagon 78-107-amide) inhibits gastric and pancreatic functions in man. Dig Dis Sci 1993;38(4):665–73.

11. Drucker DJ, Nauck MA. The incretin system: glucagon-like peptide-1 receptor agonists and dipeptidyl peptidase-4 inhibitors in type 2 diabetes. Lancet 2006;368(9548):1696–705.

12. Perfetti R, Merkel P. Glucagon-like peptide-1: a major regulator of pancreatic beta-cell function. Eur J Endocrinol 2000;143(6):717–25.

13. Xu G, Stoffers DA, Habener JF, et al. Exendin-4 stimulates both beta-cell replication and neogenesis, resulting in increased beta-cell mass and improved glucose tolerance in diabetic rats. Diabetes 1999;48(12):2270–6.

14. Orskov C, Poulsen SS, Moller M, et al. Glucagon-like peptide I receptors in the subfornical organ and the area postrema are accessible to circulating glucagon-like peptide I. Diabetes 1996;45(6):832–5.

15. Larsen PJ, Tang-Christensen M, Holst JJ, et al. Distribution of glucagon-like peptide-1 and other preproglucagon-derived peptides in the rat hypothalamus and brainstem. Neuroscience 1997;77(1):257–70.

16. Treiman M, Elvekjaer M, Engstrom T, et al. Glucagon-like peptide 1- a cardiologic dimension. Trends Cardiovasc Med 2010;20(1):8–12.

17. Irwin N, Flatt PR. Therapeutic potential for GIP receptor agonists and antagonists. Best Pract Res Clin Endocrinol Metab 2009;23(4):499–512.

18. Nauck MA, Heimesaat MM, Orskov C, et al. Preserved incretin activity of glucagon-like peptide 1 [7-36 amide] but not of synthetic human gastric inhibitory polypeptide in patients with type-2 diabetes mellitus. J Clin Invest 1993;91(1):301–7.

19. Vilsboll T, Krarup T, Madsbad S, et al. Defective amplification of the late phase insulin response to glucose by GIP in obese Type II diabetic patients. Diabetologia 2002;45(8):1111–9.

20. Hojberg PV, Vilsboll T, Rabol R, et al. Four weeks of near-normalisation of blood glucose improves the insulin response to glucagon-like peptide-1 and glucose-dependent insulinotropic polypeptide in patients with type 2 diabetes. Diabetologia 2009;52(2):199–207.

21. Meier JJ, Gallwitz B, Siepmann N, et al. Gastric inhibitory polypeptide (GIP) dose-dependently stimulates glucagon secretion in healthy human subjects at euglycaemia. Diabetologia 2003;46(6):798–801.

22. Widenmaier SB, Kim SU, Yang GK, et al. A GIP receptor agonist exhibits β-cell anti-apoptotic actions in rat models of diabetes resulting in improved β-cell function and glycemic control. PLoS One 2010;5(3):e9590.

23. Orskov C, Wettergren A, Holst JJ. Biological effects and metabolic rates of glucagonlike peptide-1 7-36 amide and glucagonlike peptide-1 7-37 in healthy subjects are indistinguishable. Diabetes 1993;42(5):658–61.

24. Campbell RK. Clarifying the role of incretin-based therapies in the treatment of type 2 diabetes mellitus. Clin Ther 2011;33(5):511–27.

25. Meier JJ. GLP-1 receptor agonists for individualized treatment of type 2 diabetes mellitus. Nat Rev Endocrinol 2012;8:728–42.

26. Byetta (exenatide) [package insert]. Princeton, NJ: Bristol-Myers Squibb Company; 2013.

27. Victoza (liraglutide) [package insert]. Plainsboro, NJ: Novo Nordisk, Inc; 2013.
28. Bydureon (exenatide extended-release for injectable suspension) [package insert]. Wilmington, DE: AstraZeneca Pharmaceuticals LP; 2014.
29. Tanzeum (albiglutide) [package insert]. Wilmington, DE: GlaxoSmithKline, LLC; 2014.
30. DeFronzo RA, Ratner RE, Han J, et al. Effects of exenatide (exendin-4) on glycemic control and weight over 30 weeks in metformin-treated patients with type 2 diabetes. Diabetes Care 2005;28(5):1092–100.
31. Buse JB, Henry RR, Han J, et al. Effects of exenatide (exendin-4) on glycemic control over 30 weeks in sulfonylurea-treated patients with type 2 diabetes. Diabetes Care 2004;27(11):2628–35, 3.
32. Kendall DM, Riddle MC, Rosenstock J, et al. Effects of exenatide (exendin-4) on glycemic control over 30 weeks in patients with type 2 diabetes treated with metformin and a sulfonylurea. Diabetes Care 2005;28(5):1083–91.
33. Zinman B, Hoogwerf BJ, Dúran Garcia S, et al. The effect of adding exenatide to thiazolidinedione in suboptimally controlled type 2 diabetes: a randomized trial. Ann Intern Med 2007;146(7):477–85.
34. Marre M, Shaw J, Brändle M, et al. Liraglutide, a once-daily human GLP-1 analogue, added to a sulphonylurea over 26 weeks produces greater improvements in glycaemic and weight control compared with adding rosiglitazone or placebo in subjects with Type 2 diabetes (LEAD-1 SU). Diabet Med 2009;26(3):268–78.
35. Nauck M, Frid A, Hermansen K, et al. Efficacy and safety comparison of liraglutide, glimepiride, and placebo, all in combination with metformin in type 2 diabetes: the LEAD (liraglutide effect and action in diabetes)-2 study. Diabetes Care 2009;32(1):84–90.
36. Zinman B, Gerich J, Buse JB, et al. Efficacy and safety of the human glucagon-like peptide-1 analog liraglutide in combination with metformin and thiazolidinedione in patients with type 2 diabetes mellitus (LEAD-4 Met + TZD). Diabetes Care 2009;32(7):1224–30.
37. Russell-Jones D, Vaag A, Schmitz O, et al. Liraglutide vs insulin glargine and placebo in combination with metformin and sulfonylurea therapy in type 2 diabetes mellitus (LEAD-5 met + SU): a randomized controlled trial. Diabetologia 2009; 52(10):2046–55.
38. Drucker DJ, Buse JB, Taylor K, et al. Exenatide once weekly versus twice daily for the treatment of type 2 diabetes: a randomized, open-label, non-inferiority study. Lancet 2008;372(9645):1240–50.
39. Buse JB, Drucker DJ, Taylor KL, et al. DURATION 1: exenatide once weekly produces sustained glycemic control and weight loss over 52 weeks. Diabetes Care 2010;33(6):1255–61.
40. Bergenstal RM, Wysham C, Macconell L, et al. Efficacy and safety of exenatide once weekly versus sitagliptin or pioglitazone as an adjunct to metformin for treatment of type 2 diabetes (DURATION-2): a randomized trial. Lancet 2010; 376(9739):431–9.
41. Diamant M, Van Gaal L, Stranks S, et al. Once weekly exenatide compared with insulin glargine titrated to target in patients with type 2 diabetes (DURATION-3): an open-label randomised trial. Lancet 2010;375(9733):2234–43.
42. Blevins T, Pullman J, Malloy J, et al. DURATION-5: exenatide one weekly resulted in greater improvements in glycemic control compared with exenatide twice daily in patients with type 2 diabetes. J Clin Endocrinol Metab 2011;96(5):1301–10.
43. Reusch J, Stewart M, Perkins C, et al. HARMONY 1 week 52 results: albiglutide vs. placebo in patients with type 2 diabetes mellitus not controlled on

pioglitazone ± metformin [abstract 57-LB]. In: Programs and abstracts of the 73rd Annual Scientific Sessions of the American Diabetes Association. Chicago, Illinois. June 21–25, 2013.

44. Nauck M, Stewart M, Perkins C, et al. HARMONY 2 Wk 52 results: albiglutide monotherapy in drug naïve patients with type 2 diabetes mellitus [abstract 55-LB]. In: Programs and abstracts of the 73rd Annual Scientific Sessions of the American Diabetes Association. Chicago, Illinois. June 21–25, 2013.

45. Reinhardt R, Nauck MA, Stewart M, et al. HARMONY 2 results at week 52 primary endpoint: once-weekly albiglutide monotherapy for patients with type 2 diabetes mellitus inadequately controlled with diet and exercise [abstract 903]. In: Programs and abstracts of the 49th Annual Meeting of the European Association for the Study of Diabetes. Barcelona, Spain. September 23–27, 2013.

46. Ahren B, Stewart M, Cirkel D, et al. HARMONY 3: 104 week (wk) efficacy of albiglutide (Albi) compared to sitagliptin (Sita) and glimepiride (SU) in patients (pts) with type 2 diabetes mellitus (T2DM) on metformin (Met) [abstract 52-LB]. In: Programs and abstracts of the 73rd Annual Scientific Sessions of the American Diabetes Association. Chicago, Illinois. June 21–25, 2013.

47. Johnson S, Ahren B, Stewart M, et al. HARMONY 3: 104 week efficacy of albiglutide compared to sitagliptin and glimepiride in patients with type 2 diabetes mellitus on metformin [abstract 5]. In: Programs and abstracts of the 49th Annual Meeting of the European Association for the Study of Diabetes. Barcelona, Spain. September 23–27, 2013.

48. Home P, Stewart M, Yang F. 52-week efficacy of albiglutide vs placebo and vs pioglitazone in triple therapy (background metformin and glimepiride) in people with type 2 diabetes: HARMONY 5 Study [abstract 58-LB]. In: Programs and abstracts of the 73rd Annual Scientific Sessions of the American Diabetes Association. Chicago, Illinois. June 21–25, 2013.

49. Mudaliar S, Henry RR. Incretin therapies: effects beyond glycemic control. Eur J Intern Med 2009;20:S319–28.

50. Olansky LQ. Do incretin drugs for type 2 diabetes increase the risk of acute pancreatitis? Cleve Clin J Med 2010;77(8):503–5.

51. Noel RA, Braun DK, Patterson RE, et al. Increased risk of acute pancreatitis and biliary disease observed in patients with type 2 diabetes: a retrospective cohort study. Diabetes Care 2009;32(5):834–8.

52. U.S. Food and Drug Administration (FDA). Byetta (exenatide)—renal failure. Available at: http://www.fda.gov/safety/MedWatch/SafetyInformation/Safety AlertsforHumanMedicalProducts/ucm188703.htm. Accessed June 1, 2014.

53. Buse JB, Rosenstock J, Sesti G, et al. Liraglutide once a day versus exenatide twice a day for type 2 diabetes: a 26-week randomised, parallel-group, multinational, open-label trial (LEAD-6). Lancet 2009;374(9683):39–47.

54. Parks M, Rosebraugh C. Weighing risks and benefits of liraglutide—The FDA's review of a new antidiabetic therapy. N Engl J Med 2010;362(9):774–7.

55. US Food and Drug Administration. NDA 22-341 Victoza (liraglutide [rDNA origin] injection) risk evaluation and mitigation strategy (REMS). Available at: http://www.fda.gov/downloads/Drugs/DrugSafety/PostmarketDrugSafetyInformationfor PatientsandProviders/UCM202063.pdf. Accessed June 1, 2014.

56. Tzefos M, Harris K, Brackett A. Clinical efficacy and safety of once-weekly glucagon-like peptide-I agonists in development for treatment of type 2 diabetes mellitus in adults. Ann Pharmacother 2012;46:68–78.

57. Poole RM, Nowlan ML. Albiglutide: first global approval. Drugs 2014. http://dx.doi.org/10.1007/s40265-014-0228-2.

58. Pratley RE, Nauck MA, Barnett AH, et al. Once-weekly albiglutide versus once-daily liraglutide in patients with type 2 diabetes inadequately controlled on oral drugs (HARMONY 7): a randomised, open-label, multicentre, non-inferiority phase 3 study. Lancet Diabetes Endocrinol 2014;2(4):289–97.

59. Ahren B. Clinical results of treating type 2 diabetic patients with sitagliptin, vildagliptin or saxagliptin—diabetes control and potential adverse events. Best Pract Res Clin Endocrinol Metab 2009;23(4):487–98.

60. Deacon CF. Therapeutic strategies based on glucagon-like peptide 1. Diabetes 2004;53(9):2181–9.

61. Fadini GP, Avogaro A. Cardiovascular effects of DPP-4 inhibition: beyond GLP-1. Vascul Pharmacol 2011;55:10–6.

62. Januvia (sitagliptin) [package insert]. Whitehouse Station, NJ: Merck & Co., Inc; 2014.

63. Onglyza (saxagliptin) [package insert]. Princeton, NJ: Bristol-Myers Squibb Company; 2013.

64. Tradjenta (linagliptin) [package insert]. Ridgefield, CT: Boehringer Ingelheim Pharmaceuticals, Inc; 2014.

65. Nesina (alogliptin) [package insert]. Deerfield, IL: Takeda Pharmaceuticals American, Inc; 2013.

66. Aschner P, Kipnes M, Lunceford M, et al. Effect of the dipeptidyl peptidase-4 inhibitor sitagliptin as monotherapy on glycemic control in patients with type 2 diabetes. Diabetes Care 2006;29(12):26327.

67. Charbonnel B, Karasik A, Liu J, et al. Efficacy and safety of the dipeptidyl peptidase-4 inhibitor sitagliptin added to ongoing metformin therapy in patients with type 2 diabetes inadequately controlled with metformin alone. Diabetes Care 2006;29(12):2638–43.

68. Hermansen K, Kipnes M, Luo E, et al. Efficacy and safety of the dipeptidyl peptidase-4 inhibitor, sitagliptin, in patients with type 2 diabetes mellitus inadequately controlled on glimepiride alone or on glimepiride and metformin. Diabetes Obes Metab 2007;9(5):733–45.

69. Rosenstock J, Brazg R, Andryuk PJ, et al. Efficacy and safety of the dipeptidyl peptidase-4 inhibitor sitagliptin added to ongoing pioglitazone therapy in patients with type 2 diabetes: a 24 week, multicenter, randomized, double-blind, placebo-controlled, parallel-group study. Clin Ther 2006; 28(10):1556–68.

70. Rosenstock J, Aguilar-Salinas C, Klein E, et al. Effect of saxagliptin monotherapy in treatment-naive patients with type 2 diabetes. Curr Med Res Opin 2009; 25(10):2401–11.

71. DeFronzo RA, Hissa MN, Garber AJ, et al. The efficacy and safety of saxagliptin when added to metformin therapy in patients with inadequately controlled type 2 diabetes on metformin alone. Diabetes Care 2009;32(9):1649–55.

72. Hollander P, Li J, Allen E, et al. Saxagliptin added to a thiazolidinedione improves glycemic control in patients with type 2 diabetes and inadequate control on thiazolidinedione alone. J Clin Endocrinol Metab 2009;94(12): 4810–9.

73. Del Prato S, Barnett AH, Huisman H, et al. Effect of linagliptin monotherapy on glycaemic control and markers of beta-cell function in patients with inadequately controlled type 2 diabetes: a randomized controlled trial. Diabetes Obes Metab 2011;13(3):258–67.

74. Taskinen MR, Rosenstock J, Tamminen I, et al. Safety and efficacy of linagliptin as add-on therapy to metformin in patients with type 2 diabetes: a randomized,

double-blind, placebo-controlled study. Diabetes Obes Metab 2011;13(1): 65–74.

75. Owens DR, Swallow R, Dugi KA, et al. Efficacy and safety of linagliptin in persons with type 2 diabetes inadequately controlled by a combination of metformin and sulfonylurea: a 24-week randomized study. Diabet Med 2011;28(11): 1352–61.

76. Gomis R, Espadero RM, Jones R, et al. Efficacy and safety of initial combination therapy with linagliptin and pioglitazone in patients with inadequately controlled type 2 diabetes: a randomized, double-blind, placebo-controlled study. Diabetes Obes Metab 2011;13(7):653–61.

77. Nauck MA, Ellis GC, Fleck PR, et al. Efficacy and safety of adding the dipeptidyl peptidase-4 inhibitor alogliptin to metformin therapy in patients with type 2 diabetes inadequately controlled with metformin monotherapy: a multicentre, randomised, double-blind, placebo-controlled study. Int J Clin Pract 2009; 63(1):46–55.

78. Seino Y, Miyata Y, Hiroi S, et al. Efficacy and safety of alogliptin added to metformin in Japanese patients with type 2 diabetes: a randomized, double-blind, placebo-controlled trial with an open-label, long-term extension study. Diabetes Obes Metab 2012;14(10):927–36.

79. Kaku K, Itayasu T, Hiroi S, et al. Efficacy and safety of alogliptin added to pioglitazone in Japanese patients with type 2 diabetes: a randomized, double-blind, placebo-controlled trial with an open-label long-term extension study. Diabetes Obes Metab 2011;13(11):1028–35.

80. Pratley RE, Reusch JE, Fleck PR, et al. Efficacy and safety of the dipeptidyl peptidase-4 inhibitor alogliptin added to pioglitazone in patients with type 2 diabetes: a randomized, double-blind, placebo-controlled study. Curr Med Res Opin 2009;25(10):2361–71.

81. U.S. Food and Drug Administration. Safety: Sitagliptin (marketed as Januvia and Janumet)—acute pancreatitis. Available at: http://www.fda.gov/Safety/MedWatch/ SafetyInformation/SafetyAlertsforHumanMedicalProducts/ucm183800.htm. Accessed June 1, 2014.

82. Dore DD, Seeger JD, Arnold Chan K. Use of a claims-based active drug safety surveillance system to assess the risk of acute pancreatitis with exenatide or sitagliptin compared to metformin or glyburide. Curr Med Res Opin 2009; 25(4):1019–27.

83. U.S. Food and Drug Administration. Controlled phase 2b/3 pooled population— day 120 update: stratified analyses of FDA-defined MACE. Available at: http:// www.fda.gov/downloads/advisorycommittees/committeesmeetingmaterils/drugs/ endocrinologicandmetabolicdrugsadvisorycommittee/ucm149589. Accessed June 1, 2014.

84. Hüttner S, Graefe-Mody EU, Withopf B, et al. Safety, tolerability, pharmacokinetics, and pharmacodynamics of single oral doses of BI 1356, an inhibitor of dipeptidyl peptidase 4, in healthy male volunteers. J Clin Pharmacol 2008; 48(10):1171–8.

85. Graefe-Mody U, Friedrich C, Port A, et al. Effect of renal impairment on the pharmacokinetics of the dipeptidyl peptidase-4 inhibitor linagliptin. Diabetes Obes Metab 2011;13(11):939–46.

86. Nissen SE, Wolski K. Effect of rosiglitazone on the risk of myocardial infarction and death from cardiovascular causes. N Engl J Med 2007;356(24):2457–71.

87. Feinglos MN, Bethel MA. Therapy of type 2 diabetes, cardiovascular death, and the UGDP. Am Heart J 1999;138(5 Pt 1):S346–52.

88. Nissen SE, Wolski K, Topol EJ. Effect of muraglitazar on death and major adverse cardiovascular events in patients with type 2 diabetes mellitus. JAMA 2005;294:2581–6.

89. Food and Drug Administration, Center for Drug Evaluation and Research. Guidance for industry: diabetes mellitus-evaluating cardiovascular risk in new antidiabetic therapies to treat type 2 diabetes. Available at: http://www.fda.gov/downloads/Drugs/GuidanceComplianceRegulatoryInformation/Guidances/ucm 071627.pdf. Accessed July 28, 2014.

90. Scirica BM, Bhatt DL, Braunwald E, et al. Saxagliptin and cardiovascular outcomes in patients with type 2 diabetes mellitus. N Engl J Med 2013;369:1317–26.

91. Monami M, Dicembrini I, Mannucci E. Dipeptidyl peptidase-4 inhibitors and heart failure: a meta-analysis of randomized clinical trials. Nutr Metab Cardiovasc Dis 2014;24(7):689–97.

92. Pratley R, Nauck M, Bailey T, et al. Liraglutide versus sitagliptin for patients with type 2 diabetes who did not have adequate glycaemic control with metformin: a 26-week, randomised, parallel-group, open-label trial. Lancet 2010;375(9724): 1447–56.

93. ClinicalTrials.gov. Available at: http://clinicaltrials.gov. Accessed July 28, 2014.

94. Inzucchi SE, Bergenstal RM, Buse JB, et al. Management of hyperglycemia in type 2 diabetes: a patient-centered approach. Diabetes Care 2012;35:1364–79.

95. Garber AJ, Abrahamson MJ, Barzilay JI, et al. American Association of Clinical Endocrinologists' comprehensive diabetes management algorithm 2013 consensus statement. Endocr Pract 2013;19(Suppl 2):1–48.

96. Kirkman MS, Briscoe VJ, Clark N, et al. Diabetes in older adults: a consensus report. J Am Geriatr Soc 2012;35(12):2650–64.

Sodium Glucose Cotransporter 2 Inhibitors

John R. White Jr, PA-C, PharmD

KEYWORDS

- Sodium glucose cotransporter 2 • SGLT2 • SGLT2 inhibitors • Type 2 diabetes
- Antihyperglycemic agents

KEY POINTS

- Sodium glucose cotransporter 2 (SGLT2) inhibition offers a novel mechanism to mitigate hyperglycemia in patients with diabetes.
- SGLT2 inhibitors are generally associated with a reduction in hemoglobin A1c of between 0.5% and 1%.
- The mechanism of action and efficacy of SGLT2 inhibitors are not linked to insulin and are associated with an exceedingly low incidence of hypoglycemia when used independently of exogenous insulin or secretagogues.
- SGLT2 inhibitors are associated with an increased incidence of urinary tract and genital infections but these infections are typically mild, responsive to treatment, and are not use limiting.

INTRODUCTION

For much of the history of modern medicine the kidney has been thought of as primarily an organ of elimination of waste materials and a regulator of ion balance.[1] The impact of the kidney on glucose homeostasis was for the most part unrecognized until it was incorrectly implicated as the structural cause of diabetes in the late 1800s. It is now known that the kidney plays other roles and is involved intimately in glucose metabolism and homeostasis. Advances in the recognition of the role that the kidney plays in glucose homeostasis and metabolism has over the past few decades fueled an interest in modulation of these systems for therapeutic reasons. One area of particular interest has been the sodium glucose cotransporters (SGLTs). At present, several medications for the management of type 2 diabetes are on the market that inhibit SGLTs (specifically SGLT2).

This article reviews the role of the kidney in glucose regulation in nondiabetic and diabetic patients. It also discusses the therapeutic modulation of SGLT for therapeutic

Disclosure: None.

Department of Pharmacotherapy, Washington State University, Health Sciences Building, Suite 210, PO Box 1459, Spokane, WA 99210, USA

E-mail address: whitej@wsu.edu

Med Clin N Am 99 (2015) 131–143

http://dx.doi.org/10.1016/j.mcna.2014.08.020

medical.theclinics.com

reasons and specifically review the development of the SGLT2 inhibitors. Individual SGLT2 inhibitors, their use in patients with renal disease, and drug-drug interactions with these agents are discussed, as well as the overall potential benefits and adverse effects.

THE KIDNEY AND GLUCOSE REGULATION

The kidney has not always been thought of as one of the major organs responsible for glucose homeostasis. However, the kidney plays a major role in glucose metabolism and homeostasis via at least 3 processes: (1) gluconeogenesis, (2) glucose use, and (3) glomerular filtration and reabsorption of glucose in the proximal convoluted tubules.[2] In addition, there are significant perturbations in each of these key processes in patients who have diabetes.

Renal Gluconeogenesis

The endogenous production and release of glucose into the circulation occurs either by gluconeogenesis (GNG) or glycogenolysis. In individuals who have fasted for greater than 14 hours, about half of the endogenously produced glucose released into the circulation comes from the production of glucose by the kidney or liver (GNG) and about half comes from the breakdown of glycogen stores in the liver (glycogenolysis).[2,3] It has also been suggested that the small intestines may play role in GNG in some species.[4] In humans, the liver and the kidney are the only organs that possess sufficient quantities of glucose-6-phosphatase and other enzymes needed to drive gluconeogenesis. The kidney is important in this regard because renal glucose production accounts for about 20% to 25% of glucose released into the circulation after a fast of 12 to 16 hours. The kidney is responsible for one-fifth of overall endogenous glucose release and is responsible for approximately 40% of glucose released specifically by gluconeogenesis.[2,3]

Endogenous glucose liberation is reduced by about 60% overall in the postprandial state.[5] Hepatic glycogenolysis is essentially extinguished several hours after a meal and hepatic gluconeogenesis reduced by about 80%. In the postprandial state, renal gluconeogenesis is increased by 100% and accounts for 60% of endogenous glucose release. One theory suggests that this increase in postprandial renal gluconeogenesis is directed toward building hepatic glycogen stores.

The role of gluconeogenesis as a factor in worsening hyperglycemia in patients with both types 1 and 2 diabetes has been documented.[3] Significant increases in renal gluconeogenesis have been shown in animal diabetes models and in human studies. Studies in patients with type 1 and type 2 diabetes have shown that renal glucose release increases in about the same proportion as hepatic glucose production does in these patients. In patients with type 2 diabetes an increase (compared with people with normal glucose tolerance) in both fasting and postprandial gluconeogenesis has been shown.[2]

Renal Glucose Use

The kidneys have an important role in glucose use. In the fasting state the kidneys use approximately 10% of all the glucose used by the body for energy. The amount of glucose used increases significantly (approximately 3-fold) in the fed state but proportionally is still about 10% of all of the glucose used.[5] Patients with type 2 diabetes have significantly increased renal glucose uptake compared with nondiabetic individuals in both the fasting and postprandial states. Glucose use is approximately 3-fold higher in the fasting state and 2-fold higher in the postprandial state in patients with type 2 diabetes versus nondiabetic individuals.[5]

Filtration, Reabsorption of Glucose, and Sodium Glucose Cotransporter 2

Although the kidney is involved in glucose homeostasis via several mechanisms, the primary influence of the kidney on glucose homeostasis is by glomerular filtration and reabsorption.[3] Urine glucose excretion (UGE) is calculated by subtracting the amount of glucose that is reabsorbed from the amount filtered. Normal healthy adults filter approximately 180 g of glucose daily.[1] In nondiabetic individuals most of this glucose is reabsorbed, with less than 1% being excreted in the urine.[6]

Several transport mechanisms are involved in the multistep reabsorption of glucose. The filtered glucose must be transported out of the tubule, through the tubular epithelial cells, and then across the basolateral membrane into the peritubular capillary (**Fig. 1**). Under normal nondiabetic conditions, when the tubular glucose load is normal little to no glucose is lost in the urine. However, when the renal glucose threshold is exceeded, UGE occurs. The plasma glucose value required to exceed the renal glucose threshold is not a set value in humans but is a range. One study published about 45 years ago evaluating this process reported that the required blood glucose concentration needed to exceed the renal glucose threshold ranged from as low as 130 mg/dL in young subjects to as high as 300 mg/dL in elderly subjects.[7] It is estimated that this threshold in most individuals is approximately 200 mg/dL.[8]

The reabsorption of glucose from the urine begins with the transport of glucose from the tubule (lumen) into the tubular epithelial cells. This step is governed by SGLTs (see **Fig. 1**). SGLTs include several membrane proteins that transport many compounds including glucose, amino acids, vitamins, ions, and osmolytes across the lumen membrane of renal tubules as well as from the lumen of the intestine across the intestinal epithelium.[9] The 2 most well characterized members of this family of transporters are SGLT1 and SGLT2. SGLT1 is a low-capacity, high-affinity Na+/glucose transporter that is located in the

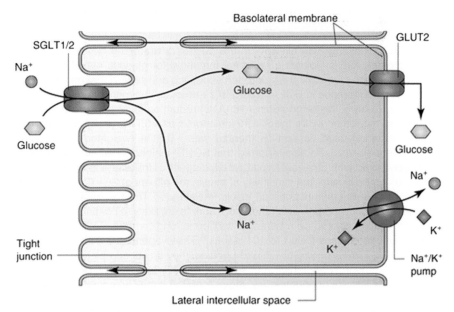

Fig. 1. Glucose reabsorption from glomerular filtrate through the proximal tubule epithelial cell into the blood. GLUT, glucose transporter protein. (*From* Bakris GL, Fonseca V, Sharma K, et al. Renal sodium-glucose transport: role in diabetes mellitus and potential clinical implications. Kidney Int 2009;75:1273; with permission.)

gastrointestinal tract and in the S3 segment of the proximal tubule. Although SGLT1 accounts for only about 10% of glucose reabsorption in the kidney it is the key transporter for glucose absorption in the gastrointestinal tract. SGLT2 is a high-capacity, low-affinity transporter found primarily in the kidney. It is the most prevalent and functionally important SGLT transporter in the kidney and accounts for approximately 90% of glucose reabsorption. This transporter is found at a high density on the lumen (brush border) membrane of the S1 segment of the proximal convoluted tubule (PCT).[1] SGLT2 binds with glucose and Na^+ in the tubular filtrate and actively transports glucose across the membrane via coupling with the transport of Na^+. This process is driven by the electrochemical Na^+ gradient between the tubular filtrate and the cell (secondary active transport).[6]

After glucose is transported via SGLT2 into the luminal epithelium it is then transported through the basolateral membrane and back into the peritubular capillary. This process of facilitated diffusion of glucose depends on another family of glucose transporter proteins (GLUTs).[3] This basolateral membrane–peritubular capillary transfer uses GLUT1 transporters in the late proximal tubule and GLUT2 transporters in the early proximal tubule.

One study evaluating the maximum rate of renal glucose reabsorption in insulin-treated patients with diabetes reported that most of the patients with diabetes (10 of 12) had higher rates of glucose reabsorption than healthy subjects.[10] One study has also suggested that there is an increase in both expression and activity of SGLT2 transporters in renal proximal tubular cells from patients with type 2 diabetes.[11]

Other SGLTs include SGLT3, SGLT4, SGLT5, and SGLT6.[1] SGLT3 is found throughout the body in skeletal muscle and the nervous system and is thought to act as a glucose sensor. Other members of this family have been identified (SGLT4, SGLT5, and SGLT6) but their function in humans is still being elucidated.

THERAPEUTIC MODULATION OF SODIUM GLUCOSE COTRANSPORTER 2 AND POTENTIAL NON-ANTIHYPERGLYCEMIC BENEFITS

Several SGLT2 inhibitors are already on the market or are being developed. These agents increase UGE by lowering the renal threshold for glucose excretion.[8] There are several reasons that make this approach appealing and several that may be cause for concern. This increase in UGE is linked to a reduction in hyperglycemia, as is discussed later. Overall, the hemoglobin A1c (A1C) reduction (difference from placebo) when used as monotherapy for the SGLT2 inhibitors was −0.79% (weighted mean difference) and when used as add-on therapy was −0.61% (weighted mean difference).[12] This meta-analysis also reported that SGLT2 inhibitors had similar glycemic efficacy compared with other antihyperglycemic agents. Unlike agents that stimulate secretion of insulin or alter the sensitivity of insulin the effects of SGLT2 inhibitors are independent of beta cell function and insulin resistance.[2] Thus as beta cell function and insulin resistance worsen over time, these agents are likely to continue to be effective, which would prove to be a benefit if verified in long-term studies. Studies have shown continued efficacy for up to 104 weeks.[8] These agents are also less likely to be linked directly to hypoglycemia, in part because they do not completely block renal glucose reabsorption. They inhibit reabsorption of 30% to 50% of filtered glucose.[8] The reasons for this are not completely understood but it may be caused by a saturation in the transport mechanism that delivers the medication to the active site. Very low rates of hypoglycemia have been reported in clinical trials with SGLT2 inhibitors except in patients receiving background insulin or sulfonylureas (SUs). A meta-analysis reported that the odds ratio for hypoglycemia in patients treated with SGLT2 inhibitors was 0.44 compared with other antihyperglycemic medications.[12]

The SGLT2 inhibitors have also been linked to weight loss. The loss in weight has been reported to be as much as 4.7 kg. Although the magnitude of weight loss varies depending on the trial, a positive effect on weight (ie, loss) has been consistently observed in multiple studies. In a trial with the thiazolidinedione (TZD) pioglitazone (which is linked to weight gain), dapagliflozin was reported to attenuate this side effect.[13] A study evaluating weight loss with SGLT2 inhibitors reported that about 66% of the weight loss linked to dapagliflozin was from fat (both visceral and subcutaneous fat).[14] The beneficial implications of weight loss in this milieu that is rich in cardiovascular disease and insulin resistance are obvious. Another potential positive aspect of SGLT2 inhibition is a mild reduction in blood pressure. A range in reduction of systolic blood pressure from 2 to 10 mm Hg has been reported in clinical trials with these agents.[8] A meta-analysis reported a weighted mean difference of -3.77 mm Hg compared with placebo and -4.45 mm Hg in evaluation against active comparators.[12]

COMMON ADVERSE EVENTS

The primary adverse events associated with SGLT2 inhibitors are urinary tract infections (UTIs), vulvovaginitis, and balanitis. In addition, because of the mechanisms of action of these agents, there was anticipation of and vigilance regarding their potential for causing hypotension secondary to osmotic diuresis.

Side effects that have been encountered in patients with glucosuria include urinary tract and other genital infections. These potential adverse events were anticipated with the SGLT2 inhibitors and have been documented. UTIs have occurred at a higher rate in patients treated with SGLT2 inhibitors in most studies.[2,8,12,15,16] The incidence of UTIs in patients treated with SGLT2s varied greatly across the published studies and was similar to placebo in some.[8] A meta-analysis of SGLT2 studies reported an odds ratio of 1.34 for the development of UTIs in patients treated with SGLT2 inhibitors versus placebo and an odds ratio of 1.42 in patients treated with SGLT2 inhibitors versus other antihyperglycemic agents.[12] Another study evaluated the overall rates of UTIs reported in 12 randomized placebo controlled trials involving dapagliflozin. The overall rates of UTIs in 3152 patients treated with dapagliflozin 2.5, 5, 10 mg, or placebo were 3.6%, 5.7%, 4.3%, and 3.7% respectively.[17] The overall rates of UTIs in 2313 patients treated with canagliflozin 100 mg, 300 mg, or placebo were 5.9%, 4.3%, and 4% respectively.[16] Across the SGLT2 inhibitors, women are linked to a higher incidence of UTIs than are men.[8] Genital infections (vulvovaginitis, balanitis, and others) also occur at a higher rate in patients treated with SGLT2 inhibitors than in those treated with placebo.[2,8,12,15,16] A meta-analysis of SGLT2 inhibitors reported an odds ratio of 3.5 for the development of genital infections in patients treated with SGLT2 inhibitors versus placebo and an odds ratio of 5.06 for the development of genital infections in patients treated with SGLT2 inhibitors versus active comparators.[12] The overall rates of genital infections in 3152 patients treated with dapagliflozin 2.5 mg, 5 mg, 10 mg, or placebo were 4.1%, 5.7%, 4.8%, and 0.9% respectively.[18] The overall rates of genital infections in 2313 patients treated with canagliflozin 100 mg, 300 mg, or placebo were 10.4%, 11.4%, and 3.2% respectively in women and 4.2%, 3.7%, and 0.6% respectively in men.[16] Overall, both UTIs and genital infections were mild and rarely resulted in discontinuation of participation from trials.[15,16]

Volume depletion leading to hypotension has also been a concern with these medications. Both package inserts from the currently marketed SGLT2 inhibitors contain warnings about this potential adverse event and suggest care with patients at high risk for side effects related to intravascular volume contraction.[15,16] The greatest increase in incidence of volume contraction–related events occurred in patients 75 years of age or older, in patients with reduced glomerular filtration rates (GFRs), and in patients treated with loop diuretics.

CANAGLIFLOZIN AND HEMOGLOBIN A1C

Canagliflozin was approved by the US Food and Drug Administration (FDA) in March 2013 and was the first SGLT2 inhibitor to be approved in the United States.[2] Canagliflozin is indicated as an adjunct to improve glycemic control in adult patients with type 2 diabetes.[16] It has been studied in patients with type 2 diabetes as monotherapy, as an add-on to metformin, in a comparison trial versus glimepiride as an add-on to metformin, as an add-on to sulfonylurea, as an add-on to sulfonylurea and metformin, in a comparison trial versus sitagliptin, as an add-on to sulfonylurea and metformin, as an add-on to metformin and pioglitazone, and as an add-on to insulin (with and without other antihyperglycemic agents). The A1C level–lowering results of some of those trials are listed in **Table 1**.[16] The baseline A1C in these trials varied but was approximately 8% in all of these phase III trials. In general, canagliflozin monotherapy as a first-line pharmacotherapeutic agent lowered A1C levels approximately 1% (compared with placebo), whereas the A1C level lowering encountered when canagliflozin was added to other agents was between 0.6% and 0.9% (compared with placebo). Its A1C level lowering was similar to that observed with glimepiride (added to metformin) and greater (−0.37% difference from sitagliptin) than that of sitagliptin

Table 1 A1C reduction: adjusted means			
Monotherapy	—	Canagliflozin 100 mg	Canagliflozin 300 mg
A1C difference from placebo (%)	—	−0.91	−1.16
Canagliflozin added to metformin	—	Canagliflozin 100 mg + metformin	Canagliflozin 300 mg + metformin
A1C difference from placebo (%)	—	−0.62	−0.77
Comparison of Glimepiride with Canagliflozin combined with Metformin	Glimepiride + metformin	Canagliflozin 100 mg + metformin	Canagliflozin 300 mg + metformin
A1C difference from glimepiride (%)	—	−0.01	−0.12
Canagliflozin vs placebo added to SU	Placebo added to SU	Canagliflozin 100 mg + SU	Canagliflozin 300 mg + SU
A1C difference from placebo (%)	—	−0.74	−0.83
Canagliflozin vs placebo added to metformin + SU	Placebo + metformin + SU	Canagliflozin 100 mg + metformin + SU	Canagliflozin 300 mg + metformin + SU
A1C difference from placebo (%)	—	−0.71	−0.92

Data from INVOKANA-canagliflozin tablet, film coated [package insert]. Janssen Pharmaceuticals; 2014. Available at: https://www.invokanahcp.com/prescribing-information.pdf. Accessed June 19, 2014.

(added to metformin and SU). It effectively lowered glycemic indices in all of the iterations of combinations studied in phase III trials.

DAPAGLIFLOZIN AND HEMOGLOBIN A1C

Dapagliflozin was approved by the FDA in January 2014 for use in adults with type 2 diabetes.[2] This compound has been approved and in use in Europe since 2012. Dapagliflozin is indicated for use as an adjunct to diet and exercise in the management of type 2 diabetes. It has been studied as monotherapy and in combination with pioglitazone, metformin, glimepiride, sitagliptin (with or without metformin), and insulin (with or without other antihyperglycemic therapy). In addition, it has been evaluated in a comparison with an SU, each added to metformin. A1C results from some of these studies are presented in **Table 2**. The baseline A1C levels in these trials varied and ranged from 7.9 to 9.2 in the phase III trials. Dapagliflozin monotherapy as a first-line pharmacotherapeutic agent lowered A1C levels by approximately 0.6% (compared with placebo), whereas the A1C reduction encountered when dapagliflozin was added to other agents ranged from 0.4% to 0.7% (compared with placebo or comparator). It effectively lowered glycemic indices in all of the iterations of combinations studied in phase III trials.

EMPAGLIFLOZIN

Empagliflozin has been extensively studied in the management of type 2 diabetes. It is the most recently approved SGLT2 inhibitor. Empagliflozin was approved for use in the European Union in May 2014 and by the FDA in August 2014.[19,20] Several of the phase III clinical trials have been published.[21–24] The A1C reduction associated with

Table 2
A1C reduction: adjusted means

Monotherapy	—	Dapagliflozin 5 mg	Dapagliflozin 10 mg
A1C difference from placebo (%)	—	−0.5	−0.7
Dapagliflozin or dapagliflozin plus metformin XR compared with metformin XR	—	Dapagliflozin 10 mg + metformin XR	Dapagliflozin 10 mg
A1C difference from metformin XR (%)	—	−0.5	−0.0
Comparison of glipizide with dapagliflozin combined with metformin	Glipizide + metformin	Dapagliflozin (up to 10 mg) mg + metformin	—
A1C difference from glipizide plus metformin (%)	—	−0.0	—
Dapagliflozin vs placebo added to SU	Placebo added to SU	Dapagliflozin 5 mg + SU	Dapagliflozin 10 mg + SU
A1C difference from placebo + SU (%)	—	−0.5	−0.7
Dapagliflozin vs placebo added to pioglitazone	Placebo + pioglitazone	Dapagliflozin 5 mg + pioglitazone	Dapagliflozin 10 mg + pioglitazone
A1C difference from placebo (%)	—	−0.4	−0.6

Abbreviation: XR, extended release.
    Data from FARXIGA-dapagliflozin propanediol table, film coated [package insert]. E.R. Squibb & Sons, LLC; 2014. Available at: http://packageinserts.bms.com/pi/pi_farxiga.pdf. Accessed June 19, 2014.

empagliflozin in these trials is similar to reductions observed with other SGLT2 inhibitors.

SODIUM GLUCOSE COTRANSPORTER 2 INHIBITORS AND RENAL DISEASE

Dapagliflozin was evaluated in patients with varying degrees of renal function.[2,15] It is not recommended for patients with moderate to severe renal disease, end-stage renal disease, or patients being managed with dialysis. In patients with significant disease, dapagliflozin is not an effective glucose level–lowering agent. A 24-week trial in 252 patients with type 2 diabetes with estimated glomerular filtration rate (eGFR) in the range of 30 to 59 mL/min/1.73 m^2 (mean 45 mL/min/1.73 m^2) it did not show efficacy as measured by A1C level for either the 5-mg or 10-mg dose. The placebo-corrected mean A1C level change was 0.1% for both doses. The presumptive reason for this lack of efficacy is that because of renal disease these patients lack an adequate renal filtered glucose load, which in turn renders the SGLT2 inhibitor ineffective.[25] Dapagliflozin may be used without dose adjustment in patients with eGFR greater than or equal to 60 mL/min/1.73 m^2.[15]

Canagliflozin was evaluated in 269 patients with type 2 diabetes with eGFR in the range of 30 to less than 50 mL/min/1.73 m^2 (mean 39 mL/min/1.73 m^2). This trial added canagliflozin (100 mg or 300 mg daily) or placebo to existing antihyperglycemic medication. At the conclusion of the trial, canagliflozin 100 mg and 300 mg resulted in reductions in A1C relative to placebo (-0.3 and -0.4, respectively).[16] However, patients with stage 3 chronic kidney disease achieved less glycemic reduction than did patients with normal renal function. In addition, these subjects experienced a higher incidence of hypovolemia and hyperkalemia. This medication has not been studied in patients with eGFR less than 30 mL/min/1.73 m^2, or end-stage renal disease, or dialysis.[2] Canagliflozin package insert guidelines suggest a dose of 100 mg daily for patients with eGFR 46 to 59 mL/min/1.73 m^2 and it is not recommended for patients with an eGFR less than 45 mL/min/1.73 m^2.[16] A dose increase to 300 mg is recommended in patients taking 100 mg per day with eGFR greater than or equal to 60 mL/min/1.73 m^2 who are also on a uridine diphosphate glucuronic acid glucuronyltransferase (UGT) inducer (discussed later) and require additional glycemic control. Patients with an eGFR of 45 to 59 mL/min/1.73 m^2 who require a UGT inducer should be treated with a different antihyperglycemic agent.

Empagliflozin pharmacokinetics were evaluated in a trial that included 40 patients with type 2 diabetes and varying levels of renal function from mild to end-stage renal disease.[26] The study concluded that a single 50-mg dose of empagliflozin was well tolerated in all subjects with normal renal function or with any degree of renal impairment. However, like other SGLT2 inhibitors, empagliflozin's glucose level–lowering efficacy is reduced as renal function declines. In patients with severe renal impairment or end-stage renal disease, UGE was changed very little after the administration of empagliflozin.

The potential for a renal protective effect associated with the use of SGLT2 inhibitors has been suggested.[27] This suggestion is based primarily on the notion that patients show a renal hyperfiltration phase with an increase in GFR that is associated with glomerular death and ultimately results in the decline of renal function. Reversing this process by use of angiotensin-converting enzyme inhibitors via reduction in glomerular pressure is used therapeutically to slow down the progression of renal decline. One study evaluated the impact of the initial decrease in GFR by angiotensin-converting enzyme inhibitors on renal outcome. There was a correlation between the magnitude of initial reduction in GFR and improved long-term renal outcomes.[28] Animal studies have shown that the nonspecific SGLT inhibitor phlorizin can reduce glomerular hyperfiltration.[27] One study in 40 patients with type 1 diabetes showed that empagliflozin was associated with a reduction in GFR in hyperfiltering patients but was associated with no change in GFR in normal-filtering patients.[29] The investigators suggested that SGLT2 inhibition may be useful in the management of diabetes-related renal disease. The SGLT2 inhibitors may be useful in this regard for several reasons. First, as mentioned earlier, they are associated with a reduction in glomerular hyperfiltration (similar to but via a different mechanism than angiotensin-converting enzyme inhibitors). Second, they are typically associated with a modest reduction in blood pressure. Third, by reducing the uptake of glucose they may protect the proximal convoluted tubules.[30] This line of investigation probably warrants more clinical trials in order to evaluate the potential efficacy and safety of this approach.

SODIUM GLUCOSE COTRANSPORTER 2 INHIBITORS AND DRUG INTERACTIONS

SGLT2 inhibitors are likely to be frequently used with multiple other medications thus the potential for drug-drug interactions (as with all medications) is present. The 3 most salient SGLT2 inhibitors (canagliflozin, dapagliflozin, and empagliflozin) have been evaluated for potential interactions with multiple medications. A review of this work was recently published.[31] These studies were in most cases performed on healthy volunteers and evaluated the potential impact of interactions after the administration of a single dose of an SGLT2 inhibitor. The exposure (as shown by concentration maximum [C_{max}] and area under the curve [AUC]) to each SGLT2 inhibitor tested was not clinically significantly altered by the concomitant administration of cardiovascular agents or antihyperglycemic medications commonly encountered in patients with type 2 diabetes (ie, metformin, glimepiride, pioglitazone, sitagliptin, linagliptin, voglibose, simvastatin, valsartan, ramipril, hydrochlorothiazide, torasemide, verapamil, warfarin; note that not all of these medications was evaluated with all three SGLT2 inhibitors). In contrast, the SGLT2 inhibitors studied did not significantly affect the pharmacokinetic parameters of the second drug studied. Dapagliflozin undergoes its primary metabolism through the UGT1A9 pathway. Because of this, dapagliflozin pharmacokinetics were evaluated with 2 potential UGT1A9 pathway modulators: rifampicin, an inducer, and mefenamic acid, an inhibitor. Rifampin coadministration with dapagliflozin resulted in a significant reduction in dapagliflozin exposure (AUC reduction of 22%). Mefenamic acid coadministration with dapagliflozin resulted in a significant increase in dapagliflozin exposure (AUC increase of 51%). Canagliflozin was evaluated in combination with rifampicin (600 mg/d for 8 days). Canagliflozin exposure was significantly reduced (AUC reduction, 51%; C_{max} reduction, 28%) after exposure to rifampin. Canagliflozin was shown to increase the AUC (20%) and the C_{max} (36%) of digoxin when the two were coadministered.[16]

   In general, the SGLT2 inhibitors seem to be subject to clinically significant interactions (except for canagliflozin and digoxin) with commonly used medications. However, care should be taken when coadministering these agents with modulators of UGT1A9. Upper-dose adjustment of the SGLT2 inhibitors dapagliflozin and canagliflozin may be needed if the patient is also treated with UGT1A9 inducers such as rifampin, phenytoin, phenobarbital, or ritonavir. It is unclear at this time whether or not UGT is involved in the metabolism of empagliflozin.

SODIUM GLUCOSE COTRANSPORTER 2 INHIBITORS AND CARDIOVASCULAR OUTCOMES TRIALS

As with all new antihyperglycemic medications the FDA is requiring that SGLT2 inhibitors undergo cardiovascular outcomes trials. Dapagliflozin is being evaluated in the

DECLARE-TIMI58 (Multicenter Trial to Evaluate the Effect of Dapagliflozin on the Incidence of Cardiovascular Events) study, which is a trial to evaluate the effect of this SGLT2 inhibitor when added to a patient's preexisting diabetes therapy on risk of CV events such as CV death, myocardial infarction, or ischemic stroke compared with placebo.[32] This is a randomized, double-blind, placebo controlled study that is expected to include more than 17,000 patients and is anticipated to be completed in 2019. CANVAS (Canagliflozin Cardiovascular Assessment Study) is a study that evaluated patients who were at risk of cardiovascular disease. The FDA allowed this study to be continued to provide evidence of cardiovascular safety. The results of this study, which will include 4330 patients, are expected to be available in 2015.[33] Some clinicians have expressed concerns about this approach (allowing interim data from a trial to be part of an initial submission and then continuing the same trial after approval for the purpose of evaluating cardiovascular safety). In addition, the impact of empagliflozin treatment on cardiovascular safety is being investigated in a dedicated cardiovascular outcomes trial (BI 10773 [Empagliflozin] Cardiovascular Outcomes Event Trial in Type 2 Diabetes Mellitus Patients). The study has enrolled 7000 patients and is expected to be completed in 2015.[34]

SODIUM GLUCOSE COTRANSPORTER 2 INHIBITION AND INTERFERENCE WITH SERUM 1,5-ANHYDROGLUCITROL

The measurement of 1,5-anhydroglucitrol (1,5-AG; GlycoMark) may be confounded by the coadministration of SGLT2 inhibitors.[35] Under usual conditions (without SGLT2 inhibition) of hyperglycemia there is an inverse relationship between mean glucose levels and 1,5-AG levels. High serum glucose levels result in significant glucose in the renal tubules. This glucose competes with 1,5-AG for reabsorption via SGLT4 transporters. High glucose levels result in greater renal excretion of 1,5-AG and hence lower serum concentrations of 1,5-AG. When patients treated with canagliflozin were evaluated their 1,5-AG concentrations were lower than those observed in the placebo group.[35] These findings of low 1,5-AG concentrations were incongruent with the improved glycemic indices observed in the patients. The study concluded that there was interference with the 1,5-AG test when used in the context of SGLT2 inhibition. It is likely that all SGLT2 inhibitors cause this interference with the interpretation of the 1,5-AG test.

OTHER SODIUM GLUCOSE COTRANSPORTER INHIBITORS IN DEVELOPMENT

In addition to the SGLT2 inhibitors mentioned earlier, several others are in development. Ipragliflozin and ertugliflozin are currently in phase III trials.[34] Three so far unnamed compounds (LX 4211, EGT0001442, GW 869682) are in phase II trials and 1 compound (ISIS 388626) is in phase 1 of development. LX 4211 is a novel agent that inhibits both SGLT1 and SGLT2.[2] Its dual mechanism, inhibition of small intestine glucose absorption and/or glucose reabsorption in the kidney, may offer benefits to SGLT2 inhibition if it is well tolerated. Studies thus far have suggested that it is well tolerated.[36,37]

SUMMARY

SGLT2 inhibition offers a novel mechanism to mitigate hyperglycemia in patients with diabetes and the introduction of SGLT2 has added a significant new tool to the antihyperglycemic armamentarium. At present, 2 agents are approved for use in the United States and several more are in development. SGLT2 inhibitors are generally associated with a reduction in A1C of between 0.5% and 1%. SGLT2 inhibitors are associated with an increased incidence of urinary tract and genital infections but these infections are typically mild, responsive to treatment, and are not use limiting.

REFERENCES

1. White J. Apple trees to sodium glucose co-transporter inhibitors: a review of SGLT2 inhibition. Clin Diabetes 2010;28(1):5–10.
2. Hasan F, Alsahli M, Gerich J. SGLT2 inhibitors in the treatment of type 2 diabetes. Diabetes Res Clin Pract 2014;104:297–322. http://dx.doi.org/10.1016/j.diabres.2014.02.014.
3. Gerich J, Woerle H. Renal gluconeogenesis: its importance in human glucose homeostasis. Diabetes Care 2001;24(2):382–91.
4. Mithieux G, Rajas F, Gautier-Stein A. A novel role for glucose 6-phosphatase in the small intestine in the control of glucose homeostasis. J Biol Chem 2004;279:44231–4.
5. Meyer C, Stumvoll M, Dostou J, et al. Renal substrate exchange and gluconeogenesis in normal postabsorptive humans. Am J Physiol Endocrinol Metab 2002;282:E428–34.
6. Wright EM. Renal N+-glucose transporters. Am J Physiol Renal Physiol 2001;280:F10–8.
7. Butterfield WJ, Keen H, Whichelow MJ. Renal glucose threshold variations with age. BMJ 1967;4:505–7.
8. Chao E. SGLT-2 inhibitors: a new mechanism for glycemic control. Clin Diabetes 2014;32(1):4–11.
9. Bakris GL, Fonseca V, Sharma K, et al. Renal sodium-glucose transport: role in diabetes mellitus and potential clinical implications. Kidney Int 2009;75:1272–7.
10. Farber S, Berger E, Earle D. Effect of diabetes and insulin on the maximum capacity of the renal tubules to reabsorb glucose. J Clin Invest 1951;30:125–9.
11. Rahmoune H, Thompson P, Ward J, et al. Glucose transporters in human renal proximal tubular cells isolated from the urine of patients with non-insulin-dependent diabetes. Diabetes 2005;54:3427.
12. Vasilakou D, Karagiannis T, Athanasiadou E, et al. Sodium-glucose cotransporter 2 inhibitors for type 2 diabetes: a systematic review and meta-analysis. Ann Intern Med 2013;159:262–74.
13. Rosenstock J, Vico M, Wei L, et al. Effects of dapagliflozin, an SGLT2 inhibitor, on HbA1c, body weight, and hypoglycemia risk in patients with type 2 diabetes inadequately controlled on pioglitazone monotherapy. Diabetes Care 2012;35:1473–8.
14. Bolinder J, Ljunggren O, Kullberg J, et al. Effects of dapagliflozin on body weight, total fat mass, and regional adipose tissue distribution in patients with type 2 diabetes mellitus with inadequate glycemic control on metformin. J Clin Endocrinol Metab 2012;97:1020–31.
15. FARXIGA- dapagliflozin propanediol table, film coated [package insert]. E.R. Squibb & Sons, LLC; 2014. Available at: http://packageinserts.bms.com/pi/pi_farxiga.pdf. Accessed June 19, 2014.
16. INVOKANA- canagliflozin tablet, film coated [package insert]. Janssen Pharmaceuticals, Inc; 2014. Available at: https://www.invokanahcp.com/prescribing-information.pdf. Accessed June 19, 2014.
17. Johnson K, Pataszynska A, Schmitz B, et al. Urinary tract infections in patients with diabetes treated with dapagliflozin. J Diabetes Complications 2013;27:473–8.

18. Johnson K, Pataszynska A, Schmitz B, et al. Vulvovaginitis and balanitis in patients with diabetes treated with dapagliflozin. J Diabetes Complications 2013; 27:479–84.

19. European Medicines Agency. EMEA/H/C/002677- Jardiance: EPAR-product information. 2014. Available at: http://www.ema.europa.eu/docs/en_GB/document_library/EPAR_-_Product_Information/human/002677/WC500168592.pdf. Accessed June 19, 2014.

20. FDA. Prescribing information: Jardiance (empagliflozin) tablets, for oral use. 2014. Available at: http://www.accessdata.fda.gov/drugsatfda_docs/label/2014/204629s000lbl.pdf. Accessed June 19, 2014.

21. Roden M, Weng J, Eilbracht J, et al. Empagliflozin monotherapy with sitagliptin as an active comparator in patients with type 2 diabetes: a randomized, double-blind, placebo-controlled, phase 3 trial. Lancet Diabetes Endocrinol 2013;1: 208–19.

22. Haring HU, Merker L, Seewaldt-Becker E, et al. Empagliflozin as add-on to metformin in patients with type 2 diabetes: a 24-week, randomized, double-blind, placebo controlled trial. Diabetes Care 2014;37(6):1650–9.

23. Haring HU, Merker L, Seewaldt-Becker E, et al. Empagliflozin as add-on to metformin plus sulfonylurea in patients with type 2 diabetes: a 24-week, randomized, double-blind, placebo-controlled trial. Diabetes Care 2013;36:3396–404.

24. Kovacs CS, Seshiah V, Swallow R, et al. Empagliflozin improves glycaemic and weight control as add-on therapy to pioglitazone or pioglitazone plus metformin in patients with type 2 diabetes: a 24-week, randomized, placebo-controlled trial. Diabetes Obes Metab 2013;16(2):147–58.

25. Kohan D, Fioretto P, List J. Efficacy and safety of dapagliflozin in patients with type 2 diabetes and moderate renal impairment. J Am Soc Nephrol 2011;232A [abstract no: TH-PO542].

26. Macha S, Mattheus M, Halabi A, et al. Pharmacokinetics, pharmacodynamics and safety of empagliflozin, a sodium glucose cotransporter 2 (SGLT2) inhibitor, in subjects with renal impairment. Diabetes Obes Metab 2014;16:215–22.

27. Stanton R. Sodium glucose transport 2 (SGLT2) inhibition decreases hyperfiltration: is there a role for SGLT2 inhibitors in diabetic kidney disease? Circulation 2014;129:542–4. http://dx.doi.org/10.1161/CIRCULATIONAHA.113.007071.

28. Holtkamp FA, de Zeeuw D, Thomas MC, et al. An acute fall in estimated glomerular filtration rate during treatment with losartan predicts a slower decrease in long-term renal function. Kidney Int 2011;80:282–7.

29. Cherney D, Perkins BA, Soleymanlou N, et al. The renal hemodynamic effect of SGLT2 inhibition in patients with type 1 diabetes. Circulation 2014. http://dx.doi.org/10.1161/CIRCULATIONAHA.113.005081.

30. Vallon T. The proximal tubule in the pathophysiology of the diabetic kidney. Am J Physiol Regul Integr Comp Physiol 2011;200:1009–22.

31. Scheen A. Drug-drug interactions with sodium-glucose cotransporters type 2 (SGLT2) inhibitors, new oral glucose-lowering agents for the management of type 2 diabetes mellitus. Clin Pharmacokinet 2014;53:295–304.

32. BMS. FDA Advisory Committee recommends the investigational SGLT2 inhibitor dapagliflozin for the treatment of type 2 diabetes in adults. 2013. Available at: http://news.bms.com/press-release/rd-news/fda-advisory-committee-recommends-investigational-sglt2-inhibitor-dapagliflozi. Accessed June 19, 2014.

33. Medscape. Experts express mixed thoughts on canagliflozin approval. 2013. Available at: http://www.medscape.com/viewarticle/782712. Accessed June 19, 2014.

34. ClinicalTrials.gov. Available at: http://clinicaltrials.gov/. Accessed June 19, 2014.
35. Balis DA, Tong C, Meininger G. Effect of canagliflozin, a sodium-glucose cotransporter 2 inhibitor, on measurement of serum 1,5-anhydroglucitol. J Diabetes 2014;6:378–81.
36. Zambrowicz B, Freiman J, Brown P, et al. LX4211, a dual SGLT1/SGLT2 inhibitor, improved glycemic control in patients with type 2 diabetes in a randomized, placebo-controlled trial. Clin Pharmacol Ther 2012;92(2):158–69.
37. Zambrowicz B, Ding ZM, Ogbaa J, et al. Effects of LX4211, a dual SGLT1/SGLT2 inhibitor, plus sitagliptin in postprandial active GLP-1 and glycemic control in type 2 diabetes. Clin Ther 2013;35(3):273–85.e7. http://dx.doi.org/10.1016/j.clinthera.2013.01.010.

Insulin Therapy in Type 1 Diabetes

Elizabeth Stephens, MD

KEYWORDS

- Insulin • Diabetes • Glucose monitoring • Hypoglycemia • Carbohydrate counting

KEY POINTS

- Intensive glucose control reduces microvascular and cardiovascular complications in those with type 1 diabetes.
- Management of type 1 diabetes requires a combination of basal and bolus insulin, administered either by injection or by continuous insulin infusion.
- Adequate glucose control requires education around the relationship between insulin, activity, food, and blood glucose levels.
- An interdisciplinary team keeps patients motivated and engaged and provides the greatest likelihood of attaining optimal glucose control.

INTRODUCTION

Multiple factors underlie the increasing importance for primary care physicians to expand their knowledge and skills in managing patients with type 1 diabetes mellitus. First, The National Health and Nutrition Examination Survey (NHANES) estimates that type 1 and type 2 diabetes now affects 21 million people in the United States; this number represents an increase in diabetes prevalence from 6.2% to 9.9% between the periods of 1988 to 1994 and 2005 to 2010 respectively.[1] The incidence of type 1 diabetes was estimated to be 40% higher in 2010 compared with 1997.[2] Because of the anticipated workforce shortage of endocrinologists, primary care physicians, who already manage nearly 40% of patients with type 1 diabetes in the United States,[3] will fill an expanded role both in initial diagnosis and care and in long-term prevention and management of diabetic complications.

Another factor important in primary care relates to the understanding of dosing of insulin in type 1 diabetes in light of the increasing complexity of insulin and delivery mechanisms. As an autoimmune disorder, type 1 diabetes destroys pancreatic beta cells, which causes children to present typically with complete beta cell failure and acute, severe hyperglycemia. In contrast, individuals with type 1 diabetes who present

Providence Medical Group NE-Medical Education, 5050 Northeast Hoyt, Suite 540, Portland, OR 97213, USA; Department of Internal Medicine, Oregon Health and Sciences University, Portland, OR, USA
E-mail address: Elizabeth.Stephens@providence.org

Med Clin N Am 99 (2015) 145–156
http://dx.doi.org/10.1016/j.mcna.2014.08.016
0025-7125/15/$ – see front matter © 2015 Elsevier Inc. All rights reserved.

in adulthood often follow a smoldering course with adequate glucose control maintained if physicians can carefully adjust low-dose insulin regimens. Eventually, however, complete insulin deficiency requires insulin replacement therapy with the twin goals of normalizing blood glucose levels while avoiding hypoglycemic episodes. The Diabetes Complications and Control Trial (DCCT) underscored the critical importance of precise insulin dosing to achieve these goals.[4] The study randomized subjects with type 1 diabetes to intensive control (target A1c 7%) or conventional treatment (target A1c 9%). After 6.5 years, the intensive therapy group had a reduced relative risk of diabetic retinopathy of 76%; for nephropathy, the same group had a reduced relative risk of 56%, and for neuropathy, it was 69%.[5] Long-term follow up of these subjects for an additional 11 years reported in the Epidemiology of Diabetes Interventions and Complications (EDIC) trial found that intensive therapy during the initial 6.5 years resulted in a long-term 42% risk reduction for any cardiovascular event and a 57% risk reduction of nonfatal myocardial infarction, stroke, or death from cardiovascular disease.[6] Unfortunately, these gains need to be balanced against the risk of hypoglycemia, which is a critical limiting factor in attaining tight glucose control in those with type 1 diabetes. Although the benefits of the DCCT were impressive, it is important to note that participants were relatively new to the diagnosis of diabetes. Severe hypoglycemia leading to seizure and loss of consciousness is strongly associated with diabetes duration[7] and necessitates less stringent glycemic targets in those with limited symptoms of hypoglycemia, especially if diabetes has been present for over 20 years.

The insulin regimens used in the DCCT and EDIC studies require primary care physicians to understand how to replicate normal insulin secretory patterns using multiple daily injections (MDI) or insulin pumps. Although these approaches are variably termed basal–bolus therapy, intensive insulin therapy (IIT), and physiologic insulin therapy, they share a common goal of dosing insulin based on glucose levels and food intake in addition to other variables, such as activity, stress, and absorption of insulin. Although seemingly complex, primary care physicians can master these advanced regimens in order to normalize glucose levels while avoiding hypoglycemia.

MANAGEMENT FRAMEWORK

Essential components of care provide a framework for developing a management strategy and a shared understanding for primary care physicians and patients with type 1 diabetes. These components include

1. A combination of basal and bolus insulin, either as a part of MDI or continuous subcutaneous insulin infusions (CSII)
2. Monitoring, including self-monitored blood glucose (SMBG) with or without continuous glucose monitoring (CGM) and hemoglobin A1c with individualized glucose targets that balance effectiveness and the risk of hypoglycemia
3. Patient education around the relationship between insulin, SMBG, activity, and food, specifically carbohydrates; issues of risk with insulin therapy also need to be discussed
4. An experienced interdisciplinary team that can facilitate overall management, insulin adjustments, goal setting, safety, education, and support

INSULIN THERAPY

Insulin replacement represents a cornerstone of management for patients with type 1 diabetes, because progressive beta cell destruction ultimately leads to total insulin deficiency. Early in the disease, patients may require total daily doses (TDD) of only .2 to .4 U/kg/d of insulin, to supplement partially impaired insulin secretion. The longer patients remain able to secrete endogenous insulin, the less subject they are to hypoglycemic episodes and the development of retinopathy.[8] Time to complete loss of insulin secretion varies. When it occurs, patients require a TDD .5 to 1.0 U/kg/d.[9] To mimic physiologic insulin secretion, both long- and short-acting insulins are used. Long-acting insulin suppresses glucose output from the liver overnight and provides basal insulin between meals; bolus doses of short-acting insulin modulate glucose excursions associated with carbohydrate consumption. See **Table 1** and **Fig. 1** for a description of currently available basal and bolus insulins and their action profiles.

Basal Insulin

The availability of multiple basal insulin formulations with varied pharmacokinetic features requires a clear understanding of their use to allow safe and effective glucose control. Although lente and ultralente were previously mainstays of therapy, they are no longer manufactured because of variable absorption and glucose effects, and the advent of more effective basal insulins. Available since 1946,[10] neutral protamine Hagedorn (NPH) remains in use, although primarily for those with type 2 diabetes. As an intermediate-acting insulin with a peak effect 6 to 10 hours after injection, NPH serves as both bolus and basal insulin. Morning NPH injections affect breakfast and lunchtime glucose levels and glucose release between meals. Evening injections provide overnight basal control, with bedtime administration reducing the risk of nocturnal hypoglycemia, as well as hyperglycemia associated with the dawn phenomenon.[11,12] Many challenges exist with NPH, including midday hypoglycemia if lunch is delayed, hyperglycemia with excessive ingestion of carbohydrate at mid-day, and predinner hyperglycemia due to the waning effect of morning NPH injection. Despite these limitations, NPH remains an acceptable alternative for patients who cannot afford newer insulin analogs. The introduction to the United States in 2001 of glargine as a basal insulin provided a more stable and physiologic insulin effect as compared with NPH. The onset of action occurs 2 to 3 hours after injection, but glargine is notable for not having a peak effect, thereby reducing risk of nocturnal hypoglycemia, especially when dosed at bedtime.

Table 1
Currently available insulin options

	Onset	Peak	Duration	Cost[a]-Vial (10 mL)	Cost-Pens (5 Pens/15 mL)
Basal insulin options					
NPH	1–2 h	4–10 h	10–16 h	$100 ($25 at Walmart)	$330
Detemir	2–4 h	No peak	14–20 h	$203	$318
Glargine	2–4 h	No peak	20–24 h	$207	$337
Bolus insulin options					
Regular	30–60 min	2–4 h	4–8 h	$100 ($25 at Walmart)	N/A
Aspart, glulisine, lispro	5–15 min	1–2 h	3–5 h	$180	$340

[a] Costs are approximate from Costco.com and GoodRx.com.
   Courtesy of Jonathan R. White, PharmD, BCPS, BCACP, Clinical Pharmacy Specialist, Providence Medical Group.

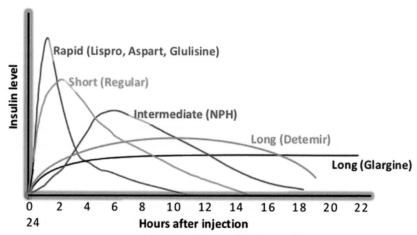

Fig. 1. Action profiles of insulins. (*From* Inzucchi SE, Bergenstal RM, Buse JB, et al. Management of hyperglycemia in type 2 diabetes: A patient-centered approach. Diabetes Care 2012;35:1364–79 [data supplement]; with permission.)

Compared with NPH, studies of subjects with type 1 diabetes note decreased frequency of hypoglycemia and less weight gain with glargine[13-16] but similar effects on A1c.[13] Insulin glargine's peakless profile provides a cleaner basal effect, which probably limits weight gain by decreasing a need for snacking between meals and at bedtime, which is needed in response to the relative hyperinsulinemia from NPH.

Insulin detemir is the second available long-acting insulin analog, which also reduces hypoglycemia risk compared with NPH.[17] Acylated with a fatty acid chain, insulin detemir binds to albumin, prolonging its effect compared with other analogs,[18] while also leading to weaker effects on glucose and lipid metabolism compared with glargine.[19] The binding of detemir leads to a shorter effect and higher dosing requirements; some patients may need twice-daily administration.[20]

Bolus Insulin

Many options exist for bolus insulin. Regular insulin has been a mainstay for decades but has significant limitations. Hampered by its tendency to self-associate into hexamers after injection, regular insulin diffuses slowly into the circulation,[21] necessitating injections 20 to 30 minutes before meals in order to match insulin action to carbohydrate absorption. In real life, this 30-minute lag time is inconvenient for patients who do not adhere to consistent mealtimes, which is the reality for 30% to 70% of patients.[22,23]

Consequently, the rapid-acting insulin analogs, which include insulins lispro, aspart, and glulisine, are generally preferred in type 1 diabetes. These insulins, by virtue of their amino acid structural changes, remain monomeric following injection, giving them a more rapid onset of effect that allows their injection 10 to 15 minutes before, during, or immediately after meals.[21] One meta-analysis of 1400 patients demonstrated that insulin lispro reduces the frequency of severe hypoglycemic events by 25% compared with regular insulin.[24] Insulins lispro and aspart also provide better control of postprandial hyperglycemia and glucose variability compared with regular insulin.[21] Interestingly, despite these improvements in convenience and glucose control, meta-analyses have reported only a small benefit in A1c with use of rapid-acting insulin analogs.[25]

Dosing Regimens

Determination of initial insulin doses for a newly diagnosed patient with type 1 diabetes starts with estimation of the TDD, provided as 50% basal and 50% bolus insulin.[26] Initially, most patients require low doses of .2 to .4 U/kg/d, which increase over time as endogenous insulin secretion declines so that ultimately doses of .5 to 1.0 U/kg/d comprise the average TDD. Basal insulin with insulin glargine or detemir is dosed once or twice daily. Previously administered at night to better match glucose elevations with the dawn phenomenon, recent studies note that basal dosing can be equally effective when given either in the morning, evening, or as a split dose,[27] providing flexibility of dosing and promoting adherence. For insulin-sensitive patients, splitting basal insulin into twice-daily dosing may reduce the risk of hypoglycemia that could occur with a single larger dose. When transitioning from NPH to a long-acting analog, decreasing the basal dose by 20% to reduce the risk of hypoglycemia is worth considering.[3] Physicians must remind patients that the long-acting analogs cannot be mixed with other bolus insulins.

Many alternative strategies exist for determining bolus insulin doses. One option is carbohydrate counting, which is the most physiologic approach. Using this method, individuals are taught how to estimate carbohydrate content in certain foods by either reading labels or measuring. Estimation of a carbohydrate ratio is the next step, where insulin is taken for a certain number of carbohydrate grams. A typical algorithm uses a factor of 1 U of insulin for every 15 g of carbohydrate consumed, with the patient then dividing the total amount of carbohydrate in a meal by the factor to determine the dose of insulin. Dosing insulin in this manner provides flexibility to meet variation in meal timing and content and has been shown to reduce A1c by 0.7%, and the frequency of severe hypoglycemic events.[28] For patients who find this strategy too complex, an alternative approach is to maintain a consistent carbohydrate diet and match the meal insulin dose to the carbohydrate consumed. This method has also been shown to improve glucose control.[29]

Patients should also receive education around on how to add an extra amount of bolus insulin to their calculated premeal insulin doses in response to elevated blood glucose levels measured before meals or snacks. Commonly this extra dose, called supplemental or correctional insulin, is a ratio of 1 U for every 50 mg/dL. Effective use of supplemental insulin also requires a targeted premeal glucose goal, which is often set at 100 mg/dL. See **Table 2** for an example of dosing insulin using these factors.

Patients should also receive education in avoiding insulin stacking, which is the administration of any insulin doses at too short of intervals in response to between meal elevations in blood glucose.[26] Generally, glucose levels increase 30 to 50 mg/dL above the premeal level in the 2 hours after eating if the insulin dose is correct for the meal. When the measured glucose between meals is higher than anticipated, patients may incorrectly administer a full dose of supplemental insulin calculated by the desired reduction in blood glucose. Because the insulin administered before the meal has a duration of action of 4 to 6 hours, this supplement after the meal may stack onto the residual premeal insulin dose, causing hypoglycemia. Patients may reduce this risk by decreasing the calculated correctional insulin dose by 50% when it is administered less than 3 hours after the premeal bolus dose.[3] **Table 2** includes an example of this adjustment for review.

Exercise presents a special challenge in type 1 diabetes, because strenuous activity during severe insulin deficiency can cause hyperglycemia due to release of counter-regulatory hormones, as well as delayed hypoglycemia due to increased insulin

Table 2
Examples of insulin dosing calculations

Case	Factors	Calculations	Doses
Eating meal of 45 g of carbohydrate, and premeal glucose value 200 mg/dL	Carbohydrate ratio: 1 U meal insulin for every 15 g of carbohydrate	For carbohydrate: 45 ÷ 15 = 3	The patient would need 3 U for carbohydrate and 2 U for supplemental insulin, leading to a total premeal dose of 5 U
	Supplemental factor: 1 U meal insulin lowers glucose level by 50 mg/dL, with premeal target of 100 mg/dL	For supplemental: 200 − 100 = 100; 100 ÷ 50 = 2	
Checking glucose 2-h after eating out at a restaurant, and uncertain about carbohydrate content; blood glucose now is 300 mg/dL	Correction factor: 1 U meal insulin lowers glucose level by 50 mg/dL, premeal goal of 100 mg/dL	Current SMBG 300 − 100 = 200 200 ÷ 50 = 4 U, reduced by 50% since between meals to 2 U	Because 2 h after eating, patient would take 50% of recommended correction to reduce stacking risk, it would take 2 U bolus insulin

sensitivity in the hours after activity.[30] Because patients are encouraged to exercise for better glucose control, they may become frustrated by these exercise-related glucose excursions. Weight loss can also be a struggle due to more frequent hypoglycemia following exercise. Adjustments in meal insulin can be helpful, with 1 option being a decrease in the premeal dose by 50% to 75% if the exercise occurs in the 1 to 3 hours after a meal. No adjustment may be necessary if the activity is later in the postprandial period.[31,32]

Insulin Pump Therapy

Insulin pumps or CSII are attractive alternatives for type 1 diabetes management, because they deliver insulin in a more physiologic and accurate manner compared with MDI.

CSII consists of small, portable devices that provide insulin delivery 24 hours a day though a catheter placed subcutaneously by the patient or family member. Changed every 2 to 3 days, the catheter is inserted in the same areas where injections are usually administered, including the abdomen, buttocks, thighs, and upper arms.[33] Insulins aspart, lispro, and glulisine are most commonly infused. The pump delivers both basal and bolus, with the option to adjust basal doses to meet variable needs and administer bolus insulin before meals using carbohydrate counting and calculated glucose corrections. The bolus calculator is a useful feature of CSII, which incorporates carbohydrate ratios and correction factors, to calculate a suggested insulin dose based on carbohydrate eaten and glucose levels.[34] The active insulin feature assists to recommend adjustments in doses based on previous boluses, in an effort to reduce the risk of stacking.

CSII has many advantages, but success with pump therapy depends on a careful matching of the patient with the right technology. A history of poor glucose control represents the main indication for pump therapy. The technology can be especially effective for patients with higher baseline A1c values,[35] but less so for those with tighter glucose control. One review noted CSII lowered A1c values by .3% to .6% compared with MDI, and also resulted in a 10% to 20% reduction in insulin doses.[34,36] Hypoglycemia frequency is reduced with CSII,[37] likely because of more consistent insulin absorption from infusion sites compared with MDI,[38] as well as the ability to deliver more accurate, small insulin doses for insulin-sensitive patients. Pumps may also better match insulin dosing with changing schedules, activity, and mealtimes.[38] A 2010 Cochrane review noted that CSII showed improvements in quality of life, overall health, and satisfaction compared with MDI.[39] A review of indications for pump therapy is listed in **Box 1**.

Before making the transition to a pump, patient expectations need clarification. Blood glucose monitoring still needs to occur, and patients need to carry supplies in the event of pump malfunction. Concerns regarding an increased risk for diabetic ketoacidosis with pump diminish with appropriate patient education. Infusion site infections are uncommon with adequate site preparation.[40] Cost of insulin pump therapy represents is a prominent limitation, with current insulin pumps costing $5000 to $7000, and pump supplies costing up to $2500 per year.[34] Despite this, compared with MDI, CSII has been shown to be a cost-effective option.

Risks of Intensive Therapy

Although clinical trials demonstrate IIT reduces diabetic complications, use of MDI or CSII to achieve this level of control presents risks for hypoglycemia, weight gain, and worsening of retinopathy. Hypoglycemia has become increasingly problematic now that patients survive longer with their diabetes. IIT can lower glucose levels closer to normal, thereby reducing the glucose level at which hypoglycemia becomes symptomatic. As the glucose levels persist near normal, the brain becomes more efficient in extracting glucose. Although this response is desirable, it may impair catecholamine release in response to hypoglycemia and the patient's recognition of early symptoms.[41] Moreover, frequent episodes of hypoglycemia can lead to hypoglycemia unawareness (HU), in which symptoms are diminished or absent, leading to crises with loss of consciousness or seizures. Observation of adults with type 1 diabetes in the T1D Exchange Registry[7] have noted higher frequency of severe hypoglycemia associated with lower socioeconomic status and diabetes duration, especially when present for over 20 years. Hypoglycemia has been associated with death in 6% to 10% of patients with type 1 diabetes, likely because of arrhythmias.[42]

Glucose monitoring, especially before activities like driving, should be encouraged in those with more frequent hypoglycemia. Increasing blood glucose goals can also be helpful to decrease frequency and severity of hypoglycemia. Symptoms of hypoglycemia can often be restored by avoiding low glucose levels for 2 to 3 weeks, allowing recovery of autonomic axes.[43]

Weight gain due to a combination of reduced glycosuria and hypoglycemia can present a barrier to IIT. In the DCCT, intensively treated participants gained on average 4.5 kg more than those in the conventional arm.[4] To manage weigh gain, education

---

Box 1
Indications for insulin pump therapy in type 1 diabetes

1. Persistent elevation in A1c despite adjustments in MDI and ongoing patient education

2. Continued hypoglycemia despite adjustments in MDI and ongoing patient education

3. Significant insulin sensitivity, where .5 to 1 U dosing amounts often result in significant glucose excursions/hypoglycemia

4. To get to glucose/A1c goal in those attempting pregnancy, who are unable with MDI

is provided about food choices, reduction in hypoglycemia frequency, and use of insulin analogs such as insulin detemir, which has been associated with slightly less weight gain.[16]

Diabetic retinopathy may progress after rapid correction of hyperglycemia, with the greatest risk seen in those with A1c greater 10% when there is underlying retinopathy. To prevent deterioration of retinopathy, a gradual correction in A1c by 2% per year and twice-yearly evaluation by an ophthalmologist to monitor for changes should be considered.[3]

MONITORING

Monitoring allows patients to achieve their glucose goals. The American Diabetes Association (ADA) recommends that individuals on MDI or CSII consider monitoring glucose levels before meals and snacks, occasionally postprandially, at bedtime, prior to exercise, in response to suspected hypoglycemia, and prior to tasks such as driving.[44] Adherence to these recommendations may require monitoring glucose levels up to 6 to 10 times per day. To ensure the value of this time-consuming and expensive effort, patients need to know how to respond to the glucose data. The ADA guidelines recommend a preprandial glucose goal of 70 to 130 mg/dL, and a glucose goal 1 to 2 hours after a meal of less than 180 mg/dL. Controversy exists however, regarding postprandial monitoring. Although postprandial hyperglycemia is associated with endothelial dysfunction, which is a surrogate marker for vascular disease,[45] glucose corrections with supplemental insulin after meals often lead to hypoglycemia. Encouraging patients to eat more complex carbohydrates may reduce the postprandial hyperglycemia associated with eating simple starches. Also, patients should consider postprandial glucose monitoring when they are uncertain about the carbohydrate amount in a meal, and administer supplemental insulin cautiously.

Variability of glucose levels can be identified and managed more efficiently with the use of CGM. CGM includes a sensor that is inserted subcutaneously to measure interstitial glucose levels every 5 minutes and transmits the data either to a separate receiver or insulin pump. These data are available to the user, who can anticipate changes missed with traditional SMBG, and respond to set alarms when glucose levels rise above or drop below preset targets. Studies comparing these devices with SMBG report variable results, with A1c improvements of .53% shown in 1 study,[46] and a small, but significant reduction of A1c by .26% without reductions in hypoglycemia frequency in another meta-analysis.[47] Currently a CGM-augmented pump is available, bringing a closed-loop system closer. This device will suspend insulin delivery for up to 2 hours, when persistent hypoglycemia occurs. Use of these augmented pumps has been shown to be effective in reducing the duration and frequency of severe hypoglycemia.[48,49]

Finally, in regards to monitoring, the A1c should be measured 2 to 4 times per year depending on patient status, glucose levels, and changes in therapy. A goal of less than 7% is recommended for most patients with type 1 diabetes given the findings from the DCCT and EDIC that showed reductions in complications with this level of control.[6] A higher A1c target for patients with frequent hypoglycemia and longer duration of diabetes should be considered.[7]

EDUCATION AND WORKING WITH A TEAM

A diabetes team assists in the management of patients with type 1 diabetes. Ideally the team should include a provider with experience in IIT, a dietitian to provide education around carbohydrate counting, and a mental health provider to identify and manage depression, which is commonly associated with diabetes.[50] Diabetes teams also include family members, interested friends, and/or a support group to motivate patients to maintain the higher level of self-care required and assist when life challenges interfere. The Internet may provide assistance for patients in rural areas who are distant from teams. Organizations such as the ADA (http://www.diabetes.org) and the Juvenile Diabetes Research Foundation (http://jdrf.org) have resources specific to type 1 diabetes, as well as active online communities and blogs. A listing of useful sites is available at www.healthline.com. Phone apps can assist with record keeping and carbohydrate counting in addition to other details in management.

SUMMARY

Although not curable, type 1 diabetes is eminently controllable. IIT, as guided by the results of landmark studies such as the DCCT, provides primary care providers with a blueprint for reducing the frequency of the devastating complications of diabetes that were all too common in the recent past. Considering the remarkable advances in contemporary therapy, including MDI and CSII, the likelihood of even greater future improvements in quality of life and survivability can be anticipated. Success requires patient engagement and education, an informed primary care provider, and an interdisciplinary team to maximize the benefits of insulin therapy and avoid the risks of hypoglycemia.

REFERENCES

1. Selvin E. Trends in prevalence and control of diabetes in the United States, 1988-1994 and 1999-2010. Ann Intern Med 2014;160(8):517–25.
2. Onkamo P. Worldwide increase in incidence of type I diabetes—the analysis of the data on published incidence trends. Diabetologia 1999;42(12):1395–403.
3. DeWitt DE, Hirsch IB. Outpatient insulin therapy in type 1 and type 2 diabetes mellitus: scientific review. JAMA 2003;289(17):2254–64.
4. The effect of intensive treatment of diabetes on the development and progression of long-term complications in insulin-dependent diabetes mellitus. The Diabetes Control and Complications Trial Research Group. N Engl J Med 1993; 329(14):977–86.
5. Writing team for the Diabetes, Control and Complications Trial/Epidemiology of Diabetes Interventions, and Complications Research Group. Effect of intensive therapy on the microvascular complications of type 1 diabetes mellitus. JAMA 2002;287(19):2563–9.
6. Nathan DM. Intensive diabetes treatment and cardiovascular disease in patients with type 1 diabetes. N Engl J Med 2005;353(25):2643–53.
7. Weinstock RS. Severe hypoglycemia and diabetic ketoacidosis in adults with type 1 diabetes: results from the T1D Exchange clinic registry. J Clin Endocrinol Metab 2013;98(8):3411–9.
8. Steffes MW. Beta-cell function and the development of diabetes-related complications in the diabetes control and complications trial. Diabetes Care 2003; 26(3):832–6.
9. Hirsch IB. Intensive treatment of type 1 diabetes. Med Clin North Am 1998; 82(4):689–719.
10. Deckert T. Intermediate-acting insulin preparations: NPH and lente. Diabetes Care 1980;3(5):623–6.
11. Fanelli CG. Administration of neutral protamine Hagedorn insulin at bedtime versus with dinner in type 1 diabetes mellitus to avoid nocturnal hypoglycemia

and improve control. A randomized, controlled trial. Ann Intern Med 2002; 136(7):504–14.

12. Pampanelli S. Long-term intensive insulin therapy in IDDM: effects on HbA1c, risk for severe and mild hypoglycaemia, status of counterregulation and awareness of hypoglycaemia. Diabetologia 1996;39(6):677–86.

13. Ratner RE. Less hypoglycemia with insulin glargine in intensive insulin therapy for type 1 diabetes. U.S. Study Group of Insulin Glargine in Type 1 Diabetes. Diabetes Care 2000;23(5):639–43.

14. Vague P. Insulin detemir is associated with more predictable glycemic control and reduced risk of hypoglycemia than NPH insulin in patients with type 1 diabetes on a basal-bolus regimen with premeal insulin aspart. Diabetes Care 2003;26(3):590–6.

15. Rosenstock J. Basal insulin therapy in type 2 diabetes: 28-week comparison of insulin glargine (HOE 901) and NPH insulin. Diabetes Care 2001;24(4):631–6.

16. De Leeuw I. Insulin detemir used in basal-bolus therapy in people with type 1 diabetes is associated with a lower risk of nocturnal hypoglycaemia and less weight gain over 12 months in comparison to NPH insulin. Diabetes Obes Metab 2005;7(1):73–82.

17. Owens DR, Bolli GB. Beyond the era of NPH insulin–long-acting insulin analogs: chemistry, comparative pharmacology, and clinical application. Diabetes Technol Ther 2008;10(5):333–49.

18. Havelund S. The mechanism of protraction of insulin detemir, a long-acting, acylated analog of human insulin. Pharm Res 2004;21(8):1498–504.

19. Porcellati F. Comparison of pharmacokinetics and dynamics of the long-acting insulin analogs glargine and detemir at steady state in type 1 diabetes: a double-blind, randomized, crossover study. Diabetes Care 2007;30(10): 2447–52.

20. Heller S, Koenen C, Bode B. Comparison of insulin detemir and insulin glargine in a basal–bolus regimen, with insulin aspart as the mealtime insulin, in patients with type 1 diabetes: a 52-week, multinational, randomized, open-label, parallel-group, treat-to-target noninferiority trial. Clin Ther 2009;31(10):2086–97.

21. Hirsch IB. Insulin analogues. N Engl J Med 2005;352(2):174–83.

22. Lean ME, Ng LL, Tennison BR. Interval between insulin injection and eating in relation to blood glucose control in adult diabetics. Br Med J (Clin Res Ed) 1985;290(6462):105–8.

23. Sackey AH, Jefferson IG. Interval between insulin injection and breakfast in diabetes. Arch Dis Child 1994;71(3):248–50.

24. Brunelle BL. Meta-analysis of the effect of insulin lispro on severe hypoglycemia in patients with type 1 diabetes. Diabetes Care 1998;21(10):1726–31.

25. Siebenhofer A. Short acting insulin analogues versus regular human insulin in patients with diabetes mellitus. Cochrane Database Syst Rev 2006;(2):CD003287.

26. DeWitt DE, Dugdale DC. Using new insulin strategies in the outpatient treatment of diabetes: clinical applications. JAMA 2003;289(17):2265–9.

27. Garg SK. Improved glycemic control without an increase in severe hypoglycemic episodes in intensively treated patients with type 1 diabetes receiving morning, evening, or split dose insulin glargine. Diabetes Res Clin Pract 2004;66(1): 49–56.

28. Samann A. Glycaemic control and severe hypoglycaemia following training in flexible, intensive insulin therapy to enable dietary freedom in people with type 1 diabetes: a prospective implementation study. Diabetologia 2005; 48(10):1965–70.

29. Rabasa-Lhoret R. Effects of meal carbohydrate content on insulin requirements in type 1 diabetic patients treated intensively with the basal-bolus (ultralente-regular) insulin regimen. Diabetes Care 1999;22(5):667–73.

30. Guelfi KJ. Effect of intermittent high-intensity compared with continuous moderate exercise on glucose production and utilization in individuals with type 1 diabetes. Am J Physiol Endocrinol Metab 2007;292(3):E865–70.

31. Rabasa-Lhoret R. Guidelines for premeal insulin dose reduction for postprandial exercise of different intensities and durations in type 1 diabetic subjects treated intensively with a basal-bolus insulin regimen (ultralente-lispro). Diabetes Care 2001;24(4):625–30.

32. Tuominen JA. Exercise-induced hypoglycaemia in IDDM patients treated with a short-acting insulin analogue. Diabetologia 1995;38(1):106–11.

33. Scheiner G. Insulin pump therapy: guidelines for successful outcomes. Diabetes Educ 2009;35(Suppl 2):29S–41S [quiz: 28S, 42S–43S].

34. Pickup JC. Insulin-pump therapy for type 1 diabetes mellitus. N Engl J Med 2012;366(17):1616–24.

35. Pickup JC. Determinants of glycaemic control in type 1 diabetes during intensified therapy with multiple daily insulin injections or continuous subcutaneous insulin infusion: importance of blood glucose variability. Diabetes Metab Res Rev 2006;22(3):232–7.

36. Switzer SM. Intensive insulin therapy in patients with type 1 diabetes mellitus. Endocrinol Metab Clin North Am 2012;41(1):89–104.

37. Pickup JC, Sutton AJ. Severe hypoglycaemia and glycaemic control in type 1 diabetes: meta-analysis of multiple daily insulin injections compared with continuous subcutaneous insulin infusion. Diabet Med 2008;25(7):765–74.

38. Weissberg-Benchell J, Antisdel-Lomaglio J, Seshadri R. Insulin pump therapy: a meta-analysis. Diabetes Care 2003;26(4):1079–87.

39. Misso ML. Continuous subcutaneous insulin infusion (CSII) versus multiple insulin injections for type 1 diabetes mellitus. Cochrane Database Syst Rev 2010;(1):CD005103.

40. Bruttomesso D, Costa S, Baritussio A. Continuous subcutaneous insulin infusion (CSII) 30 years later: still the best option for insulin therapy. Diabetes Metab Res Rev 2009;25(2):99–111.

41. Boyle PJ. Adaptations leading to hypoglycaemia in type 1 diabetes mellitus and comparison with type 2 diabetes mellitus. Int J Clin Pract Suppl 2000;(112):39–44.

42. Cryer PE. Death during intensive glycemic therapy of diabetes: mechanisms and implications. Am J Med 2011;124(11):993–6.

43. Seaquist ER. Hypoglycemia and diabetes: a report of a workgroup of the American Diabetes Association and the Endocrine Society. Diabetes Care 2013;36(5):1384–95.

44. American Diabetes Association. Standards of medical care in diabetes–2014. Diabetes Care 2014;37(Suppl 1):S14–80.

45. Ceriello A. Evidence for an independent and cumulative effect of postprandial hypertriglyceridemia and hyperglycemia on endothelial dysfunction and oxidative stress generation: effects of short- and long-term simvastatin treatment. Circulation 2002;106(10):1211–8.

46. Tamborlane WV, Beck RW. Continuous glucose monitoring in type 1 diabetes mellitus. Lancet 2009;373(9677):1744–6.

47. Yeh HC. Comparative effectiveness and safety of methods of insulin delivery and glucose monitoring for diabetes mellitus: a systematic review and meta-analysis. Ann Intern Med 2012;157(5):336–47.

48. Bergenstal RM. Threshold-based insulin-pump interruption for reduction of hypoglycemia. N Engl J Med 2013;369(3):224–32.
49. Ly TT. Effect of sensor-augmented insulin pump therapy and automated insulin suspension vs standard insulin pump therapy on hypoglycemia in patients with type 1 diabetes: a randomized clinical trial. JAMA 2013;310(12):1240–7.
50. Anderson RJ. The prevalence of comorbid depression in adults with diabetes: a meta-analysis. Diabetes Care 2001;24(6):1069–78.

Insulin Tactics in Type 2 Diabetes

Farah Meah, DO, Rattan Juneja, MBBS, MD, MRCP (UK)*

KEYWORDS

- Type 2 diabetes • Insulin secretion • Exogenous insulin profiles
- Insulin administration • Insulin adjustment • Noninsulin therapy

KEY POINTS

- Type 2 diabetes is a multifactorial disease comprising insulin resistance, relative insulin deficiency, increased hepatic glucose output, and increased renal glucose reabsorption, which together result in failure to maintain normal glucose homeostasis.
- Therapeutic interventions for Type 2 diabetes include lifestyle modifications, noninsulin drugs, and insulin therapy.
- Although insulin can be used as stand-alone therapy, it is more commonly used as add-on to other noninsulin agents.
- Insulin treatment in Type 2 diabetes is generally instituted with basal insulin alone and intensified to basal plus bolus insulin regimens if glycemic goals are not achieved.
- Self-monitored blood glucose (SMBG) testing is critical in guiding the titration of insulin treatment.
- The addition of newer noninsulin drugs to previous insulin treatment may allow for partial or complete reduction of the insulin.
- Patient education by a multidisciplinary treatment team that includes diabetes educators is helpful in maximizing efficacy and minimizing adverse events related to the use of insulin.

INTRODUCTION

Type 2 diabetes (T2D) is a heterogeneous disorder in which multiple pathophysiologic defects result in an imbalance between the rate of glucose production (which is increased) and its disposal (which is decreased) resulting in hyperglycemia (**Fig. 1**). Among the defects is insulin resistance, leading to decreased glucose uptake by peripheral tissues (predominantly the muscles) and an increase in hepatic glucose production (gluconeogenesis). Compounding this are defects in incretin hormones,

Disclosures: Past speaker for Astra Zeneca, Boehringer Ingelheim, Eli Lilly, Merck, Janssen (R. Juneja); Nothing to disclose (F. Meah).
Division of Endocrinology, Indiana University School of Medicine, 541 Clinical Drive, CL 365, Indianapolis, IN 46202, USA
* Corresponding author.
E-mail address: rajuneja@iu.edu

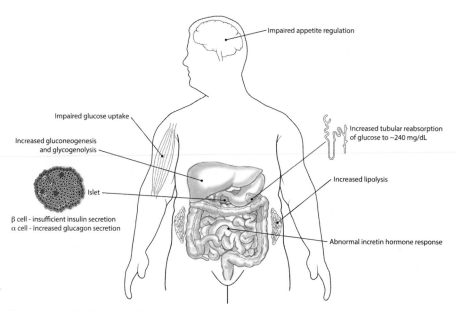

Fig. 1. Pathophysiologic defects in T2D.

resulting in decreased postprandial insulin release by the beta (β) cells accompanied by a failure to suppress glucagon by the alpha (α) cells, resulting in postprandial hyperglycemia and continued release of glucose from hepatic glycogen stores (glycogenolysis).[1] Furthermore, there is increased renal tubular reabsorption of glucose due to upregulation of sodium glucose co-transporters-2 (SGLTs-2) and a β-cell deficiency secondary to a decrease in its numbers, mass, and function.[1,2] All these factors together increase the workload of the β cell, which can, over time, lead to its exhaustion, implying that insulin therapy might be an inevitable consequence of long-standing T2D.[3–5]

Therapy with insulin, however, has challenges, because unlike most other drugs, it needs to be dosed in synergy with the peaks and troughs of glucose. Commercially available insulin, however, does not share the physiologic properties of endogenous insulin. It is therefore important to understand the pharmacokinetic properties of insulin preparations and to time the dose of the insulin to meet the needs of the patient. In this article, we discuss strategies of how to introduce insulin as a treatment option in patients with T2D and how to decrease it when other noninsulin drugs are added to the treatment.

Physiology of Insulin Production

Insulin secretion in the nondiabetic individual

Following an overnight fast, the liver of nondiabetic individuals produces glucose at a rate of approximately 2.0 mg/kg/min (**Fig. 2**).[1] The kidneys reabsorb most of this glucose, based on a physiologically set renal threshold of approximately 180 mg/dL, resulting in less than 0.5 g of glucose being excreted per day.[1,6] This glucose (referred to as basal glucose) is metabolized by a steady production of basal insulin by the β cell and euglycemia is maintained. With an oral load of glucose, such as during a meal, additional bolus (also referred to as prandial) insulin is secreted by the β cells (**Fig. 3**) to help in its metabolism.

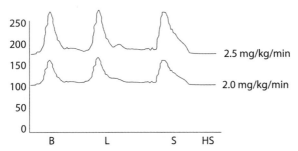

Fig. 2. Endogenous glucose production of the nondiabetic and the diabetic individual. Compared with nondiabetic individuals who produce glucose at a rate of 2.0 mg/kg/min, hepatic glucose output in diabetic individuals is increased to a rate of 2.5 mg/kg/min. In addition, in response to an oral glucose load, diabetic individuals experience a greater rise in glucose related to insufficient insulin production. B, breakfast; L, lunch; S, supper/dinner; HS, bedtime.

As seen in **Fig. 4**, insulin (along with C-peptide) packaged in membrane-bound storage granules in the pancreatic β cell, is released into the portal circulation in a pulsatile and biphasic manner when stimulated by rising glucose.[7] The first phase of insulin release (FPIR) is steep, with an onset in 1 minute and lasting 5 to 10 minutes.[8] It is believed that this FPIR reflects the immediate discharge of primed and docked insulin from secretory vesicles due to direct stimulation by glucose and indirectly through the production of intestinal incretin hormones.[1] This first phase is followed by a second phase of insulin release, which is gradual, and most likely requires mobilization of secretory insulin granules to the cell membrane before their discharge.[7] Once released, insulin enters the portal circulation and is cleared by the liver. The concentration of insulin in the portal vein therefore is twofold to fourfold higher than in the peripheral circulation.[9] This higher concentration of insulin in the portal vein is important in suppressing hepatic glucose production; an important attribute of endogenously produced insulin. When administered exogenously (ie, as a drug), insulin enters the peripheral circulation directly, bypassing the portal circulation, creating an insulin gradient in which peripheral hyperinsulinemia is necessary to suppress hepatic

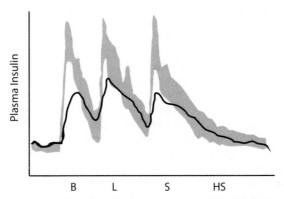

Fig. 3. Endogenous insulin production of the nondiabetic and the diabetic individual. Pulsatile endogenous insulin production in the nondiabetic individual (*gray shaded areas*) closely maintains euglycemia during and between meals. In the diabetic individual (*black lines*), FPG is elevated, as there is insufficient basal insulin production by the pancreatic β cell. In addition, there is insufficient mealtime insulin production due to a blunted FPIR and incretin hormone defects. B, breakfast; L, lunch; S, supper/dinner; HS, bedtime.

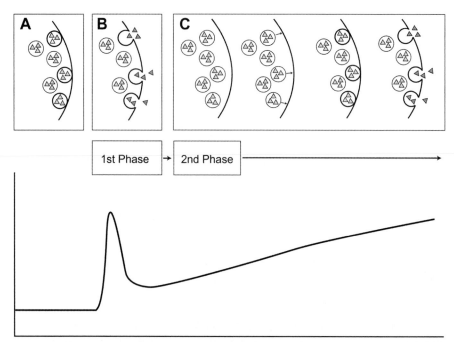

Fig. 4. The first and second phases of insulin secretion. Insulin (Δ) is packaged in membrane-bound insulin secretory granules in the pancreatic β cell. (*A, B*) The steep first-phase insulin response reflects the immediate discharge of primed and docked insulin from secretory vesicles due to direct stimulation by glucose and indirectly through intestinal incretin hormones. The second phase of insulin release is gradual and requires mobilization of insulin secretory granules to the cell membrane before their discharge (*C*).

glucose production.[9] This explains why high doses of exogenous insulin are often required in patients with insulin resistance.

Insulin secretion in individuals with type 2 diabetes

In patients with T2D, hepatic glucose output is increased to 2.5 mg/kg/min secondary to multiple defects, as discussed previously (see **Figs. 2** and **3**).[1] In addition, the renal threshold in T2D can be increased up to 240 mg/dL due to upregulation of SGLT-2 transporters,[6,10] resulting in the kidneys reabsorbing excessive amounts of glucose (see **Fig. 1**), further adding to the hyperglycemia.

Normally, the β cell responds to an increment change in glucose (ΔG) with an increment change in insulin (ΔI). With increasing insulin resistance, the β cell increases its secretion. This changing insulin response to changing insulin sensitivity forms a hyperbolic relationship termed the disposition index and can be used to provide an assessment of β-cell function (**Fig. 5**).[11–13] At any given insulin sensitivity, the capacity of the β cell can be measured by exposing it to an intravenous glucose challenge: the Acute Insulin Response to Glucose (AIR$_{glucose}$). As seen in **Fig. 5**, patients who can maintain adequate β-cell secretion, such as those with polycystic ovarian syndrome might not progress to hyperglycemia despite substantial insulin resistance.[12,13] If, however, the AIR$_{glucose}$ decreases with increasing insulin resistance, patients progress from normal glucose tolerance to impaired glucose tolerance and eventually T2D. Relative insulin deficiency is therefore a key pathophysiological defect in T2D and exogenous insulin therapy becomes a therapeutic option for all patients.

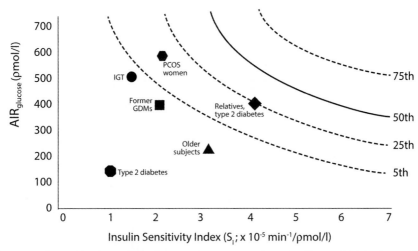

Fig. 5. Insulin sensitivity and insulin secretion. At any given insulin sensitivity, the residual capacity of the β cell can be measured by exposing it to an intravenous glucose challenge called the Acute Insulin Response to Glucose (AIRglucose). If the AIRglucose decreases with increasing insulin resistance, patients progress from normal glucose tolerance to impaired glucose tolerance, and eventually T2D. Patients who can maintain adequate β-cell secretion, such as those with polycystic ovarian syndrome, might not progress to hyperglycemia despite substantial insulin resistance. (*From* Kahn SE. The relative contributions of insulin resistance and beta-cell dysfunction to the pathophysiology of Type 2 diabetes. Diabetologia 2003;46(1):7; with permission.)

GUIDELINES FOR INITIATION OF INSULIN IN TYPE 2 DIABETES

Before one can initiate insulin (or any drug therapy) in a patient with diabetes, it is critical that goals of treatment are established. The first of these goals is the trigger for initiation of a new drug. The second goal is to set parameters under which therapy needs to be advanced either with the same drug or with the addition of new agents.

The trigger to initiate drug therapy can be either the hemoglobin A1c (HbA1c) or self-monitored blood glucose values (SMBG). In general, it is easiest to use HbA1c as the trigger for initiation of therapy; a parameter used by most guidelines. SMBG can then be used to modify the initiated therapy.

The most commonly used guidelines for the treatment of T2D used in the United States come from the American Diabetes Association (ADA) (**Fig. 6**)[14] and the American Association of Clinical Endocrinologists (AACE) (**Fig. 7**).[15] The ADA guidelines recommend a target HbA1c of 7.0% or lower in most patients. More stringent HbA1c targets of 6.0% to 6.5% are recommended in patients with short disease duration, long life expectancy, and no significant history of cardiovascular disease; provided these goals can be achieved without adverse effects (particularly hypoglycemia). Less-stringent HbA1c targets of 7.5% to 8.0% are recommended in patients with long disease duration, short life expectancy, history of severe hypoglycemia, advanced complications, extensive comorbid conditions, and in patients difficult to control despite intensive education (see **Fig. 6**). With these guidelines, following metformin (MET) monotherapy as first line, the addition of a second drug is recommended if HbA1c is not at goal after 3 months. Importantly, besides HbA1c-lowering ability, the ADA guidelines recommend consideration to cost, effect on weight, hypoglycemia risk, and potential for side effects when making the choice of second agent, with basal

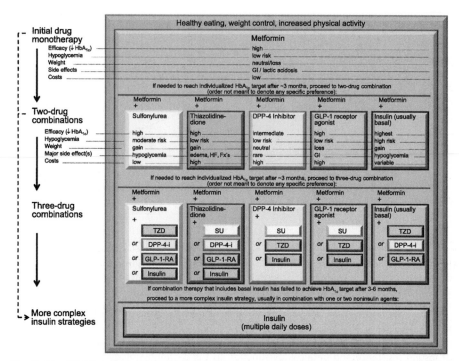

Fig. 6. The ADA treatment algorithm for T2D. These guidelines recommend MET monotherapy followed by addition of agents every 3 months if HbA1c is not at goal. Basal insulin can be used as a second-line agent. The guidelines recommend taking into consideration efficacy, hypoglycemia risk, effect on weight, side-effect profile, and cost when making a choice of drug. (*From* the American Diabetes Association. Standards of medical care in diabetes—2014. Diabetes Care 2014;37(Suppl 1):S14; with permission.)

insulin being one of the choices (see **Fig. 6**). After 3 to 6 months of a 2-drug regimen, if HbA1c targets are still not achieved, the guidelines recommend addition of a third noninsulin agent or intensification of insulin therapy if already initiated.[14]

The AACE treatment algorithm also uses HbA1c as a guide to therapy; however, they recommend a more stringent goal of 6.5% or lower for most patients. In addition, these guidelines use baseline HbA1c itself as *the trigger for choosing the number of drugs* with which to start therapy (see **Fig. 7**). With the AACE guidelines, for patients with baseline HbA1c less than 7.5%, monotherapy with any of the approved noninsulin agents is considered appropriate. For patients with baseline HbA1c between 7.5% and 9.0%, these guidelines recommend a 2-drug approach with MET plus another agent from a different class, including basal insulin. For patients with a baseline HbA1c higher than 9.0%, the AACE guidelines recommend initiating therapy with an aggressive 2-drug or in some cases even a 3-drug approach, and in severely symptomatic patients they recommend having insulin be one of these agents. Once treatment is initiated, these guidelines go on to recommend an aggressive 3-monthly up-titration of therapy with the addition of additional drugs if HbA1c targets of 6.5% or lower are not achieved.[15]

Our own approach is a hybrid of the ADA and AACE guidelines. As initial therapy, we prefer a "MET Plus" approach; maximizing MET over a period of 1 month to 2000 mg per day or the maximum tolerated dose followed by the addition of a second noninsulin agent in 1 to 3 months irrespective of HbA1c. If MET is contraindicated or not tolerated,

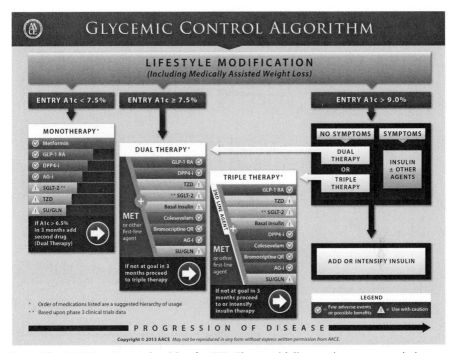

Fig. 7. The AACE treatment algorithm for T2D. These guidelines make recommendations on the choice and number of agents based on baseline HbA1c. (*From* American Association of Clinical Endocrinologists. Garber AJ, Abrahamson MJ, Barzilay JI, et al. AACE comprehensive diabetes management algorithm. Endocr Pract 2013;19:6; with permission.)

we use one of the other noninsulin oral agents from the AACE guidelines as first line.[15] We use this approach to address the multiple pathophysiological defects of T2D[1] because we have found that single-drug approaches generally fail to maintain HbA1c over time similar to what has been observed in the UK Prospective Diabetes Study and A Diabetes Outcome Progression Trial (ADOPT) Study.[16,17] Our choice of second drug is based on the criteria of cost, hypoglycemia risk, weight-losing properties, and side-effect profiles as proposed by the ADA (**Fig. 8**).[14] If a 2-drug regimen is ineffective in maintaining HbA1c, a third drug from a different class can be added. We, however, wait 6 to 12 months before proceeding from a 2-drug to a 3-drug regimen. Waiting for this period is particularly helpful when using agents that can result in weight loss; therapies that have the potential to continue to modify the diabetes disease process by reducing insulin resistance. In addition, it can take up to 6 months or longer for a newly diagnosed patient to truly affect lifestyle changes, which may also alter the need for additional medications. Unless there is severe and symptomatic hyperglycemia, we try different combinations of noninsulin agents for a period of 12 to 24 months before considering insulin. We initiate insulin therapy earlier if weight loss has stabilized but hyperglycemia persists or if weight loss continues in the setting of sustained hyperglycemia, indicating an insulin-deficient, catabolic state. We also consider insulin as a treatment option at the time of diagnosis of T2D for those patients who have severe symptoms of polyuria and polydipsia and especially those with excessive weight loss. In these individuals and in patients who do not manifest the typical features of metabolic syndrome, such as low high-density lipoprotein levels, high triglycerides, or hypertension, it may be appropriate to test for immune markers of Type 1 diabetes,

Approach to management of hyperglycemia:

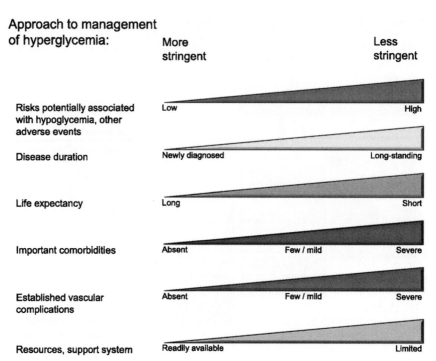

Fig. 8. ADA approach to management of hyperglycemia. Multiple factors contribute to the decision of which therapy to add to the therapeutic regimen in the treatment of T2D. Elements toward the left justify more stringent glycemic efforts, whereas those toward the right justify less-stringent efforts. (*From* the American Diabetes Association. Standards of medical care in diabetes—2014. Diabetes Care 2014;37(Suppl 1):S12; with permission.)

such as Glutamic Acid Decarboxylase (GAD) antibodies, to rule out the possibility of Latent Autoimmune Diabetes of the Adult (LADA), a condition not typically prone to ketoacidosis that can be managed initially with noninsulin therapy but may, in 6 to 12 months after diagnosis, require insulin to maintain glycemic goals.[18,19]

ROLE OF SELF-MONITORED BLOOD GLUCOSE IN ACHIEVING GLYCEMIC GOALS

Although HbA1c is typically measured every 90 days, it can be checked every 30 days in the early stages of therapy to monitor response. However, once insulin (or any non-insulin therapy) has been initiated, we find SMBG to be most helpful in guiding titration. Particularly in the early stages of insulin therapy, it is helpful for patients to monitor glucose fasting, before meals, and at bedtime to gauge an understanding of glycemic control. The ADA guidelines recommend a goal fasting plasma glucose (FPG) of less than 130 mg/dL and 2-hour post-prandial glucose (2h-PPG) less than 180 mg/dL[14] whereas the AACE guidelines recommend a goal FPG less than 110 mg/dL and 2h-PPG less than 140 mg/dL,[15] if these goals can be achieved safely without hypoglycemia. Once glycemic goals have been achieved, then checking SMBG 2 to 3 times daily (one must be fasting) may be adequate. PPG testing may be helpful in individuals on basal-bolus insulin therapy to help assess the adequacy of the chosen insulin-to-carbohydrate ratio (ICR) (discussed later).

It is important to keep in mind that SMBG goals chosen for the patient must be congruent with HbA1c targets for that patient. As seen in **Table 1**, for every 29-mg/dL

Table 1
Estimated average blood glucose (eAG) and hemoglobin A1c (HbA1c)

Hemoglobin A1c, %	Blood Glucose (range), mg/dL	Blood Glucose (range), mmol/L
5	97 (76–120)	5.4 (4.2–6.7)
6	126 (100–152)	7.0 (5.5–8.5)
7	154 (123–185)	8.6 (6.8–10.3)
8	183 (147–217)	10.2 (8.1–12.1)
9	212 (170–249)	11.8 (9.4–13.9)
10	240 (193–282)	13.4 (10.7–15.7)
11	269 (217–314)	14.9 (12.0–17.5)
12	298 (240–347)	16.5 (13.3–19.3)

Adapted from Nathan DM, Kuenen J, Borg R, et al. Translating the A1C assay into estimated average glucose values. Diabetes Care 2008;31(8):1473–8.

increase in blood glucose (BG), HbA1c goes up by approximately 1%.[20] This relationship between HbA1c and BG is referred to as the estimated Average Glucose (eAG), and most validated laboratory assays for HbA1c now report an eAG result as well. Explaining this relationship to patients is helpful, because they can correlate their SMBG data with HbA1c goals.[20]

CHOOSING AN INSULIN PREPARATION

Because the basis of insulin therapy is to try to match the onset of insulin action, its peak, and duration with the onset, peak, and duration of its need to metabolize glucose, if there is a mismatch between glucose levels and the actions of the injected insulin, either hyperglycemia persists or hypoglycemia can result. Because the pharmacokinetic properties of exogenously administered insulin (when the insulin peaks) do not always match the pharmacodynamic needs of the body (when the insulin should peak), it is critical to understand the properties of different insulin preparations and choose a product based on the glycemic needs of the patient (**Fig. 9**, **Tables 2 and 3**).[21–23]

Human Insulin Preparations

The earliest insulins were derived from animal pancreas. These extracts had significant variability in their onset, peak, and duration of action depending on purification

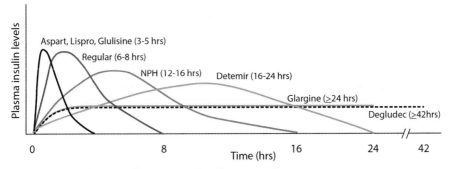

Fig. 9. Pharmacokinetics of exogenous insulin preparations.

Table 2
Pharmacokinetics of insulin preparations

Insulin	Onset	Peak	Duration of Action	Trade Name	Shelf Life (Days) After Opened	Manufacturer
Short-acting						
Human Regular	30–60 min	2–4 h	6–8 h	Humulin R	Vial (31) ΩΨ	Eli Lilly
				Novolin R	Vial (42) ΩΨ	Novo Nordisk (Bagsvaerd, Denmark)
Rapid-acting						
Lispro	5–15 min	0.5–1.5 h	3–5 h	Humalog	Vial (28)ΩΨ Pen (28)Ψ	Eli Lilly (Indianapolis, USA)
Aspart				NovoLog	Vial (28)ΩΨ Pen (28)Ψ	Novo Nordisk (Bagsvaerd, Denmark)
Glulisine				Apidra	Vial (28)ΩΨ Pen (28)Ψ	Sanofi (Bridgewater, USA)
Intermediate-acting						
NPH	1–2 h	6–12 h	12–16 h	Humulin N	Vial (31)ΩΨ Pen (14)Ψ	Eli Lilly (Indianapolis, USA)
				Novolin N	Vial (42)ΩΨ Pen (14)Ψ	Novo Nordisk (Bagsvaerd, Denmark)

	Onset	Peak	Duration	Brand	Supply	Manufacturer
Long-acting						
Glargine	1 h	Peakless	≥24 h	Lantus	Vial (28)ΩΨ Pen (28)Ψ	Sanofi (Bridgewater, USA)
Detemir	1 h	Peakless	16–≥24 h	Levemir	Vial (42)ΩΨ Pen (42)Ψ	Novo Nordisk (Bagsvaerd, Denmark)
Degludec[a]	0.5–1.5 h	Peakless	>42 h	Tresiba	Not Available in the US	Novo Nordisk (Bagsvaerd, Denmark)
Premixed						
70/30 NPH/Regular	30–60 min	Dual	10–16 h	Humulin 70/30	Vial (31)ΩΨ Pen (10)Ψ	Eli Lilly (Indianapolis, USA)
				Novolin 70/30	Vial (42)ΩΨ Pen (10)Ψ	Novo Nordisk (Bagsvaerd, Denmark)
75/25 NPL/Lispro	5–15 min	Dual	12–20 h	Humalog Mix 75/25	Vial (28)ΩΨ Pen (10)Ψ	Eli Lilly (Indianapolis, USA)
50/50 NPL/Lispro	5–15 min	Dual	12–20 h	Humalog Mix 50/50	Vial (28)ΩΨ Pen (10)Ψ	Eli Lilly (Indianapolis, USA)
70/30 NPA/Aspart	5–15 min	Dual	12–20 h	NovoLog Mix 70/30	Vial (28)ΩΨ Pen (14)Ψ	Novo Nordisk (Bagsvaerd, Denmark)
70/30 Degludec/Aspart[a]	5–15 min	Dual	>24 h	Degludec Plus 70/30	Not Available in the U.S.	Novo Nordisk (Bagsvaerd, Denmark)

Abbreviations: NPA, neutral protamine aspart; NPH, neutral protamine Hagedorn; NPL, neutral protamine Lispro; Ω, refrigerate; Ψ, room temperature.
[a] Insulin Degludec and Degludec/Aspart are not approved for use in the United States.
Adapted from Skyler JS. Insulin treatment. In: Lebovitz HE, editor. Therapy for diabetes mellitus and related disorders. 5th edition. Alexandria (Egypt): American Diabetes Association; 2009. p. 273–89.

Table 3
Important facts and caveats regarding insulin preparations

Insulin	US Trade Name	Insulin Type	Timing or Frequency of Injection	Characteristics
Short-acting insulin				
Regular	Humulin R Novolin R	Human	30–60 min before each meal	• Tends to self-associate into hexameric aggregates but subsequent to subcutaneous injection, disassociates in the interstitium to dimers, then monomers, which explains delayed absorption[25] • Activity profile is dose-dependent • Provides some basal coverage because still has activity after food has been absorbed • Can result in postprandial hypoglycemia due to sustained action
Rapid-acting insulin				
Lispro Aspart Glulisine	Humalog NovoLog Apidra	Analog	15 min before meal up to 15 min after meal	• Forms hexameric aggregates in solution; however, subsequent to subcutaneous injection, quickly disassociates into the active monomeric form[25] • No change in dose needed if switching among the rapid-acting insulins
Intermediate-acting insulin				
NPH	Humulin N Novolin N	Human	Daily-twice a day	• Delayed absorption due to the addition of protamine and zinc • Can be mixed with prandial insulins • Activity profile is dose-dependent, meaning the higher the dose, the broader the peak, and the longer the duration of action • Greater risk of afternoon and nocturnal hypoglycemia
Long-acting insulin				
Glargine	Lantus	Analog	Daily	• Solubilized in acidic pH; precipitates in neutral subcutaneous tissue pH once injected forming hexamers, which slowly disassociate, thereby prolonging action • Can sting on injection due to acidic pH (pH 4)
Detemir	Levemir	Analog	Daily-twice a day	• Omission of threonine at position B30 and acylation with a 14-carbon fatty acid to lysine at position B29 facilitates albumin binding, which prolongs action • Dose-dependent duration of action thus dosed twice daily at smaller doses (<20–30 units) but once daily at larger doses (>0.4 U/kg) • Reduced insulin receptor affinity and metabolic potency, thus slightly higher doses may be required[26]
Degludec[a]	Not available in the US	Analog	Daily	• Omission of threonine at position B30 and acylation with a 16-carbon fatty acid to lysine at position B29 facilitates albumin binding, which prolongs action[27] • Exists as dihexamers; however, forms long multihexamers subsequent to subcutaneous injection with subsequent slow release of monomers into the circulation[22] • Has displayed flexibility in that time of injection can vary from day to day[22]

[a] Insulin Degludec is not approved for use in the United States.

techniques. They also had a propensity to induce anti-insulin antibodies[24] and have since been phased out in the United States. Now, with recombinant DNA technology, the human insulin gene can be introduced into yeast or *Escherichia coli*, which then secrete insulin with the same amino acid sequence as native human insulin; this is the predominant form of insulin in the world. These recombinant DNA–produced insulins are collectively referred to as *Human Insulin* and broadly, there are 2 types: a short-acting product called human regular insulin (Regular) and an intermediate-acting product called neutral protamine Hagedorn (NPH) insulin (see **Fig. 9**, **Tables 2** and **3**).

Short-acting human regular insulin

Human regular insulin is a short-acting insulin that, when injected, tends to self-associate to form hexameric aggregates in the presence of zinc.[25] These hexamers slowly disassociate into dimers, then monomers, which are the active form of the insulin (**Fig. 10**). This disassociation takes time, which explains the need to administer this insulin approximately 30 to 45 minutes before meals. The typical activity profile of human regular insulin is displayed in **Fig. 9**. However, it is important to keep in mind that the activity profile of human regular insulin is also dose-dependent; the higher the dose, the slower is the onset of action (sometimes up to 60 minutes), the broader the peak (2–3 hours), and the longer the duration of action (up to 3–6 hours). Because the time to peak and duration of action do not replicate endogenous bolus insulin secretion, it is a disadvantage for most patients when used at mealtimes.

Intermediate-acting neutral protamine Hagedorn insulin

NPH is an intermediate-acting insulin that has delayed absorption kinetics due to the addition of protamine and zinc. It has an onset of action in 1 to 2 hours, broad peak at 6 to 12 hours, and duration of action of 12 to 16 hours. It is a cloudy suspension and, to prevent variability in its absorption, it must be gently rolled in the palms of the hands 15 to 20 times to resuspend it before injection.

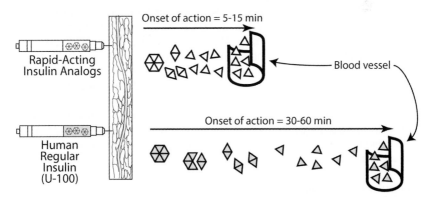

Fig. 10. Dissociation and absorption of human regular compared with rapid-acting analog insulin. Human regular insulin tends to self-associate to form hexameric aggregates in the presence of zinc. After subcutaneous injection, these hexamers slowly disassociate into dimers, then monomers, which are the active form of insulin. The onset of action is slow and human regular insulin must be administered approximately 30 to 45 minutes before meals. Rapid-acting insulin analogs also exist in hexameric aggregates in solution; however, have a low tendency to self-aggregate subsequent to subcutaneous injection. Once injected, they quickly disassociate into the active monomeric form. The onset of action is therefore quick, allowing this insulin to be given approximately 15 minutes before and up to approximately 15 minutes after the meal is consumed.

NPH should typically be dosed twice daily, once with breakfast and again with dinner or at bedtime to provide continuous basal coverage, although it is sometimes used only once a day in clinical practice. When used twice a day, the morning dose peaks in the afternoon, which can result in hypoglycemia, particularly if lunch is delayed or skipped. The dinner or bedtime dose peaks during sleep. This nocturnal peak is a reason to recommend SMBG testing at approximately 3 AM, especially when a dose change is made.

Analog Insulin Preparations

Because recombinant human insulins do not replicate physiologic insulin production, with amino acid substitutions in the human insulin molecule, insulin pharmacokinetics can be modified to facilitate more physiologic action profiles. These modified peptides are called analog insulins, of which there are 2 types: rapid-acting analogs, generally used for meal coverage (and insulin pump therapy), and long-acting products for basal coverage (see **Fig. 9**, **Tables 2** and **3**).

Rapid-acting analog insulins

The main objective with a rapid-acting analog insulin is to make the onset of action quick. This allows the insulin to be injected closer to the meal or in some cases even immediately after the meal has been consumed. Unlike human regular insulin, with rapid-acting analogs, active monomers are formed quickly after subcutaneous injection, allowing this insulin to be given approximately 15 minutes before and up to approximately 15 minutes after the meal is consumed, (see **Fig. 10**). This profile better matches the time course of carbohydrate absorption from the gut thus overcoming the main disadvantage of human regular insulin, which needs to be dosed well in advance of the meal. There are 3 rapid-acting analog products available in the United States, which are interchangeable with each other (see **Tables 2** and **3**).

Long-acting (basal) analog insulins

For basal insulin coverage, a key requirement is to have an insulin that does not have a peak and lasts at least 24 hours. Two analog basal insulin products are available in the United States: glargine and detemir.[26] With amino acid changes that are made to create insulin glargine, it has to be solubilized at an acidic pH of 4.0. This creates microprecipitates of the insulin when injected into neutral pH subcutaneous tissue, slowly releasing monomeric insulin, thus prolonging and flat lining its action over 24 hours (see **Fig. 9**). Detemir on the other hand is acylated with a 14-carbon fatty acid, facilitating albumin binding, which prolongs its action.[27] An ultra-long-acting basal insulin analog, degludec, with a duration of action greater than 24 hours, is also available in some countries, but is currently not approved for use in the United States (see **Tables 2** and **3**).[22,27]

Other Insulin Preparations

Premixed insulin

Premixed insulin is a combination product of intermediate-acting insulin with human regular or a rapid-acting analog in fixed proportions. The main advantage of these insulins is the convenience of fewer injections in patients on basal-bolus therapy. However, titration is not easy because changes occur in both the intermediate and short/rapid-acting insulin when doses are titrated. Human insulin containing premixed products must be injected 30 to 40 minutes before a meal, whereas the analog insulin containing premixed products can be injected in the 15-minute window around the meal (see **Table 2**).[28,29]

Highly concentrated (U-500) insulin

When first isolated from animal pancreatic extract in 1922, 1 unit of insulin (US Pharmacopeia) was defined as the amount of insulin that will lower the glucose of a healthy 2-kg (4.4-lb) rabbit that has fasted for 24 hours to 45 mg/dL (2.5 mmol/L) within 4 hours.[30] When first commercialized in 1923, the concentration of insulin was 20 units in 1 mL (U-20). Subsequently, more concentrated insulins were produced: U-40, U-80, and currently U-100, which is the most common concentration worldwide. A U-200 concentration of degludec is also available, but not in the United States.[22]

For patients with severe insulin resistance, very high doses of insulin could be needed. The large volume of U-100 insulin required for such patients may be painful and impractical. In such a circumstance, a highly concentrated insulin containing 500 units/mL (Humulin R U-500; Eli Lilly and Company, Indianapolis, USA) is available. This preparation is made from human regular insulin and should be reserved for patients requiring more than 200 units of insulin per day and those with a good understanding of self-management principles. It should be prescribed only by providers who are trained in its safe use. Special caution is required for this insulin to be used in the hospital due to the possibility of an error.

INSULIN-DELIVERY DEVICES

Insulin can be dispensed in vials, pens, or with pumps. When dispensed in a vial, there is usually 1000 units/10 mL; whereas in pens, 300 units per device. **Table 4** summarizes the advantages and disadvantages of the various insulin-administration devices.[31,32]

INITIATING INSULIN THERAPY IN TYPE 2 DIABETES

The overarching goal with insulin therapy is to mimic physiologic insulin profiles, with basal insulin to suppress overnight and between-meal hepatic glucose production and bolus insulin to account for meal excursions (**Figs. 11–17**).[33] Much of the actual insulin tactics discussed here are anecdotal, although more recently some guidelines are evolving from experience in clinical trials.[14,15,34,35]

Approaches Using Basal Insulin

We generally follow the ADA guidelines for the introduction of basal insulin after failure of 2 or more noninsulin agents, as discussed previously, and AACE guidelines on titration/intensification, as shown in **Fig. 11**.[14,15] These guidelines have been developed from studies such as the treat-to-target trial, which showed that the addition of a single dose of basal insulin (NPH or glargine) was effective in achieving a target HbA1c of less than 7.0%. One critical element of the treat-to-target trial was a forced titration algorithm,[36] which highlighted the importance of regular and sustained efforts at adjusting doses of the insulin to predetermined glycemic goals. We prefer a long-acting basal analog over NPH insulin because of its sustained action over 24 hours and less risk of afternoon and nocturnal hypoglycemia (see **Figs. 12** and **13**). If there is concern for nocturnal hypoglycemia, 3 AM SMBG values should be checked, especially when using NPH insulin. In most circumstances, at the time of basal insulin initiation, ongoing noninsulin therapies are not discontinued. Although there is some controversy whether secretagogues, especially sulfonylureas should be continued when insulin is started, our approach is to stop these medications only when we introduce bolus insulin.

Numerous studies have shown that glycemic goals can be achieved when patients are given guidance and autonomy in managing their own insulin dose titration.[37–39] We strongly endorse such empowerment. We however feel the 2-day to 3-day schedule suggested in the AACE guidelines (see **Fig. 11**)[15] is too aggressive for self-titration

Table 4
Advantages and disadvantages of insulin delivery devices

Delivery Device	Advantages	Disadvantages	Additional Information
Vials/Syringes	• Least-expensive insulin delivery device	• Patient has to draw up insulin before injection with a syringe, which requires good visual acuity and dexterity	• U-100 vials are available in 10 mL (containing 1000 units of insulin) or less commonly in 3 mL (containing 300 units). The latter is primarily for hospital use • Syringe sizes: 3/10 mL (30 units) with $1/_2$-unit markings, 3/10 mL (30 units) with 1-unit markings, $1/_2$-mL (50 units) syringe with 1-unit markings, and 1-mL (100 units) syringe with 1-unit markings • Needle lengths: 5 mm, 8 mm, 12 mm
Pens	• Easy to use, dose set by turning the dial, more consistent subcutaneous insulin delivery than syringe • Preferred device for most patients	• More expensive than insulin vials	• U-100 pens are available in 3 mL (containing 300 units of insulin) • Pen needle lengths: 4 mm, 5 mm, 8 mm, 12 mm • Maximum dose of insulin per injection is 60–80 units (depending on pen)
Insulin pump	• Useful for patients who desire very tight control of BG • Fewer injections	• No basal insulin depot, so high risk of DKA if pump fails requires meticulous monitoring of BG and self-management skills on the part of the patient	• Some pumps connect to the body with tubing (such as Medtronic, Animas, Accucheck); however, a tubeless pump is available (OmniPod)[32]
Insulin patch	• Disposable, 24-h use • No batteries, syringes, or needles needed	• Fixed doses, therefore tight glycemic control may not be possible	• Only 1 product V-Go produced by Valeritas[31] • Available in 3 preset basal insulin devices: the V-Go 20 (20 units/24 h or 0.83 U/h), the V-Go 30 (20 units/24 h or 1.25 U/h), and the V-Go 40 (40 units/h or 1.67 U/h) • Each push of the bolus button releases 2 units of insulin with a maximum of 36 units per use

Abbreviations: BG, blood glucose; DKA, diabetic ketoacidosis.

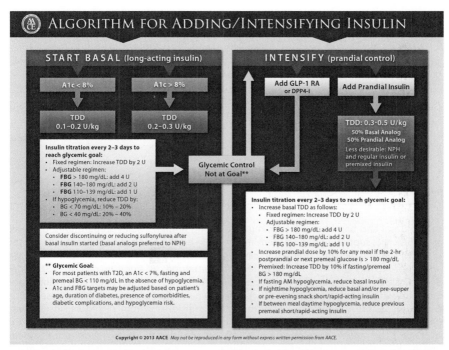

Fig. 11. AACE algorithm for initiation and modification of insulin therapy. These guidelines provide guidance on the starting dose of basal insulin based on body weight. In the event of hypoglycemia, a decrease of the total daily dose is recommended. If glycemic goals are being achieved, intensification to a basal-bolus regimen with titration based on SMBG is the next step. (*From* American Association of Clinical Endocrinologists, Garber AJ, Abrahamson MJ, Barzilay JI, et al. AACE comprehensive diabetes management algorithm. Endocr Pract 2013;19:7; with permission.)

and prefer a 5-day to 7-day schedule instead. Like the treat-to-target trial, we use a mean of the last 3 days of FPG as a guide to dose adjustment.[36] Once insulin is initiated, it is important for the physician to monitor the patient's progress every 1 to 2 weeks for the first month and then biweekly for the next 1 to 2 months, at which time the patient should be reevaluated in the clinic. We pick a maximum daily basal insulin dose, generally 30 to 40 units a day, at which time if FPG goals have not been achieved, we ask the patient to return to the clinic for an evaluation. At the visit, we reassess the patient's understanding of self-management, with particular attention to insulin-injection techniques and compliance. We then determine if therapy needs to be modified with the addition of or changes to noninsulin drugs or if the addition of bolus insulin is necessary.

Approaches Using Bolus Insulin

It is uncommon to use bolus insulin alone in the treatment of T2D; such therapy is usually added on to basal insulin. Some of the triggers[15,40,41] that can be used to consider adding bolus insulin include 50% of the total daily dose of insulin (TDD) is reached with basal insulin alone but before-meal targets are still not being achieved; FPG is at target, however HbA1c is still above target; FPG is at target, but 2h-PPG after breakfast is elevated; there is sustained bedtime hyperglycemia (BG >180 mg/dL); or high-dose glucocorticoid therapy is added in individuals with uncontrolled T2D (see **Fig. 14**).

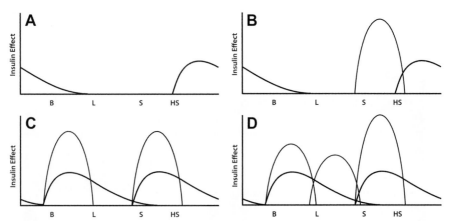

Fig. 12. Basal and basal-bolus insulin regimens using human insulin preparations. B, break-fast; L, lunch; S, supper/dinner; HS, bedtime. (*A*) NPH insulin alone at bedtime. As seen in this figure, NPH alone has the potential to cause nocturnal hypoglycemia at its peak action and it does not provide coverage for the entire 24-hour period. (*B*) Addition of 1 dose of human regular insulin with the largest meal to bedtime NPH. This regimen helps cover dinner and also helps with bedtime targets. However, the human regular insulin must be dosed 30 to 45 minutes before the meal. (*C*) Addition of 2 fixed doses of human regular insulin with NPH before breakfast and supper. As seen in the figure, this regimen produces a gap in coverage if the patient were to consume lunch. In addition, because the dose of the meal-time insulin is fixed, the amount of carbohydrate consumed also needs to be fixed to match the injected insulin dose. (*D*) Addition of flexible (carbohydrate-based) doses of human regular insulin with each meal with NPH before breakfast and supper. Although this regimen allows for variable amounts of carbohydrates with each meal, the protracted duration of action of the regular insulin results in an overlap (stacking) of the insulin doses. Patients also need to learn to count carbohydrates.

Generally, the total daily dose consists of 50% basal and 50% bolus insulin. With the initiation of bolus insulin, therefore, the basal insulin may need to be decreased by 10% to 20% to prevent fasting hypoglycemia. If FPG is already at target, a greater reduction in the basal insulin may be necessary.

There are 2 broad approaches to bolus insulin therapy in T2D. The first approach is to start with fixed doses of mealtime insulin and then adjust based on 2h-PPG or the blood glucose immediately before the next meal. For this fixed dose approach, we follow AACE guidelines for initiation, as shown in **Fig. 11**. The second approach is based on counting carbohydrates, which is more complex but provides more precise mealtime insulin dosing and allows patients the flexibility to adjust insulin to varying amounts of carbohydrates (see **Figs. 12**D and **13**D). Although the complexity of the carbohydrate-counting approach has been called into question in patients with T2D, in our clinical experience it remains a valuable tool for patients and both this approach and the fixed-dose approach can achieve similar glycemic goals.[42] With either approach it is important to assess meal patterns so as to choose the best initial regimen.

Dose with largest meal or high carbohydrate-containing meals
For patients who consume 1 large meal or 1 carbohydrate-rich meal, a single dose of prandial insulin can be added to the meal with the greatest glucose excursion (see **Figs. 12**B and **13**B).

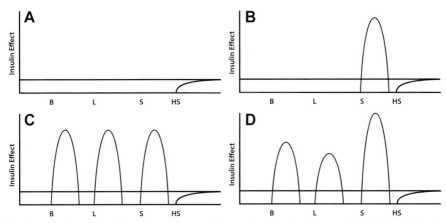

Fig. 13. Basal and basal-bolus regimens using analog insulin preparations. B, breakfast; L, lunch; S, supper/dinner; HS, bedtime. (*A*) Long-acting basal insulin analog alone at bedtime. As seen in this figure, unlike with NPH insulin (see **Fig. 12**A), a single dose of a long-acting analog insulin given once a day has the potential to provide consistent basal insulin coverage for the entire day. (*B*) Addition of 1 dose of rapid-acting analog insulin with the largest meal to bedtime long-acting analog insulin. Unlike with human regular insulin (see **Fig. 12**B), a rapid-acting analog can be administered with the meal and also helps achieve bedtime targets. (*C*) Addition of fixed doses of rapid-acting analog insulin with each meal to bedtime long-acting analog insulin. Due to the shorter duration of action of rapid-acting analogs, this regimen highlights the need for continuous basal insulin coverage. There is, however, less potential for insulin stacking. (*D*) Addition of flexible (carbohydrate-based) doses of rapid-acting analog insulin with each meal to bedtime long-acting analog insulin. This is the ideal basal-bolus insulin regimen with multiple daily injections. The analog rapid-acting insulin can be dosed with meals based on carbohydrates consumed again with little risk for insulin stacking. However, this regimen does require the patient to be well versed with self-management skills, including carbohydrate counting.

Fixed dose with each meal

This regimen is ideal for patients who consume meals similar in size and carbohydrate content. Because the doses of insulin are fixed in this regimen, hyperglycemia could result if patients eat more than they usually do or hypoglycemia if less food is consumed (see **Figs. 12**C and **13**C).

Carbohydrate-counting approach

The patient learns how to count carbohydrates using an Insulin:Carbohydrate Ratio (ICR). An ICR is calculated using the formula 500/TDD of insulin. For example, if the TDD is 50 units, 1 unit of rapid-acting analog insulin is required for every 10 g of carbohydrates consumed (500/50 = 10). Another method is to use TDD/3 to approximate the amount of bolus insulin for each meal. This is particularly helpful for patients who eat fixed amounts of carbohydrates with each meal.

With the addition of rapid-acting insulin, a correction dose, known as the Insulin Sensitivity Factor (ISF) should be added to the insulin regimen. The ISF is a dose of rapid-acting insulin *given at meal times* along with the meal dose of the same rapid-acting insulin to account for glucose that is out of target before the meal is consumed. This corrective dose of insulin is calculated using the "1800 rule," (1800/TDD) for rapid-acting analogs, or the "1500 rule" (1500/TDD) for human regular insulin. The actual calculation can be written for the patient as follows: X − (Target BG)/ISF; X

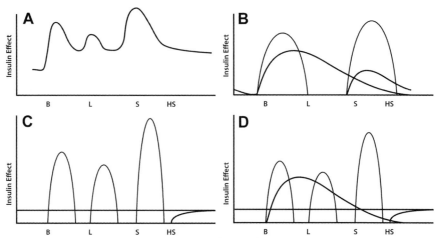

Fig. 14. Insulin regimen for exogenous glucocorticoids. B, breakfast; L, lunch; S, supper/dinner; HS, bedtime. (*A*) The addition of exogenous glucocorticoids leads to postprandial hyperglycemia, thus more insulin is required with meals. (*B*) One solution with human insulin preparations is to use NPH and regular insulin with breakfast and dinner. In this regimen, 60% of the NPH dose is administered with breakfast and 40% with dinner. For the regular insulin, the proportions are reversed, with 40% of the dose given 30 to 45 minutes before breakfast and 60% of the dose 30 to 45 minutes before dinner to try to match the expected glucose excursions, as seen in (*A*). (*C*) Another solution with analog insulin is to give 1 dose of long-acting analog basal insulin with breakfast and mealtime analog rapid-acting insulin with each meal, the highest dose administered with dinner again to match glucose excursions, as shown in (*A*). We prefer to administer the long-acting basal with breakfast in patients on steroids, because their glucose nadir occurs in the morning just before breakfast. (*D*) For patients already on a basal-bolus insulin with analog long-acting basal insulin at bedtime and mealtime, analog rapid-acting insulin, insulin NPH can be added at breakfast to account for the afternoon BG rise that occurs with glucocorticoids.

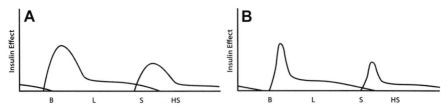

Fig. 15. Premixed insulin-based regimens. B, breakfast; L, lunch; S, supper/dinner; HS, bedtime. (*A*) Human premixed insulin products administered twice a day, 30 to 45 minutes before breakfast and supper. Typically 60% of the dose is administered before breakfast and 40% before supper. As seen in this figure, there is inadequate coverage in the middle of the day, with some stacking at dinner. The risk for nocturnal hypoglycemia persists from the evening dose of the NPH. (*B*) Analog premixed insulin products administered twice a day with breakfast and supper. Typically 60% of the dose is administered with breakfast and 40% with supper. Although this insulin offers the advantage of mealtime administration, the shorter duration of action of the rapid-acting analog manifests itself as longer periods of insulin deficiency during the day.

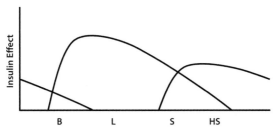

Fig. 16. Humulin R U-500 insulin-based regimens. As seen in the figure, U-500 insulin injected twice has the effect of overlapping of the doses. In effect, therefore, the pharmacokinetic profile of this insulin is similar to basal insulin. Typically 60% of the dose is administered before breakfast and 40% before supper. B, breakfast; L, lunch; S, supper/dinner; HS, bedtime.

represents the patient's BG. For example, with a premeal BG of 230 mg/dL, target BG of 130 mg/dL, and an ISF of 50, the patient will require $(230 - 130)/50 = 2$ units of rapid-acting insulin added to the meal dose.

Titration of bolus insulin
With either the fixed-dose approach or a carbohydrate-counting–based approach, bolus insulin is titrated based on the 2h-PPG or preprandial BG at the following meal (eg, breakfast bolus insulin dose is adjusted based on the 2h-post breakfast BG or prelunch BG) (see **Fig. 11**). It is important to emphasize that insulin doses in general, and prandial insulin in particular, should not be titrated based on HbA1c values, which proved a long-term measure of glycemic control and is not useful for the purpose of titrating a medication on a weekly or more frequent basis. As discussed earlier, we prefer to titrate every 5 to 7 days instead of 2 to 3 days, as recommended by the AACE guidelines. If correction doses are required for almost all meals, it would suggest that the basal insulin dose needs to be increased or the ICR needs to be changed or both. One strategy is to add up all the corrective doses used for a day and incorporate all or a significant proportion of the total into the basal insulin dose and then reassess patient response after another 5 to 7 days.

Insulin stacking
Insulin stacking refers to situations in which a previously injected insulin still has a residual effect due to its protracted duration of action. It is generally a problem with short-acting human regular insulin (see **Fig. 12**C, D), because these are dosed more

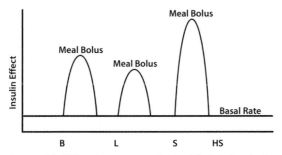

Fig. 17. Insulin regimen with CSII, using a pump. B, breakfast; L, lunch; S, supper/dinner; HS, bedtime. CSII therapy uses only rapid-acting analog insulin, delivered at preset "basal" rates with a mealtime "bolus" based on the ICR plus the ISF.

frequently, although it can occur with any type of insulin. If a subsequent short-acting insulin injection does not take the residual insulin from the previous dose into account, the two can add on to each other, resulting in hypoglycemia.[43] For this reason, short-acting insulins are typically administered at least 4 hours apart.

Approaches Using Premixed Insulin

As discussed earlier, premixed insulin has numerous drawbacks. However, it could be an option in poorly controlled T2D in patients poorly compliant with multiple daily injections, in elderly individuals who need assistance with injections, and those with less-stringent HbA1c goals (see **Fig. 15**). We generally follow the AACE calculation guidelines for the initiation of bolus insulin to dose premixed insulins (see **Fig. 11**)[15] with 60% of the TDD before breakfast and 40% of the TDD before supper. The breakfast dose of premixed insulin is titrated based on presupper BG values and the supper dose is titrated based on FPG.

Approaches Using Highly Concentrated (U-500) Insulin

The triggers, advantages, and disadvantages of Humulin R U-500 insulin (U-500) have been described earlier. Typically, the initial U-500 dose is calculated based on the U-100 insulin requirements. **Table 5** shows the U-500 dose in units (with a U-100 syringe) and in milliliters (with a tuberculin syringe).[44] Initial dosing includes administration of 60% of the TDD 30 minutes before breakfast and 40% of the TDD 30 minutes before supper (see **Fig. 16**).[44] For example, an individual on 300 units of U-100 would be transitioned to 0.36 mL (180 units) of U-500 insulin 30 minutes before breakfast and 0.24 mL (120 units) of U-500 insulin before supper. Carbohydrate counting is not done with this insulin unless used in a pump, but an ISF can be added typically in intervals of 5 units (0.01 mL). Except sulfonylureas and meglitinides, other noninsulin agents are generally continued when treating with U-500 insulin. When dosed twice daily, the breakfast dose of this insulin is titrated based on presupper BG values and the supper dose is titrated based on FPG.

Given that there is no special device for its injection, special precautions must be undertaken when using this insulin. It can be dispensed with either a U-100 insulin

Table 5
Calculating U-500 insulin dose (mL) based on U-100 insulin dosage (Units)

U-500 Regular Insulin Dose, Units	U-100 Syringe, Markings in Units	Tuberculin Syringe, Volume in mL
25	5	0.05
50	10	0.1
75	15	0.15
100	20	0.2
125	25	0.25
150	30	0.3
175	35	0.35
200	40	0.4
225	45	0.45
250	50	0.5

Adapted from Lane WS, Cochran EK, Jackson JA, et al. High-dose insulin therapy: is it time for U-500 insulin? Endocr Pract 2009;15(1):71–9.

syringe or a tuberculin syringe. Care should be taken in using only 1 of these 2 injection devices and patients should be retrained in the use of the device even if they have used a U-100 syringe before. *The prescription for U-500 insulin should always clearly state the device type to be used*. If prescribed with a U-100 insulin syringe, the amount of insulin drawn into the syringe should be written in units and if prescribed with a tuberculin syringe the amount should be written in milliliters (see **Table 5**). In the case of the patient described previously who is transitioning from 300 units of U-100 to U-500 insulin, the prescription should read: Humulin R U-500 (500 units/mL), inject 36 units 30 minutes before breakfast and 24 units before supper with an insulin syringe. If using a tuberculin syringe, the same prescription should read: Humulin R U-500 (500 units/mL), inject 0.36 mL 30 minutes before breakfast and 0.24 mL before supper with a tuberculin syringe. Our preferred administration device is the tuberculin syringe with dose written in milliliters so there is no confusion of the actual insulin dose administered with the unit markings of an insulin syringe.

Approaches Using Continuous Subcutaneous Insulin Infusion

For the highly motivated patient who frequently monitors BG, is on at least 2 daily insulin injections, and requires tighter control and fewer injections, continuous subcutaneous insulin infusion (CSII) may be an option (see **Fig. 17**).[45] It is, however, important that patients have a full evaluation with diabetes educators addressing all aspects of self-management skills before initiating pump therapy to maximize its success. An initial 1:1 dose switch from multiple daily injections to CSII can be used in patients switching to CSII.[45] We usually recommend starting with 1 basal rate, 1 ISF, and 1 ICR. These can then be modified based on response. It is prudent to follow-up with the patient either in-clinic or on the phone on a weekly basis for the first month of therapy.

ADVERSE EFFECTS OF INSULIN THERAPY

Although insulin is the most powerful agent to correct hyperglycemia, its use is not without risk. Besides weight gain, treatment with insulin can produce lipohypertrophy (deposition of fat) at the site of injections due to local anabolic effects of the drug. The absorption, and hence the kinetics, of insulin action can become erratic if the drug is injected into these hypertrophied areas. It is, therefore, important to rotate injection sites.

By far, however, the greatest risk associated with insulin use is that of hypoglycemia. Individuals should be counseled on the clinical manifestations of hypoglycemia, as well as treatment. We educate patients on "the rule of 15"; on noting the symptoms of hypoglycemia, the patient performs a BG to confirm hypoglycemia. If hypoglycemia is confirmed, the patient is to consume 15 g of carbohydrates (eg, 3 glucose tablets, 4 oz fruit juice) and then recheck BG 15 minutes later to ensure BG is trending up. The process should be repeated until the BG is greater than 100 mg/dL. Because of the potential risk of hypoglycemia with insulin therapy, we believe that all patients prescribed this drug should be given a prescription for glucagon and a family member or person who has close and constant contact with the patient should be trained in its use. All patients on insulin therapy should also be encouraged to wear a medical alert bracelet and always check their BG before driving and frequently when driving for long periods of time. In certain high-risk occupations (eg, drivers of commercial vehicles, pilots, and those operating dangerous machinery), workers who use insulin must provide detailed glucose logs and paperwork from their physicians regarding their history of diabetes and its management. Awareness of the risk of hypoglycemia is also important when using combination therapy with multiple medications in patients with T2D as discussed later in this article.

DEESCALATING INSULIN THERAPY IN TYPE 2 DIABETES

There are circumstances in which a need to deescalate previously started insulin therapy might arise. One such circumstance is following a new diagnosis of T2D with glucose toxicity, where insulin was initiated at the time of diagnosis. As glucose toxicity abates with treatment, it may be possible to taper off insulin while at the same time introducing other noninsulin therapy. Similarly, insulin-sparing agents, such as incretin mimetics or SGLT-2 inhibitors, might be introduced in patients already on insulin. The introduction of these agents could precipitate hypoglycemia if the insulin (or sulfonylurea) doses are not adjusted downward. Because there are no published guidelines on strategies for reducing insulin in such circumstances, we present our approach to insulin adjustment in the presence of such agents.[16,46-63] The approach presented is an amalgamation of our clinical experience and insulin dose titrations used in clinical trials where new therapeutic agents were used on a background of insulin therapy. We have summarized the mechanism of action of drugs from different therapeutic classes used for T2D in **Table 6** to help determine when insulin deescalation might be appropriate to consider.

For patients on basal insulin alone:

In such circumstances, our strategy is to reduce the basal insulin as follows:
- HbA1c ≤8%: Basal insulin is reduced by 20% on initiation of the new agent.
- HbA1c >8%: Basal insulin is reduced by 0% to 10% on initiation of the new agent.

The patient continues to monitor SMBG, and if any 2 values in 1 week are less than 100 mg/dL (or <80 mg/dL if tighter control is desired), basal insulin should be reduced by another 10% to 20%. Such reductions occur weekly until the patient is taking less than 10 to 20 units of basal insulin. At this time, the need for continuing basal insulin needs to be reassessed. For the management of hyperglycemia, if 3 BG values in 1 week are greater than 250 mg/dL, we recommend the patient contact the physician to assess if the dose of the newly introduced agent or insulin needs modification.

For patients on basal + bolus insulin (or bolus insulin alone):

In such circumstances, our strategy is to reduce the bolus insulin first, as follows:
- HbA1c ≤8%: Bolus insulin is reduced by 30% to 50% on initiation of the new agent.
- HbA1c >8%: Bolus insulin is reduced by 0% to 20% on initiation of the new agent.

The patient continues to monitor SMBG, and if any 2 values in 1 week are less than 100 mg/dL (or <80 mg/dL if tight control is desired), bolus insulin should be reduced by another 30% to 50%. Such reductions occur weekly until adequate glycemic control is achieved or the bolus insulin is tapered off entirely. Once bolus insulin has been tapered off completely and if the patient continues to have any 2 SMBG values in a week less than 100 mg/dL, we recommend basal insulin reductions as described previously. For the management of hyperglycemia, if 3 SMBG values in 1 week are greater than 250 mg/dL, we recommend that the patient contact the physician to assess if therapy with the noninsulin agent or insulin needs modification.

For patients on premixed insulin, we generally follow the parameters for basal insulin alone. For patients on insulin plus a sulfonylurea, our approach is to try to reduce the insulin before the sulfonylurea, because in our experience patients prefer to remain on oral agents over injectable ones.

Table 6
Mechanisms of action of currently available agents for type 2 diabetes

Class	Agents	Mechanism of Action							Effect on Glycemia		Adverse Effects	
		Decrease Hepatic Glucose Production	Increase Insulin Secretion	Increase Peripheral Insulin Intake (Insulin Sensitizer)	Slows Gastric Emptying	Decrease Renal Glucose Absorption	Decrease Intestinal Glucose Absorption	Evidence Supporting Improvement in β-Cell Function	Decrease Fasting Plasma Glucose (FPG)	Decrease 2-h Postprandial Plasma Glucose (2h-PPG)	Weight Effect	Risk of Hypoglycemia as Monotherapy
Biguanide	Metformin	+++	0	+	0	0	0	0[16]	+++	+	Neutral	No
Sulfonylurea	Glyburide Glipizide Glimepiride	0	+++	0	0	0	0	0[46,47]	+++	+	Gain	Yes
Meglitinide	Repaglinide Nateglinide	0	++	0	0	0	0	0	++	++	Gain	Yes
Thiazolidinedione	Pioglitazone Rosiglitazone	++	0	+++	0	0	0	+[51,52]	++	++	Gain	No
GLP-1 receptor agonist	Short-acting: exenatide	++	++	0	+++	0	0	+[52–54]	+	+++	Loss	No
	Long-acting: liraglutide, exenatide-QW	++							++	+		
DPP-IV inhibitor	Sitagliptin Saxagliptin Linagliptin Vildagliptin[a] Alogliptin	++	++	0	0	0	0	+[55]	++	+	Neutral	No
SGLT-2 inhibitor	Canagliflozin Dapagliflozin	0	0	0	0	+++	+	+[56]	+	+++	Loss	No
α-Glucosidase inhibitor	Acarbose Miglitol	0	0	0	0	0	+++	+[60]	+	+++	Neutral	No
Amylinomimetic	Pramlintide	+	0	0	+++	0	0	0	+	+++	Loss	N/A
Bile acid sequestrant	Colesevelam	0	0	0	0	0	+++	0	0	++	Neutral	No
Dopamine agonist	Bromocriptine	Unknown[61]	0	0	0	0	0	+[62]	+[62]	+[62]	Neutral	No

N/A, not used as monotherapy; 0, no effect; +, small effect; ++, moderate effect; +++, marked effect.
[a] Vildagliptin is not yet approved for use in the United States.

THE ABCS OF DIABETES CARE AND THE DIABETES CARE T.E.A.M. APPROACH

When managing the patient with diabetes, it is important to not only emphasize glycemic goals as measured by HbA1c, but also *B*lood Pressure and *C*holesterol targets, collectively referred to as the ABCs of diabetes.[64] Addressing these helps reduce the risk of both microvascular and macrovascular complications. This is best accomplished using what we call the T.E.A.M. approach. The most critical member of the T.E.A.M. is the patient; other members include the physician, a certified diabetes educator (CDE) dietician, nurse CDE, pharmacist, optometrist/ophthalmologist, podiatrist, behavioral psychologist, social worker, and the family of the patient. All members of the team help in achieving goals for diabetes. The T.E.A.M. approach itself consists of the following:

- *T*alking with the patient: Clearly communicating goals and roles and responsibilities of each member of the team with the patient is key in overcoming barriers to optimal glycemic control. This communication should occur with and from all team members.
- *E*xercise and nutrition: Addressing pertinent lifestyle issues.
- *A*ttitude: Help the patient deal with psychological, social, and financial issues that could become barriers to achieving control.
- *M*edications: Choosing the correct medications *in discussion with* the patient.

SUMMARY

Insulin is the most powerful glycemic control agent available. However, its use as a therapeutic modality requires education of the patient and regimentation of food intake, exercise, and frequent glucose monitoring. Such regimentation is particularly important when using a basal-bolus therapy approach.

The introduction of many novel noninsulin drugs in the past decade has resulted in better glycemic control and often a need to reduce previously instituted insulin therapy. Although many of these novel therapies by themselves do not cause hypoglycemia, by reducing the overall glycemic burden through a myriad of mechanisms, they function in an insulin-sparing fashion. The doses of exogenously administered insulin may therefore need to be reduced in the presence of these new drugs to mitigate hypoglycemia.

For insulin therapy (or any other drug treatment) to be successful, it is critical that the physician not only establish glycemic goals, but communicate these goals to the patient. The measurement of HbA1c helps in achieving a long-term goal, but on a day-to-day basis, patients need to be cognizant of their own BG goals and what they need to do if falling outside of target. The patients' understanding of self-management skills and empowerment are therefore foundational to insulin therapy.

REFERENCES

1. Defronzo RA. Banting Lecture. From the triumvirate to the ominous octet: a new paradigm for the treatment of type 2 diabetes mellitus. Diabetes 2009;58(4): 773–95.
2. Butler AE, Janson J, Bonner-Weir S, et al. Beta-cell deficit and increased beta-cell apoptosis in humans with type 2 diabetes. Diabetes 2003;52(1):102–10.
3. Weng J, Li Y, Xu W, et al. Effect of intensive insulin therapy on β-cell function and glycaemic control in patients with newly diagnosed type 2 diabetes: a multi-centre randomised parallel-group trial. Lancet 2008;371(9626):1753–60.

4. Kramer CK, Zinman B, Retnakaran R. Short-term intensive insulin therapy in type 2 diabetes mellitus: a systematic review and meta-analysis. Lancet Diabetes Endocrinol 2013;1(1):28–34.

5. Chen HS, Wu TE, Jap TS, et al. Beneficial effects of insulin on glycemic control and beta-cell function in newly diagnosed type 2 diabetes with severe hyperglycemia after short-term intensive insulin therapy. Diabetes Care 2008;31(10):1927–32.

6. Gerich JE, Meyer C, Woerle HJ, et al. Renal gluconeogenesis: its importance in human glucose homeostasis. Diabetes Care 2001;24(2):382–91.

7. White M, Copps KD, Ozcan U, et al. Mechanisms of insulin action. In: Jameson JL, Groot LJ, editors. Endocrinology, 2-Volume set: adult and pediatric. 6th edition. Philadelphia(PA): Saunders Elsevier; 2010. p. 636–59.

8. Rorsman P, Renstrom E. Insulin granule dynamics in pancreatic beta cells. Diabetologia 2003;46(8):1029–45.

9. Lebovitz HE. Insulin: potential negative consequences of early routine use in patients with type 2 diabetes. Diabetes Care 2011;34(Suppl 2):S225–30.

10. Abdul-Ghani MA, Defronzo RA. Lowering plasma glucose concentration by inhibiting renal sodium-glucose co-transport. J Intern Med 2014;276(4):352–63.

11. Kahn SE, Prigeon RL, McCulloch DK, et al. Quantification of the relationship between insulin sensitivity and beta-cell function in human subjects. Evidence for a hyperbolic function. Diabetes 1993;42(11):1663–72.

12. Ferrannini E, Gastaldelli A, Miyazaki Y, et al. Beta-cell function in subjects spanning the range from normal glucose tolerance to overt diabetes: a new analysis. J Clin Endocrinol Metab 2005;90(1):493–500.

13. Kahn SE. The relative contributions of insulin resistance and beta-cell dysfunction to the pathophysiology of Type 2 diabetes. Diabetologia 2003;46(1):3–19.

14. American Diabetes Association. Standards of medical care in diabetes–2014. Diabetes Care 2014;37(Suppl 1):S14–80.

15. Handelsman Y, Mechanick JI, Blonde L, et al. American Association of Clinical Endocrinologists Medical Guidelines for Clinical Practice for developing a diabetes mellitus comprehensive care plan. Endocr Pract 2011;17(Suppl 2):1–53.

16. Turner RC, Cull CA, Frighi V, et al. Glycemic control with diet, sulfonylurea, metformin, or insulin in patients with type 2 diabetes mellitus: progressive requirement for multiple therapies (UKPDS 49). UK Prospective Diabetes Study (UKPDS) Group. JAMA 1999;281(21):2005–12.

17. Kahn SE, Haffner SM, Heise MA, et al. Glycemic durability of rosiglitazone, metformin, or glyburide monotherapy. N Engl J Med 2006;355(23):2427–43.

18. Naik RG, Brooks-Worrell BM, Palmer JP. Latent autoimmune diabetes in adults. J Clin Endocrinol Metab 2009;94(12):4635–44.

19. Juneja R, Palmer JP. Type 1 1/2 diabetes: myth or reality? Autoimmunity 1999; 29(1):65–83.

20. Nathan DM, Kuenen J, Borg R, et al. Translating the A1C assay into estimated average glucose values. Diabetes Care 2008;31(8):1473–8.

21. Hirsch IB. Insulin analogues. N Engl J Med 2005;352(2):174–83.

22. Nordisk N. Insulin degludec and insulin degludec/insulin aspart treatment to improve glycemic control in patients with diabetes mellitus. NDAs 203314 and 203313. 2012. Available at: http://www.fda.gov/downloads/AdvisoryCommittees/CommitteesMeetingMaterials/Drugs/EndocrinologicandMetabolicDrugsAdvisoryCommittee/UCM327017.pdf. Accessed May 6, 2014.

23. Skyler JS. Insulin treatment. In: Lebovitz HE, editor. Therapy for diabetes mellitus and related disorders. 5th edition. Alexandria (Egypt): American Diabetes Association; 2009. p. 273–89.

24. Retnakaran RZ, Zinman B. Treatment of type 1 diabetes mellitus in adults. In: Jameson JL, Grott LJ, editors. Endocrinology, 2 Volume-Set: adult and pediatric. 6th edition. Philadelphia(PA): Saunders Elsevier; 2010. p. 840–57.

25. Hirsch IB. Intensive treatment of type 1 diabetes. Med Clin North Am 1998; 82(4):689–719.

26. Baxter MA. The role of new basal insulin analogues in the initiation and optimisation of insulin therapy in type 2 diabetes. Acta Diabetol 2008;45(4):253–68.

27. Owens DR, Matfin G, Monnier L. Basal insulin analogues in the management of diabetes mellitus: what progress have we made? Diabetes Metab Res Rev 2014;30(2):104–19.

28. Heise T, Weyer C, Serwas A, et al. Time-action profiles of novel premixed preparations of insulin lispro and NPL insulin. Diabetes Care 1998;21(5):800–3.

29. Weyer C, Heise T, Heinemann L. Insulin aspart in a 30/70 premixed formulation. Pharmacodynamic properties of a rapid-acting insulin analog in stable mixture. Diabetes Care 1997;20(10):1612–4.

30. Banting FG, Collip JB, MacLeod JJ, et al. The effect of pancreatic extract (insulin) on normal rabbits. Am J Phys 1922;62:162–76.

31. Rosenfeld CR, Bohannon NJ, Bode B, et al. The V-Go insulin delivery device used in clinical practice: patient perception and retrospective analysis of glycemic control. Endocr Pract 2012;18(5):660–7.

32. Neithercott T. The basics of insulin pumps: these devices are the closest thing to a pancreas–so far. Diabetes Forecast 2014;67(1):58.

33. Bergenstal RM, Buse JB, Peters AL, et al. Endocrinology (3-volume set). In: Jameson JL, Degroot LJ, editors. 4th edition. Philadelphia: W.B. Saunders; 2001.

34. Leahy JL. Insulin therapy in type 2 diabetes mellitus. Endocrinol Metab Clin North Am 2012;41(1):119–44.

35. Hirsch IB, Bergenstal RM, Parkin CG, et al. A real-world approach to insulin therapy in primary care practice. Clinical Diabetes 2005;23:78–86.

36. Riddle MC, Rosenstock J, Gerich J. The treat-to-target trial: randomized addition of glargine or human NPH insulin to oral therapy of type 2 diabetic patients. Diabetes Care 2003;26(11):3080–6.

37. Meneghini L, Koenen C, Weng W, et al. The usage of a simplified self-titration dosing guideline (303 Algorithm) for insulin detemir in patients with type 2 diabetes–results of the randomized, controlled PREDICTIVE 303 study. Diabetes Obes Metab 2007;9(6):902–13.

38. Edelman SV, Liu R, Johnson J, et al. AUTONOMY: the first randomized trial comparing two patient-driven approaches to initiate and titrate prandial insulin lispro in type 2 diabetes. Diabetes Care 2014;37(8):2132–40.

39. Davies M, Storms F, Shutler S, et al. Improvement of glycemic control in subjects with poorly controlled type 2 diabetes: comparison of two treatment algorithms using insulin glargine. Diabetes Care 2005;28(6):1282–8.

40. Monnier L, Colette C, Rabasa-Lhoret R, et al. Morning hyperglycemic excursions: a constant failure in the metabolic control of non-insulin-using patients with type 2 diabetes. Diabetes Care 2002;25(4):737–41.

41. Monnier L, Lapinski H, Colette C. Contributions of fasting and postprandial plasma glucose increments to the overall diurnal hyperglycemia of type 2 diabetic patients: variations with increasing levels of HbA(1c). Diabetes Care 2003;26(3):881–5.

42. Bergenstal RM, Johnson M, Powers MA, et al. Adjust to target in type 2 diabetes: comparison of a simple algorithm with carbohydrate counting for adjustment of mealtime insulin glulisine. Diabetes Care 2008;31(7):1305–10.

43. Heise T, Meneghini LF. Insulin stacking versus therapeutic accumulation: understanding the differences. Endocr Pract 2014;20(1):75–83.
44. Lane WS, Cochran EK, Jackson JA, et al. High-dose insulin therapy: is it time for U-500 insulin? Endocr Pract 2009;15(1):71–9.
45. Reznik Y, Cohen O. Insulin pump for type 2 diabetes: use and misuse of continuous subcutaneous insulin infusion in type 2 diabetes. Diabetes Care 2013; 36(Suppl 2):S219–25.
46. Riddle M. Combination therapies with oral agents or oral agents and insulin. In: Lebovitz HE, editor. Therapy for diabetes mellitus and related disorders. 5th edition. Alexandria (Egypt): American Diabetes Association; 2009. p. 332–41.
47. Hambrock A, de Oliveira Franz CB, Hiller S, et al. Glibenclamide-induced apoptosis is specifically enhanced by expression of the sulfonylurea receptor isoform SUR1 but not by expression of SUR2B or the mutant SUR1(M1289T). J Pharmacol Exp Ther 2006;316(3):1031–7.
48. Wright A, Burden AC, Paisey RB, et al. Sulfonylurea inadequacy: efficacy of addition of insulin over 6 years in patients with type 2 diabetes in the UK Prospective Diabetes Study (UKPDS 57). Diabetes Care 2002;25(2):330–6.
49. Johnson JA, Majumdar SR, Simpson SH, et al. Decreased mortality associated with the use of metformin compared with sulfonylurea monotherapy in type 2 diabetes. Diabetes Care 2002;25(12):2244–8.
50. Evans JM, Ogston SA, Emslie-Smith A, et al. Risk of mortality and adverse cardiovascular outcomes in type 2 diabetes: a comparison of patients treated with sulfonylureas and metformin. Diabetologia 2006;49(5):930–6.
51. Monami M, Genovese S, Mannucci E. Cardiovascular safety of sulfonylureas: a meta-analysis of randomized clinical trials. Diabetes Obes Metab 2013;15(10): 938–53.
52. Gastaldelli A, Ferrannini E, Miyazaki Y, et al. Thiazolidinediones improve beta-cell function in type 2 diabetic patients. Am J Physiol Endocrinol Metab 2007; 292(3):E871–83.
53. DeFronzo RA, Triplitt C, Qu Y, et al. Effects of exenatide plus rosiglitazone on beta-cell function and insulin sensitivity in subjects with type 2 diabetes on metformin. Diabetes Care 2010;33(5):951–7.
54. Mari A, Nielsen LL, Nanayakkara N, et al. Mathematical modeling shows exenatide improved beta-cell function in patients with type 2 diabetes treated with metformin or metformin and a sulfonylurea. Horm Metab Res 2006;38(12): 838–44.
55. Astrup A, Rossner S, Van Gaal L, et al. Effects of liraglutide in the treatment of obesity: a randomised, double-blind, placebo-controlled study. Lancet 2009; 374(9701):1606–16.
56. Mari A, Sallas WM, He YL, et al. Vildagliptin, a dipeptidyl peptidase-IV inhibitor, improves model-assessed beta-cell function in patients with type 2 diabetes. J Clin Endocrinol Metab 2005;90(8):4888–94.
57. Polidori D, Mari A, Ferrannini E. Canagliflozin, a sodium glucose co-transporter 2 inhibitor, improves model-based indices of beta cell function in patients with type 2 diabetes. Diabetologia 2014;57(5):891–901.
58. Neal B, Perkovic V, de Zeeuw D, et al. Rationale, design, and baseline characteristics of the Canagliflozin Cardiovascular Assessment Study (CANVAS)–a randomized placebo-controlled trial. Am Heart J 2013;166(2):217–23.e11.
59. Stenlof K, Cefalu WT, Kim KA, et al. Efficacy and safety of canagliflozin monotherapy in subjects with type 2 diabetes mellitus inadequately controlled with diet and exercise. Diabetes Obes Metab 2013;15(4):372–82.

60. Lavalle-Gonzalez FJ, Januszewicz A, Davidson J, et al. Efficacy and safety of canagliflozin compared with placebo and sitagliptin in patients with type 2 diabetes on background metformin monotherapy: a randomised trial. Diabetologia 2013;56(12):2582–92.

61. Chiasson JL, Josse RG, Gomis R, et al. Acarbose for prevention of type 2 diabetes mellitus: the STOP-NIDDM randomised trial. Lancet 2002;359(9323): 2072–7.

62. Weiland CM, Hilaire ML. Bromocriptine mesylate (Cycloset) for type 2 diabetes mellitus. Am Fam Physician 2013;87(10):718–20.

63. Grunberger G. Novel therapies for the management of type 2 diabetes mellitus: part 1. Pramlintide and bromocriptine-QR. J Diabetes 2013;5(2):110–7.

64. Abbate S. Expanded ABCs of Diabetes. Clinical Diabetes 2003;21(3):128–33.

Nonglycemic Targets in Diabetes

Dawn DeWitt, MD, MSc, FRACP, FRCPC[a],*, David C. Dugdale, MD[b],
William R. Adam, PhD, MBBS, FRACP[c]

KEYWORDS

- Diabetes guidelines • Diabetes treatment targets • Lipids • Hypertension
- Mental health • Nephropathy

KEY POINTS

- Blood pressure targets for all patients with diabetes are now less than 140/90 regardless of diabetic nephropathy. Geriatric guidelines concur with this target.
- All patients between 40 and 75 years of age should be considered for moderate- to high-intensity statin therapy. Patients older than 75 years should be preferentially treated with a statin if appropriate after lipid levels, risk, and longevity are considered and at doses that minimize side effects.
- Diabetes-related stress and depression has been identified as a major treatable factor that will improve outcomes.
- For medically obese patients with diabetes, there is increasing evidence that bariatric surgery decreases morbidity and mortality significantly and may be an appropriate treatment option.

INTRODUCTION

Diabetes care and, subsequently, diabetes morbidity and mortality have changed dramatically in the last decades. In addition to new agents and methods for glycemic control, newer agents to control the progression of renal disease and knowledge about interventions to improve cardiovascular outcomes are now available. Importantly, we have learned much about the importance and primacy of diet, weight loss, exercise, and mental health as they affect the risk of and progression of diabetes, the last through the critical lens of compliance and self-care. We also have better

Disclosures: None.
[a] Department of Medicine, University of British Columbia, Vancouver, British Columbia, Canada; [b] Division of Internal Medicine, Department of Medicine, University of Washington, Seattle, WA, USA; [c] Rural Health Academic Centre, Melbourne Medical School, Parkville, Graham St. Shepparton, Victoria, Australia
* Corresponding author.
E-mail address: dawn.dewitt@ubc.ca

Med Clin N Am 99 (2015) 187–200
http://dx.doi.org/10.1016/j.mcna.2014.08.014   medical.theclinics.com
0025-7125/15/$ – see front matter © 2015 Elsevier Inc. All rights reserved.

information on outcomes demonstrating the importance of team care, with patients in the center of the team.

In the last 2 years, new guidelines for nonglycemic targets in diabetes include new hypertension guidelines, new lipid target and management guidelines, and new geriatric guidelines. Importantly, the advent of new guidelines and medications has decreased the recommendations for monitoring in some instances; for example, self-monitoring of blood glucose is now recommended only intermittently for patients on oral agents, and, in an era of cost-effective care, the new lipid guidelines recommend treating with fixed doses of medications rather than to a particular lipid target per se.

This article reviews the new guidelines, summarizes the evidence for nonglycemic targets, and provides practical clinical management recommendations, including some nontraditional areas, such as depression and team-management targets.

HYPERTENSION AND RENAL DISEASE TARGETS

Diabetic renal disease commonly involves multiple primary and secondary pathologic processes that lead to a limited variety of clinical manifestations (**Box 1**). Genetic susceptibility to diabetic nephropathy, suggested by familial clustering of nephropathy,[1,2] is complex because of ill-defined pathophysiology and variable genetic expression.[3]

Classic diabetic nephropathy, with microalbuminuria progressing to macroalbuminuria and a decreased glomerular filtration rate (GFR), is common and easy to diagnose in type 1 diabetes but is responsible for less than 50% of cases of renal disease in type 2 diabetes. Renal biopsies from patients with type 2 diabetes (eg, hematuria, decreased GFR without significant albuminuria, absence of microvascular disease, and so forth) show changes consistent with diabetic nephropathy, other renal diseases, or a combination in roughly equal numbers.[4]

Indications for a renal biopsy in patients with diabetes and evidence of renal disease include the likelihood of other treatable renal disease and the patients' tolerance for any needed immunosuppressive therapy. Indications for renal biopsy include nephrotic range proteinuria in the absence of other microvascular disease or the combination of glomerular hematuria, significant proteinuria (>1 g/d), and renal impairment, particularly with clinical or serum biomarker evidence of diffuse immune-mediated diseases (antineutrophil cytoplasmic antibodies, double-stranded DNA).

The early diagnosis of diabetic nephropathy is even more problematic based as it is on the development of microalbuminuria, which is also associated with exercise, infections, and other renal diseases. These other causes of microalbuminuria probably explain transient microalbuminuria in 50% of the initial diagnoses of diabetic

---

Box 1
Pathophysiology, anatomical pathology, and clinical manifestations of renal disease in patients with diabetes

- Pathophysiology: activation of renin angiotensin aldosterone system; increased renal blood flow and intraglomerular pressure; deposition of glycosylated proteins into glomeruli, tubules, interstitium; secondary damage from hypertension, vascular disease and proteinuria

- Anatomical pathology: glomerular hypertrophy, nodular sclerosis, arteriolar hyalinosis, interstitial inflammation and fibrosis

- Clinical manifestations: albuminuria, deceased glomerular filtration rate, hematuria (less common)

nephropathy. Conversely, the lack of specificity and sensitivity of microalbuminuria in the diagnosis of diabetic nephropathy, the inability to detect damage to up to 50% of glomerular filtration surface area, and the lack of precision of GFR estimates also contribute to a significant incidence of silent diabetic nephropathy for some years before an unequivocal diagnosis, particularly in type 2 diabetes.

New blood pressure targets in patients with diabetes are the same in the presence or absence of diabetic nephropathy (see later discussion). Given the incidence of diabetic renal disease and the aforementioned issues, the case can be made that all patients with diabetes (particularly type 2) should be managed as if they had diabetic renal disease. In support of this approach, several trials have shown that early use of angiotensin-converting enzyme inhibitors (ACEI) reduces the incidence of new microalbuminuria in patients with type 2 diabetes.[5] And some of the improvement in microvascular outcomes in diabetes in the past 2 decades might be attributed to better blood pressure (and glucose) control, before the development of diabetic nephropathy.[6]

BLOOD PRESSURE TREATMENT

The control of hypertension (hyperglycemia aside) is the cornerstone of preventing/delaying the onset and progression of diabetic nephropathy. Treatment of hypertension also has a significant impact on other cardiovascular complications of diabetes. Because medication compliance is a major determinant of treatment effectiveness of hypertension, compliance should be a major determinant of treatment choices. Relevant questions include blood pressure targets and the relative importance of specific therapeutic agents or interventions, including the variable effectiveness of different antihypertensive medications in different populations (ethnicity/sex).

A 2011 study shows that, in patients who take more than one antihypertensive medication, taking at least one medication at bedtime improves control, decreases composite CV end points, and major cardiovascular (CV) events.[7]

Although there are several guidelines on the management of high blood pressure, the most recent Joint National Committee guidelines on the management of high blood pressure in adults (JNC 8)[8] provide the basis for recommendations in **Table 1**. The JNC 8 guidelines are based on a Cochrane meta-analysis and other studies showing a lack of evidence for lower targets and some evidence for harm.[8,9] However, when the JNC 8 recommendations are rated as *soft*, alternative guidelines should be considered. In patients with diabetes, the JNC 8 recommends a target blood pressure of 140/90 mm Hg or less for all adults aged 18 years and older. The JNC 8 guidelines recommend that the initial choice of, and any additional, antihypertensive medication in patients with or without diabetes should be a thiazide-type diuretic (TTD), calcium channel blocker (CCB), or one of an ACEI or angiotensin receptor blocker (ARB), except in the black population with or without diabetes, in whom initial treatment should be either a TTD or CCB. Finally the authors recommend monitoring patients with prediabetes more closely after commencement of diuretics because the nateglinide and valsartan in impaired glucose tolerance outcomes research (NAVIGATOR) trial confirms they cause 1 additional case of diabetes in every 17 patients over 5 years (Hazard Ratio 1.23) when compared to the use of other antihypertensive agents (beta-blockers, CCBs, ACEis or ARBs) (Shen and colleagues,[10] 2013). The authors recommend monitoring patients with prediabetes more closely after diuretics are started.

The Kidney Disease Improving Global Outcomes (KDIGO), the American Society of Hypertension (ASH), and the American Geriatrics Society (AGS) guidelines[11–13] recommend a lower target blood pressure (130/80 mm Hg) in patients with diabetes and evidence of kidney disease (urine microalbumin >30 mg/g), the difference

	JNC 8 BP	Alternative Approaches, When JNC 8
Patient Characteristics	**Guideline**	**Guideline** *Unhelpful or Soft*
Type 1, 18+ y, U Alb <30 mg/g	<140/90	—
Type 1, 18+ y, U Alb 30–300 mg/g	<140/90	KDIGO <130/80
Type 1, 18+ y, U Alb >300 mg/g	<140/90	KDIGO <130/80, use ACEI/ARB
Type 2, 18+ y, U Alb <30 mg/g	<140/90	Treat as if U Alb >30 mg/g (see text)
Type 2, 18+ y, U Alb 30–300 mg/g	<140/90	KDIGO <130/80. Use ACEI/ARB (see text)
Type 2, 18+ y, U Alb >300 mg/g	<140/90	KDIGO <130/80, use ACEI/ARB
Aged +/− ↓ life expectancy	<140/90	AGS & ASH <140/90, but HYVET <150/90 in >80 y (see text)[13]

Table 1
Recommendations on target BP in patients with diabetes based on JNC 8 guidelines

Alternative approaches suggested when JNC 8 guidelines rated as *soft* or *unhelpful*. JNC 8 guidelines for initial and second-line treatment in nonblack patients: a thiazide diuretic, a calcium channel blocker, or either an ACEI or angiotensin receptor blocker. Initial choice in black patients: a thiazide diuretic or calcium channel blocker (JNC 8 and American Society of Hypertension).

Abbreviations: AGS, American Geriatrics Society; ARB, angiotensin receptor blocker; ASH, American Society of Hypertension; BP, blood pressure; HYVET, Hypertension in the Very Elderly Trial; KDIGO, Kidney Disease Improving Global Outcomes; U Alb, urinary albumin.

reflecting opinion rather than compelling evidence. The justification for treating patients with type 2 diabetes and a urine microalbumin less than 30 mg/g as if they had diabetic renal disease (see **Table 1**) is based on the reduced incidence of new microalbuminuria in such patients treated with an ACEI,[5] with a likely period of silent diabetes-related renal disease before microalbuminuria.

The KDIGO guidelines also recommend an initial treatment choice of RASIs in diabetes. The rationale for the preferred use of RASIs is based on the RAS role in the development of diabetic nephropathy and the effect of RASIs on reducing the incidence of microalbuminuria,[5] the degree of proteinuria, and the rate of loss of GFR.[8] Two recent systematic reviews and meta-analyses, although supporting the preferred use of RASIs in the management of high blood pressure in diabetes, provide less compelling evidence of a specific benefit.[14,15] One of the 2 showed a reduction in mortality with ACEI compared with placebo in patients with diabetes[14]; neither trial showed a mortality benefit with an ARB. Renal outcomes were only studied in one meta-analysis,[15] which showed a reduction in the incidence of a doubling of plasma creatinine (but not the rarer event of end-stage renal disease), with ACEI and, to a lesser extent, ARB, when compared with placebo; an effect not seen with other antihypertensive; Importantly, β-blockers were considered least effective.[15] Unfortunately, the analysis did not study the differences between black and nonblack populations, leaving the JNC 8 recommendations for the black population with diabetes as the preferred option (see **Table 1**).

Recommendations for the treatment of high blood pressure in elderly diabetic patients are also problematic because of the lack of evidence. Although JNC 8,[8] ASH,[12] AGS,[13] and KDIGO[11] recommend a target of less than 140/90 mm Hg, the results of the Hypertension in the Very Elderly Trial (<10% diabetes) make a general case for a target of less than 150/80 mm Hg in patients aged greater than 80 years.[16] KDIGO also suggests that blood pressure should not be allowed to decrease much less than 140/90 mm Hg in the elderly.[17] A commonsense approach to likely long-term benefits, and the side-effect profile of individual patients, is likely to play a significant role in determining target blood pressure in the elderly with a decreased life expectancy.

If ACEI or ARB is used in the treatment of high blood pressure in diabetes, the consequent questions are as follows:

1. What is the best antihypertensive combination? There is now clear evidence that combinations of an ACEI and ARB are associated with an increased risk of hyperkalemia (3.7 cases per 100 person-years) and acute renal failure (5.5 cases per 100 person-years), without additional renal protection.[18] The choice between diuretics and CCBs as the next medication will depend on factors such as the benefits of other agents for the management of coincident issues (eg, diuretics in heart failure or hyperkalemia) and likely compliance, including the availability/affordability of combined antihypertensive tablets.

2. What is an acceptable acute deterioration in GFR when starting an ACEI or ARB? An acute decrease of 30% or less of the estimated GFR has been considered acceptable because of reversibility and an association with slower progression of kidney disease.[19] A decreased GFR may cause metabolic abnormalities and symptoms and is associated with an increased cardiovascular mortality.[20] Therefore, the life expectancy of patients, as a predictor of the likely long-term benefits in renal function compared with the possible short-term increased risk of cardiovascular or other symptoms, should influence the acceptability of an acute short-term decrease in GFR following an ACEI or ARB. There are no data to support any recommendation, but a life expectancy of less than 5 years would make one doubt the benefits of an acute decrease of 30% in GFR following an ACEI or ARB.

3. What level of hyperkalemia is acceptable on an ACEI or ARB? Hyperkalemia poses a cardiovascular risk. Surveillance after publication of the Randomized Aldactone Evaluation Study[21] showed an increased hospitalization rate and mortality for hyperkalemia (2.6 and 0.5 per 100 person-years). In dialysis patients, hyperkalemia is associated with an excess mortality of 2 per 100 person-years (plasma potassium >6 mmol/L) and 4 to 7 per 100 person-years (plasma potassium >6.5 mmol/L).[22] Consistent with other recommendations,[23] these data suggest a plasma potassium target of 6 mmol/L or less, achieved through dietary modification, diuretics, or by cessation of the ACEI or ARB.

PROTEINURIA

Microalbuminuria is associated with worse renal and cardiovascular outcomes, with greater degrees of proteinuria increasing the risk. A reduction in the degree of proteinuria by treatment with RASIs is associated with improved outcomes through control of hypertension and other mechanisms.[21] Although RASI-associated reductions in proteinuria promote their choice as preferred antihypertensives, the highest priority should be given to reaching target blood pressures.

LIPID TARGETS

In 2013, the American College of Cardiology (ACC) and the American Heart Association (AHA) jointly released new, highly controversial guidelines for lipid targets and treatment. Although the ACC/AHA's review of the evidence shows that high-intensity therapy (lowering low-density lipoprotein [LDL] by ≥50%) or moderate-intensity therapy (≥30%) changes atherosclerotic cardiovascular diseases (ASCVD) outcomes, the new guidelines focus on treatment initialization for patients with a 10-year ASCVD risk of 10% or more (with the new risk calculator) rather than target levels of lipids, with treatment, as has been common practice for the last 2 decades.[24]

The clinical bottom line is that all patients with diabetes between 40 and 75 years of age are assumed to have vascular disease and a risk of 7.5% or more, with the same treatment recommendations for this group with diabetes. In such patients, the evidence supports treatment with moderate- to high-intensity statins for primary and secondary prevention (for any LDL cholesterol [LDL-C] $\geq$70 mg/dL). It is expected that moderate-intensity statin will lower LDL-C 30% to 50% from the baseline and high-intensity statins will lower LDL-C more than 50%, including appropriate lifestyle measures in the treatment effect. Monitoring of fasting lipids should be undertaken 4 to 12 weeks after changes in therapy and every 3 to 12 months thereafter. In general, fasting LDL-C levels on treatment should only be used to assess for anticipated reductions and, thus, for adherence to medication and lifestyle changes or to signal secondary or genetic dyslipidemias for further evaluation. The ACC/AHA guidelines only give a brief mention of nonstatin therapies. However, there is a school of thought that nonfasting LDL-C values differ little from fasting levels and that nonfasting or postprandial triglycerides are a significant predictor of CV risk and may trump high-density lipoprotein for prognostic value.[25,26] Thus, clinicians should consider whether, given compliance and diagnostic issues, nonfasting lipid profiles may be indicated or even be preferable to fasting levels. Evaluation for safety (eg, transaminases) is recommended only as needed in patients with hepatic or muscle symptoms. Statins should not be prescribed for pregnant or nursing women.

Adding a nonstatin agent is only recommended for patients who do not have *expected* reductions in LDL-C ($\sim$14% of patients)[27] or have an LDL-C greater than 190 mg/dL on maximum tolerated statin therapy and who have active arteriosclerotic cardiovascular disease (ASCVD) or diabetes. Large recent studies, action to control cardiovascular risk in diabetes (ACCORD) and Aim-High Atherothrombosis intervention in metabolic syndrome with low high density lipoprotein/high triglyceride, impact on global health outcomes (AIM-HIGH), have not shown improved outcomes with added fibrates or niacin and have confirmed the well-known risk of liver function tests (LFT) elevations.[28,29] However, many patients are intolerant to statins, with patients on high-intensity statins having an adjusted odds ratio (OR) of 50% for musculoskeletal pain compared with controls[27]; no good long-term outcome data exist for other agents. An Agency for Healthcare Research and Quality–funded 2014 meta-analysis showed that the combination of a low-intensity statin with ezetimibe or a bile-acid resin could be used with fewer side effects and better LDL-C results in patients with diabetes; but there are no long-term, hard-outcome data; the data for other lipid-lowering agents were insufficient for analysis.[27] It remains to be seen whether the newer fibrates will address the fasting and/or postprandial CV risk associated with high triglycerides.[30] The ACC/AHA's report mentions safety and prescribing parameters for nonstatin agents if they are required.[24]

The 2013 guidelines also recommend shared decision making; it is important to note, for example, that the benefit of quitting smoking far outweighs the benefit from starting a statin. Thus, provider time might be better spent understanding and encouraging a patient's motivation to quit smoking as a priority before, or in parallel with, discussing and beginning another expensive medication.[31] Patients younger than 40 years or older than 75 years, with or without diabetes, should be treated using risk estimates and shared decision making.[13] When considering statin therapy, providers should be aware that the recent NAVIGATOR trial confirms that statins increase the risk of developing diabetes (number needed to harm = 1 out of 12 patients every 5 years; HR = 1.32); thus, patients with prediabetes who are started on statins should be monitored closely for hyperglycemia.

MENTAL HEALTH TARGETS

In its 2014 Standard of Care, the American Diabetes Association recommends the assessment of patients' psychological and social situation as an ongoing part of the medical management of diabetes.[32] Several mental health conditions can affect the care of patients with diabetes. In addition, some mental health conditions are associated with an increase in diabetes incidence or diabetes-related complications.

The depressive disorders have a prevalence of up to 25% in people with diabetes,[32,33] much higher than the general population prevalence of 2% to 14%. Diabetes is a risk factor for developing depression in adults, with a 24% to 43% increase in relative risk.[34,35] Conversely, depression is associated with a relative risk of incidence of diabetes of 1.37 to 2.02.[35,36] Depression is also associated with an increased incidence of the metabolic syndrome.[37]

Diabetes-related emotional distress is associated with reduced care plan adherence and worse diabetes control.[38] Depression is further associated with worse adherence to diabetes care plans, with the largest effect sizes being for missed medical appointments and a self-care composite score.[39] Depression increases the risk of diabetes-related microvascular and macrovascular complications,[40] myocardial infarction,[41] and death.[42]

Given the prevalence of depression and the well-known difficulties of recognizing it in medical practice, universal screening for depression in people with diabetes is a logical approach that will yield undiagnosed patients with active depression for whom treatment will be effective, thus, potentially decreasing morbidity. Two easily available assessment tools for measuring emotional well-being or diabetes-related distress are the World Health Organization-5 (WHO-5) Well-being Index and the Problem Areas in Diabetes Questionnaire. These tools ask a limited set of questions about mental health but are not typically used for definitive assessment of possible mental health conditions.[43] Validated screening tests are available for the common mental health conditions affecting diabetes care (**Table 2**).

The choice to treat or refer will be determined by the available resources. Most mental health conditions are initially or fully treated in primary care or general medical settings where the use of the Patient Health Questionnaire 9 and the Generalized Anxiety Disorder 7 (see **Table 2**) aid in the assessment and management of depressive and anxiety disorders. A systematic review shows that psychosocial interventions can improve A1c (−0.3%).[44] Collaborative care models for "diapression" involving mental health and medical providers in a multidisciplinary team show promise.[45] In general medical settings, the collaborative care model with colocated medical and mental health care provides superior outcomes when compared with more fragmented care systems.

WEIGHT CONTROL TARGETS

The healthy weight target of a body mass index (BMI) less than 25 is well established, but the difficulty of weight loss has been a persistent problem (see the article by Evert and Riddell elsewhere in this issue for further exploration of this topic). Although there is plentiful evidence that exercise is beneficial, the recent Look AHEAD (Action for Health in Diabetes) trial[46] was stopped early, at 9.6 years, because of futility. The bottom line from this intensive lifestyle intervention trial (cardiovascular outcomes in 5145 overweight/obese patients with type 2 diabetes undergoing 175 minutes of exercise per week and a diet with <30% fat and >15% protein, resulting in a mean weight loss of 8.6%) is that it was ineffective in reducing cardiovascular events. However, study participants had already achieved reasonable cardiovascular targets for blood

Table 2
Screening and assessment tools for well-being and mental health conditions

Condition	Assessment Tool	Reference
Depressive disorders	PHQ-2, PHQ-9	http://phqscreeners.com/pdfs/02_PHQ-9/English.pdf
Anxiety disorders	GAD-7	http://www.integration.samhsa.gov/clinical-practice/GAD708.19.08Cartwright.pdf
ADHD	Adult ADHD self-report scale	http://www.hcp.med.harvard.edu/ncs/ftpdir/adhd/18Q_ASRS_English.pdf
Obsessive-compulsive disorder	Yale-Brown Obsessive Compulsive Scale	http://healthnet.umassmed.edu/mhealth/YBOCRatingScale.pdf
Eating disorder	SCOFF	Hill LS, et al. SCOFF (Useful eating disorders screening questionnaire), the development of an eating disorder screening questionnaire. Int J Eat Disord 2010;43(4):344 (http://www.kmpt.nhs.uk/Downloads/Trust-Services/ED-primary-care-screening-tool-scoff.pdf)
General assessment	WHO-5 Well-being Index	http://www.dawnstudy.com/News_and_activities/Documents/WHO-5.pdf
General assessment, diabetes	PAID	http://www.dawnstudy.com/News_and_activities/Documents/PAID_problem_areas_in_diabetes_questionnaire.pdf

Abbreviations: ADHD, attention-deficit/hyperactivity disorder; GAD-7; Generalized Anxiety Disorder 7; PAID, Problem Areas in Diabetes; PHQ, Patient Health Questionnaire.

pressure, glycemia, lipids etc, and mean weight loss at the end of the trial differed by only 2.6% from the control group. However, study participants already had reasonable CV targets for blood pressure, glycemia, lipids, and so forth, with mean weight loss at the end of the trial differing by only 2.5%. Only a few conclusions can be drawn from the many studies on diet and weight loss (see paper on Lifestyle for details): (1) Mediterranean diets with olive oil improve cardiovascular outcomes. (2) Dietary targets of less than 30% fat and less than 20% carbohydrate intake may facilitate weight loss and improve glycemic and lipid control. (3) One trial showed that low-carbohydrate diets are probably more effective than very-low-calorie diets alone for weight loss.[47–52]

Increasing evidence points to at least 7% of body weight loss to significantly delay or prevent diabetes in those at risk. Numerous studies and several meta-analyses

Box 2
Evaluation and targets for safe driving (in any patients at risk for hypoglycemia)

- Review the driving history and risk of disruptive hypoglycemia at least every 2 years.
- Evaluate for *severe* hypoglycemia in the past 2 years and, if present, ask whether hypoglycemia is explained and correctable. The target is 3 or less disruptive hypoglycemic events per year.
- If patients are at risk for disruptive hypoglycemia, the target glucose is greater than 90 mg/dL (5.0 mmol/L) before extended driving.
- If the patients' license is suspended, reevaluate at no more than 6 months.

Box 3
Summary of nonglycemic targets for adults with diabetes

BP[8,9] and nephropathy

- <140/90 For all adults regardless of renal disease; new JNC 8 guidelines based on a Cochrane meta-analysis and other studies showing a lack of evidence for lower targets and some evidence for harm; control of BP more important than decreasing proteinuria (see text)

- ACEI or ARB for any albuminuria; new geriatric guidelines also target BP ≤140/90

Lipids[24]

- For patients aged 40–75 y with symptomatic ASCVD and/or diabetes, initiation of moderate to high-intensity statin, as tolerated, is target for LDL-C ≥70 mg/dL; check fasting lipids at 3–12 wk, then yearly if anticipated response (30%–49% reduction with moderate-intensity therapy or ≥50% reduction with high-intensity therapy)

- If LDL-C >190 mg/dL or inadequate response, consider adding a nonstatin agent; statins contraindicated in pregnant and nursing women

Foot infections[59–61]

- Confirm infected vs noninfected via ≥2 signs of infection; debride then culture and treat with antibiotics *only* if infected; classify as mild, moderate, severe; mild = oral antibiotics only; nonremovable device (complete) off-loading key to healing chronic ulcers/osteomyelitis

- 2012 antibiotic recommendations: cover only gram-positive cocci unless history of previous MRSA or specific high-risk factors for pseudomonas

Weight control/loss[32,54] via Exercise, Diet,[62,63] and Surgery[54]

- Goal BMI <25

- Patients with IFG, IGT, or prediabetes and BMI >24.9 aim for 7% weight loss

- Bariatric surgery more effective than medical treatment for weight loss, CV outcomes, and remission of diabetes

- Target of 175 min of exercise per week

- <30% Fat intake recommended

- <20% kcal As carbohydrate is more effective for short-term weight loss if overweight than very low calorie diets

Alcohol[32]

- ≤14 Standard drinks per wk for men, <7 per wk for women (2-d abstinence per wk)

Driving[55]

- Target of no disruptive hypoglycemia on assessments every 2 y

- Adequate eyesight and peripheral neuropathy assessment, particularly for accelerator/brake foot

Mental health

- Outcomes improved by screening and treating for psychological stress and other mental illness

Abbreviations: BP, blood pressure; IFG, impaired fasting glucose; IGT, impaired glucose tolerance; MRSA, methicillin-resistant *Staphylococcus aureus*.

have supported that bariatric surgery, including bypass surgery, laparoscopic band-ing, and gastric sleeve surgery, can induce remission of diabetes and improve long-term outcomes for patients with a BMI of 30 or more. Virtually all trials have shown that bariatric surgery is more effective than medical therapy, and a recent meta-analysis showed a 50% decrease in CV events and a 40% reduction in mortality compared with medical therapy, albeit with 15% of patients having malabsorptive sur-gery developing iron deficiency and 8% of patients requiring reoperation.[53,54]

DRIVING TARGETS

Targets for the evaluation of safe driving should include regular (approximately every 2 years) clinical assessments for increased risk.[55] Although driving is relatively safe for most patients with diabetes, the issue is not without controversy. Commercial drivers with diabetes are legally required to undergo medical evaluation periodically. See the National Institutes of Health's evaluation site www.diabetesdriving.com. The estimated HR for accidents while driving in those with diabetes is approximately 2, though patients with diabetes differ dramatically in their individual risk, with the great-est risks, excluding eyesight issues, being disruptive hypoglycemia (requiring the assistance of another person to normalize glucose and cognitive function) and sleep apnea (OR = 6.3 of an accident with an apnea-hypopnea index greater than 10).[56] Lesser risks include numbness in the right foot (accelerator/brake foot) (**Box 2**).[55]

SUMMARY

In conclusion, targets for patients with diabetes have actually become simpler with the release of new guidelines. The targets discussed in this article are summarized in **Box 3**. Finally, as clinicians and patients with diabetes struggle with the overwhelming burden of care, clinicians should consider the increasingly codified ethic of minimally disruptive medicine, which considers not just what patients and doctors can do but what patients' priorities, wishes, and needs are rather than the many specialist tests and treatment options available.[57,58] Finding the balance may be easier with the new evidence-based and more straightforward guidelines.

REFERENCES

1. Orchard TJ, Chang YF, Ferrell RE, et al. Nephropathy in type 1 diabetes: a mani-festation of insulin resistance and multiple genetic susceptibilities? Further evi-dence from the Pittsburgh Epidemiology of Diabetes Complication Study. Kidney Int 2002;62(3):963–70.
2. Freedman BI, Bostrom M, Daeihagh P, et al. Genetic factors in diabetic ne-phropathy. Clin J Am Soc Nephrol 2007;2(6):1306–16.
3. Divers J, Freedman BI. Genetics in kidney disease in 2013: susceptibility genes for renal and urological disorders. Nat Rev Nephrol 2014;10(2):69–70.
4. Mazzucco G, Bertani T, Fortunato M, et al. Different patterns of renal damage in type 2 diabetes mellitus: a multicentric study on 393 biopsies. Am J Kidney Dis 2002;39(4):713–20.
5. Roscioni SS, Heerspink HJ, de Zeeuw D. The effect of RAAS blockade on the progression of diabetic nephropathy. Nat Rev Nephrol 2014;10(2):77–87.
6. Gregg EW, Li Y, Wang J, et al. Changes in diabetes-related complications in the United States, 1990-2010. N Engl J Med 2014;370(16):1514–23.

7. Hermida RC, Ayala DE, Mojon A, et al. Influence of time of day of blood pressure-lowering treatment on cardiovascular risk in hypertensive patients with type 2 diabetes. Diabetes Care 2011;34(6):1270–6.
8. James PA, Oparil S, Carter BL, et al. 2014 evidence-based guideline for the management of high blood pressure in adults: report from the panel members appointed to the Eighth Joint National Committee (JNC 8). JAMA 2014;311(5): 507–20.
9. Arguedas JA, Leiva V, Wright JM. Blood pressure targets for hypertension in people with diabetes mellitus. Cochrane Database Syst Rev 2013;(10):CD008277.
10. Shen L, Shah BR, Reyes EM, et al. Role of diuretics, beta blockers, and statins in increasing the risk of diabetes in patients with impaired glucose tolerance: reanalysis of data from the NAVIGATOR study. BMJ 2013;347:f6745.
11. Blood pressure management in CKD ND patients with diabetes mellitus. Kidney Int Suppl 2012;2:363–9.
12. Weber MA, Schiffrin EL, White WB, et al. Clinical practice guidelines for the management of hypertension in the community: a statement by the American Society of Hypertension and the International Society of Hypertension. J Clin Hypertens 2014;16(1):14–26.
13. American Geriatrics Society Expert Panel on Care of Older Adults with Diabetes Mellitus, Moreno G, Mangione CM, et al. Guidelines abstracted from the American Geriatrics Society guidelines for improving the care of older adults with diabetes mellitus: 2013 update. J Am Geriatr Soc 2013;61(11):2020–6.
14. Cheng J, Zhang W, Zhang X, et al. Effect of angiotensin-converting enzyme inhibitors and angiotensin II receptor blockers on all-cause mortality, cardiovascular deaths, and cardiovascular events in patients with diabetes mellitus: a meta-analysis. JAMA Intern Med 2014;174(5):773–85.
15. Wu HY, Huang JW, Lin HJ, et al. Comparative effectiveness of renin-angiotensin system blockers and other antihypertensive drugs in patients with diabetes: systematic review and bayesian network meta-analysis. BMJ 2013;347:f6008.
16. Beckett N, Peters R, Tuolilehto J, et al. Immediate and late benefits of treating very elderly people with hypertension: results from active treatment extension to Hypertension in the Very Elderly randomised controlled trial. BMJ 2012;344:d7541.
17. Blood pressure management in elderly persons with CKD ND. Kidney Int Suppl 2012;2:377–81.
18. Fried LF, Emanuele N, Zhang JH, et al. Combined angiotensin inhibition for the treatment of diabetic nephropathy. N Engl J Med 2013;369(20):1892–903.
19. Bakris GL, Weir MR. Angiotensin-converting enzyme inhibitor-associated elevations in serum creatinine: is this a cause for concern? Arch Intern Med 2000; 160(5):685–93.
20. Go AS, Chertow GM, Fan D, et al. Chronic kidney disease and the risks of death, cardiovascular events, and hospitalization. N Engl J Med 2004;351(13): 1296–305.
21. Juurlink DN, Mamdani MM, Lee DS, et al. Rates of hyperkalemia after publication of the Randomized Aldactone Evaluation Study. N Engl J Med 2004;351(6): 543–51.
22. Adam WR. Plasma and dialysate potassium concentrations and haemodialysis associated mortality. Nephrology 2013;18(10):655–6.
23. Weir MR, Rolfe M. Potassium homeostasis and renin-angiotensin-aldosterone system inhibitors. Clin J Am Soc Nephrol 2010;5(3):531–48.
24. Stone NJ, Robinson J, Lichtenstein AH, et al. 2013 ACC/AHA guideline on the treatment of blood cholesterol to reduce atherosclerotic cardiovascular risk in adults: a

report of the American College of Cardiology/American Heart Association Task Force on Practice Guidelines. J Am Coll Cardiol 2014;63(25 Pt B):2889–934.

25. Kolovou GD, Mikhailidis DP, Kovar J, et al. Assessment and clinical relevance of non-fasting and postprandial triglycerides: an expert panel statement. Curr Vasc Pharmacol 2011;9(3):258–70.

26. Nordestgaard BG, Freiberg JJ. Clinical relevance of non-fasting and postprandial hypertriglyceridemia and remnant cholesterol. Curr Vasc Pharmacol 2011; 9(3):281–6.

27. Gudzune KA, Monroe AK, Sharma R, et al. Effectiveness of combination therapy with statin and another lipid-modifying agent compared with intensified statin monotherapy: a systematic review. Ann Intern Med 2014;160(7):468–76.

28. Linz PE, Lovato LC, Byington RP, et al. Paradoxical reduction in HDL-C with fenofibrate and thiazolidinedione therapy in type 2 diabetes: the ACCORD lipid trial. Diabetes Care 2014;37(3):686–93.

29. AIM-HIGH Investigators, Boden WE, Probstfield JL, et al. Niacin in patients with low HDL cholesterol levels receiving intensive statin therapy. N Engl J Med 2011;365(24):2255–67.

30. Kolovou GD, Kostakou PM, Anagnostopoulou KK, et al. Therapeutic effects of fibrates in postprandial lipemia. Am J Cardiovasc Drugs 2008;8(4):243–55.

31. D'Agostino RB Sr, Ansell BJ, Mora S, et al. Clinical decisions. The guidelines battle on starting statins. N Engl J Med 2014;370(17):1652–8.

32. American Diabetes Association. Standards of medical care in diabetes–2014. Diabetes Care 2014;37(Suppl 1):S14–80.

33. Sudore RL, Karter AJ, Huang ES, et al. Symptom burden of adults with type 2 diabetes across the disease course: diabetes & aging study. J Gen Intern Med 2012;27(12):1674–81.

34. Nouwen A, Winkley K, Twisk J, et al. Type 2 diabetes mellitus as a risk factor for the onset of depression: a systematic review and meta-analysis. Diabetologia 2010;53(12):2480–6.

35. Chen PC, Chan YT, Chen HF, et al. Population-based cohort analyses of the bidirectional relationship between type 2 diabetes and depression. Diabetes Care 2013;36(2):376–82.

36. Knol MJ, Twisk JW, Beekman AT, et al. Depression as a risk factor for the onset of type 2 diabetes mellitus. A meta-analysis. Diabetologia 2006;49(5):837–45.

37. Pan A, Sun Q, Okereke OI, et al. Use of antidepressant medication and risk of type 2 diabetes: results from three cohorts of US adults. Diabetologia 2012; 55(1):63–72.

38. Aikens JE. Prospective associations between emotional distress and poor outcomes in type 2 diabetes. Diabetes Care 2012;35(12):2472–8.

39. Gonzalez JS, Peyrot M, McCarl LA, et al. Depression and diabetes treatment nonadherence: a meta-analysis. Diabetes Care 2008;31(12):2398–403.

40. de Groot M, Anderson R, Freedland KE, et al. Association of depression and diabetes complications: a meta-analysis. Psychosom Med 2001;63(4):619–30.

41. Scherrer JF, Garfield LD, Chrusciel T, et al. Increased risk of myocardial infarction in depressed patients with type 2 diabetes. Diabetes Care 2011;34(8):1729–34.

42. van Dooren FE, Nefs G, Schram MT, et al. Depression and risk of mortality in people with diabetes mellitus: a systematic review and meta-analysis. PLoS One 2013;8(3):5.

43. Nicolucci A, Kovacs Burns K, Holt RI, et al. Diabetes attitudes, wishes and needs second study (DAWN2): cross-national benchmarking of diabetes-related psychosocial outcomes for people with diabetes. Diabet Med 2013;30(7):767–77.

44. Harkness E, Macdonald W, Valderas J, et al. Identifying psychosocial interventions that improve both physical and mental health in patients with diabetes: a systematic review and meta-analysis. Diabetes Care 2010;33(4):926–30.
45. Ciechanowski P. Diapression: an integrated model for understanding the experience of individuals with co-occurring diabetes and depression. Clin Diabetes 2011;29:43–50.
46. Look AR, Wing RR, Bolin P, et al. Cardiovascular effects of intensive lifestyle intervention in type 2 diabetes. N Engl J Med 2013;369(2):145–54.
47. Gardner CD, Kiazand A, Alhassan S, et al. Comparison of the Atkins, Zone, Ornish, and LEARN diets for change in weight and related risk factors among overweight premenopausal women: the A TO Z Weight Loss Study: a randomized trial. JAMA 2007;297(9):969–77.
48. Guldbrand H, Dizdar B, Bunjaku B, et al. In type 2 diabetes, randomisation to advice to follow a low-carbohydrate diet transiently improves glycaemic control compared with advice to follow a low-fat diet producing a similar weight loss. Diabetologia 2012;55(8):2118–27.
49. Krebs JD, Elley CR, Parry-Strong A, et al. The Diabetes Excess Weight Loss (DEWL) trial: a randomised controlled trial of high-protein versus high-carbohydrate diets over 2 years in type 2 diabetes. Diabetologia 2012;55(4):905–14.
50. Rock CL, Flatt SW, Pakiz B, et al. Weight loss, glycemic control, and cardiovascular disease risk factors in response to differential diet composition in a weight loss program in type 2 diabetes: a randomized controlled trial. Diabetes Care 2014;37:1573–80.
51. Salas-Salvado J, Bullo M, Estruch R, et al. Prevention of diabetes with Mediterranean diets: a subgroup analysis of a randomized trial. Ann Intern Med 2014; 160(1):1–10.
52. Schellenberg ES, Dryden DM, Vandermeer B, et al. Lifestyle interventions for patients with and at risk for type 2 diabetes: a systematic review and meta-analysis. Ann Intern Med 2013;159(8):543–51.
53. Chang SH, Stoll CR, Song J, et al. The effectiveness and risks of bariatric surgery: an updated systematic review and meta-analysis, 2003-2012. JAMA Surg 2014;149:275–87.
54. Kwok CS, Pradhan A, Khan MA, et al. Bariatric surgery and its impact on cardiovascular disease and mortality: a systematic review and meta-analysis. Int J Cardiol 2014;173(1):20–8.
55. American Diabetes Association, Lorber D, Anderson J, et al. Diabetes and driving. Diabetes Care 2014;37(Suppl 1):S97–103.
56. Teran-Santos J, Jimenez-Gomez A, Cordero-Guevara J. The association between sleep apnea and the risk of traffic accidents. Cooperative Group Burgos-Santander. N Engl J Med 1999;340(11):847–51.
57. Gallacher K, Jani B, Morrison D, et al. Qualitative systematic reviews of treatment burden in stroke, heart failure and diabetes - methodological challenges and solutions. BMC Med Res Methodol 2013;13:10.
58. Montori VM, Brito JP, Ting HH. Patient-centered and practical application of new high cholesterol guidelines to prevent cardiovascular disease. JAMA 2014; 311(5):465–6.
59. Hinchliffe RJ, Valk GD, Apelqvist J, et al. Specific guidelines on wound and wound-bed management. Diabetes Metab Res Rev 2008;24(Suppl 1):S188–9.
60. Hinchliffe RJ, Valk GD, Apelqvist J, et al. A systematic review of the effectiveness of interventions to enhance the healing of chronic ulcers of the foot in diabetes. Diabetes Metab Res Rev 2008;24(Suppl 1):S119–44.

61. Lipsky BA, Berendt AR, Cornia PB, et al. 2012 Infectious Diseases Society of America clinical practice guideline for the diagnosis and treatment of diabetic foot infections. Clin Infect Dis 2012;54(12):e132–73.

62. Sigal M. Comment on Evert et al. Nutrition therapy recommendations for the management of adults with diabetes. Diabetes care 2013;36:3821-3842. Diabetes Care 2014;37(5):e100.

63. Evert AB, Boucher JL, Cypress M, et al. Nutrition therapy recommendations for the management of adults with diabetes. Diabetes Care 2014;37(Suppl 1): S120–43.

Screening and Treatment by the Primary Care Provider of Common Diabetes Complications

Matthew P. Gilbert, DO, MPH

KEYWORDS

- Microvascular complications • Diabetic retinopathy • Diabetic nephropathy
- Macrovascular complications • Diabetic peripheral neuropathy
- Cardiovascular disease

KEY POINTS

- Diabetes is the leading cause of end-stage renal disease, blindness, and nontraumatic lower-limb amputation.
- The largest reductions in cardiovascular events are seen when multiple risk factors such as hypertension, dyslipidemia, and hyperglycemia are addressed simultaneously.
- The benefit of aspirin as secondary prevention in patients with previous stroke or myocardial infarction has been well established.
- Regular, dilated eye examinations are effective in detecting sight-threatening diabetic retinopathy and have been shown to prevent blindness.
- The combined use of appropriate tools and clinical examination/inspection has been shown to provide greater than 87% specificity in the detection of diabetic peripheral neuropathy.
- Early treatment of risk factors, including hypertension, hyperglycemia, and dyslipidemia can delay or prevent diabetic nephropathy.

INTRODUCTION

Diabetes is the leading cause of end-stage renal disease, blindness, and nontraumatic lower-limb amputation. It is also a major cause of cardiovascular morbidity and mortality and the seventh leading cause of death in the United States. The economic cost of diabetes in the United States in 2012 was estimated to be $245 billion, of which $176 billion were direct medical costs related to diabetes.[1] Much of the disability and cost associated with diabetes are related to the care of chronic complications.

Disclosure: The author has no relevant disclosures.
Division of Endocrinology and Diabetes, Department of Medicine, College of Medicine, The University of Vermont, 62 Tilley Drive, South Burlington, VT 05403, USA
E-mail address: matthew.gilbert@vtmednet.org

Med Clin N Am 99 (2015) 201–219
http://dx.doi.org/10.1016/j.mcna.2014.09.002   medical.theclinics.com

Recent advances in knowledge, therapies, and technology have enhanced the ability to effectively care for patients with diabetes. In spite of these advances, patients with diabetes still experience suboptimal glucose, blood pressure, and cholesterol levels, putting them at risk for the development of acute and chronic complications.

CARDIOVASCULAR DISEASE

Cardiovascular disease (CVD) is a major cause of morbidity and mortality in patients with diabetes mellitus and is the largest contributor to the direct and indirect costs of the disease. Patients with diabetes have a higher prevalence of coronary artery disease (CAD), a greater extent of coronary ischemia, and are more likely to have a myocardial infarction (MI).[2] In addition, patients with type 2 diabetes have a high rate of asymptomatic coronary disease and silent ischemia.[3] Recent evidence suggests an overall reduction in cardiovascular events in patients with diabetes mellitus.[4]

The largest reductions in cardiovascular events are seen when multiple risk factors, such as hypertension, dyslipidemia and hyperglycemia, are addressed simultaneously.[5,6] In all patients with diabetes, risk factors for CVD should be assessed on an annual basis. Patients with diabetes should have their blood pressure measured at every routine visit. Home blood pressure measurements may be useful in resolving discrepancies between office-based measurements and out-of-office values in selected patients. In addition to blood pressure screening, adult patients with diabetes should have a fasting lipid profile obtained on a yearly basis. Routine screening for CAD is not recommended in patients with diabetes who are asymptomatic. However, patients with typical or atypical cardiac symptoms or abnormal resting electrocardiogram are candidates for advanced or invasive cardiac testing. The effectiveness of computed tomography and cardiac MRI as screening tools for CAD in asymptomatic patients remains unclear.

The importance of glycemic control (hemoglobin A1c <7%) for the prevention of CVD has been established in patients with type 1 diabetes. The 9-year post-the diabetes control and complications trial (DCCT) follow-up trial, called the DCCT/ Epidemiology of Diabetes Interventions and Complications (EDIC) trial, showed that participants previously randomized to the intensive arm of the DCCT had a 42% reduction in CVD and a 57% reduction in the risk of nonfatal MI, stroke, or cardiovascular death compared with those subjects in the standard arm.[7] The role of glycemic control for the prevention of CVD in patients with type 2 diabetes is not as clearly defined. Most of the randomized, clinical trials have not shown a beneficial effect of intensive glycemic control on macrovascular outcomes in patients with type 2 diabetes. In The UK Prospective Diabetes Study Group (UKPDS) trial there was a 16% reduction in cardiovascular complications in the intensive glycemic control arm, but the difference was not statistically significant.[8] Despite a loss of glycemic differences between the treatment and control groups, the long-term follow-up to the UKPDS showed a continued reduction in microvascular risk and emergent risk reductions for MI during the 10-year posttrial follow-up.[9] The veterans affairs diabetes trial (VADT), action to control cardiovascular risk in diabetes (ACCORD), and action in diabetes and vascular disease—preterax and diamicron modified release controlled evaluation (ADVANCE) trials were designed to compare the effects of intensive versus standard glycemic control on CVD outcomes in high-risk patients with established type 2 diabetes.[10–12] These long-term, randomized clinical trials failed to show the benefit of intensive control on cardiovascular outcomes.

Hypertension is a major risk factor for the development of CVD in patients with type 1 and type 2 diabetes. Several studies have shown that blood pressures greater than

115/75 mm Hg are associated with increased CVD in patients with diabetes.[13–15] Several randomized clinical trials have shown a reduction in cardiovascular events, including stroke, with the lowering of systolic blood pressure to less than 140/80 mm Hg.[16–18] There remains limited evidence regarding the benefits for lower systolic blood pressure targets. All patients with diabetes and hypertension should be treated with a goal blood pressure of less than 140/80 mm Hg. Lifestyle modifications including weight loss, the dietary approaches to stop hypertension (DASH) diet, reduction in sodium intake (1500 mg/d), and increased physical activity should accompany pharmacologic treatment. Initial pharmacologic management should include an angiotensin-converting enzyme (ACE) inhibitor or angiotensin receptor blocker (ARB). Most patients with diabetes and hypertension require multiple-drug therapy to obtain treatment goals.[13]

Several large clinical trials have shown the beneficial effects of statin therapy for primary and secondary prevention of CVD.[19,20] Clinical trials in patients with diabetes have shown similar reductions.[21,22] The initial treatment goal should be to lower low-density lipoprotein (LDL) cholesterol levels to less than 100 mg/dL. In patients with known CVD, or in patients more than 40 years of age with other risk factors, pharmacologic treatment should be initiated in addition to aggressive lifestyle and dietary modifications regardless of baseline lipid values. Statins remain the drug of choice for lowering LDL cholesterol levels. Clinical trials in patients with previous cardiovascular events or known CAD have shown that aggressive therapy with statins to achieve an LDL cholesterol level of less than 70 mg/dL may lead to further reduction in cardiovascular events.[23–25] The American Diabetes Association recommends an alternative therapeutic goal of an LDL reduction of 30% to 40% from baseline in patients who have not met treatment targets on maximum tolerated statin therapy. There remains little definitive clinical evidence regarding the benefits of lipid level lowering for the prevention of CVD in patients with type 1 diabetes or in patients with type 2 diabetes less than 40 years of age. Despite lack of definitive data, similar lipid level–lowering goals should be considered for these patients. Recent guidelines published by the American Heart Association (AHA) and the American College of Cardiology (ACC) recommend high-intensity statin therapy in all patients who are 40 to 75 years of age with type 1 or type 2 diabetes and a greater than or equal to 7.5% estimated 10-year atherosclerotic cardiovascular disease (ASCVD) risk.[26]

In patients with type 2 diabetes, low levels of high-density lipoprotein (HDL) cholesterol and increased triglyceride levels are common. Several medications are available that can reduce triglyceride levels. Gemfibrozil was shown to decrease rates of CVD in a small subgroup of patients with type 2 diabetes.[27] However, Keech and colleagues[28] (2005) showed that treatment with a fenofibrate failed to reduce overall cardiovascular events. Although efficacious for the treatment of dyslipidemia, the combination of a statin, fibrate, and niacin was associated with an increased risk of abnormal liver function tests and rhabdomyolysis. In the ACCORD study, the combination of a fenofibrate and a statin medication failed to reduce the rate of cardiovascular events, nonfatal MI, or nonfatal stroke compared with statins alone in patients with type 2 diabetes.[29] The current available data suggest that combination therapy does not provide additional benefit compared with statin therapy alone and therefore is generally not recommended.

The benefit of aspirin as secondary prevention in patients with previous stroke or MI has been well established. However, the role of aspirin in primary prevention of CVD in patients with diabetes remains controversial. Baigent and colleagues[30] (2009) published a meta-analysis of the 6 largest trails of aspirin for primary prevention of CVD. The analysis included more than 4000 patients with diabetes. Aspirin was shown to reduce the risk of vascular events by 12%, with the largest reduction seen in nonfatal MI. The effect of aspirin on cardiovascular events was similar for patients with and without diabetes. Two randomized controlled clinical trials of aspirin failed to show a reduction in cardiovascular events in patients with diabetes.[31,32] Clinicians should consider treatment with aspirin (75–162 mg/d) for primary prevention of CVD in patients with type 1 and type 2 diabetes at increased cardiovascular risk (10-year risk >10%) and who are not at increased risk for bleeding. Treatment with aspirin is not recommended as primary prevention in patients with diabetes and low cardiovascular risk (10-year risk <5%). The American Diabetes Association recommends use of clinical judgment for those at intermediate risk (10-year risk 5%–10%) until further research is available regarding the risks and benefits of aspirin therapy. Aspirin therapy is recommended for all patients with diabetes and a history of CVD as secondary prevention. Aspirin use in patients less than 21 years of age is contraindicated.

Physical activity can improve insulin sensitivity and lower total cholesterol levels, LDL cholesterol levels, and triglyceride levels, as well as raising HDL cholesterol levels. In addition, exercise may further decrease the risk of CVD by improving overall cardiovascular fitness and function. Even patients with diabetes who are not obese can benefit from physical activity. Adults with diabetes should be advised to obtain at least 150 minutes per week of moderate-intensity, aerobic activity with no more than 2 consecutive days without exercise. Smoking is an independent risk factor for the development of CVD. A recent study found that smoking cessation was associated with reduction in blood pressure and albuminuria in patients with newly diagnosed type 2 diabetes.[33] All patients with diabetes should be encouraged not to smoke or use tobacco products and smoking cessation counseling should be part of routine diabetes care.

Retinopathy

Diabetic retinopathy is the most frequent cause of blindness among adults 20 to 74 years of age. The pathophysiology, natural history, and clinical presentation of diabetic retinopathy are well understood with recognizable stages of the disease. Early clinical signs of retinopathy include small outpouchings from the retinal capillaries called microaneurysms and dot intraretinal hemorrhages. As the disease progresses, macular edema, ischemic changes, collateralization, and proliferative changes may lead to visual impairment or vision loss. Risk factors for developing diabetic retinopathy include duration of diabetes,[34,35] severity of hyperglycemia,[8,36,37] hypertension,[16] and dyslipidemia.[38]

Twenty years after the diagnosis of diabetes, almost all patients with type 1 diabetes and approximately 80% of patients with type 2 diabetes have some degree of diabetic retinopathy.[35] Over the last 30 years there has been a decline in both the incidence and risk of progression of diabetic retinopathy.[39] The Wisconsin Epidemiologic Study of Diabetic Retinopathy reported a 77% decline in the annual incidence of proliferative retinopathy in patients with type 1 diabetes mellitus (T1DM) from 1980 to 2007.[40]

There are precise, safe, and accepted screening tests (ophthalmoscopy and retinal photography) for diabetic retinopathy.[41] Regular dilated eye examinations are effective in detecting sight-threatening diabetic retinopathy and have been shown to prevent blindness.[42,43] Patients with macular edema and diabetic retinopathy may be asymptomatic at the time of diagnosis, so all patients with diabetes should undergo comprehensive screening. Screening for diabetic retinopathy in patients with type 1 diabetes should be started within 5 years following the diagnosis. This screening recommendation is supported by evidence that retinopathy is estimated to take 5 years to develop after the onset of hyperglycemia.[44] Patients with newly diagnosed type 2 diabetes may have had asymptomatic hyperglycemia for several years before the diagnosis and thus have a significant risk of diabetic retinopathy at the time of diagnosis. Therefore, patients with type 2 diabetes should have an initial dilated and comprehensive eye examination at the time of diagnosis. An optometrist or an ophthalmologist with experience in the diagnosis of diabetic retinopathy should perform the comprehensive examination. Dilated and comprehensive eye examinations should be repeated on an annual basis for patients with type 1 and type 2 diabetes. However, there is evidence to suggest that, in patients with well-controlled type 2 diabetes, a comprehensive evaluation every 2 years may be cost-effective with little risk of development of diabetic retinopathy.[45]

Ophthalmoscopy remains the most common technique for monitoring diabetic retinopathy. However, the use of nondilated ophthalmoscopy by non–eye care providers has been shown to have poor sensitivity compared with retinal photography.[41] Screening for diabetic retinopathy using a nonmydriatic camera (eg, without dilating the pupils) has become more popular. Several studies have examined the efficacy of digital retinal photographs as a screening tool for retinopathy. A recent meta-analysis of 20 studies using nonmydriatic digital retinal photographs showed 82.5% sensitivity and 88.5% specificity for the diagnosis of diabetic retinopathy.[46] The use of retinal photography, with remote reading by an ophthalmologist, has been promoted as a way to improve the diagnosis and treatment of patients with retinopathy, particularly in rural areas where eye care professionals may not be readily available. Retinal photographs may be a useful screening tool for diabetic retinopathy, but should not be a substitute for a comprehensive eye examination. **Fig. 1** shows the effectiveness of retinal photographs in identifying retinopathy.

Changes in glycemic control or other hormonal factors during pregnancy may accelerate diabetic retinopathy. Patients enrolled in the DCCT had transient worsening of retinopathy during pregnancy.[47] The American Diabetes Association recommends that women with preexisting diabetes who are pregnant should have comprehensive eye examination during the first trimester with close follow-up for 1 year postpartum.

Large randomized controlled trials have shown that intensive glycemic management, with a goal of normoglycemia, can prevent the onset and delay the progression of diabetic retinopathy.[8,47–49] The UKPDS reported the effectiveness of tight (<150/ 85 mm Hg) blood pressure control in reducing the progression of diabetic retinopathy.

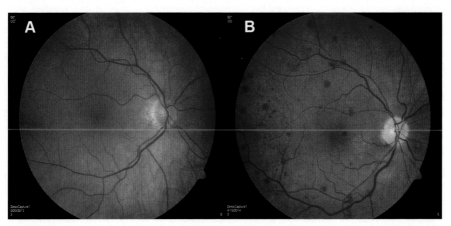

Fig. 1. (A) Normal and (B) diabetic retinopathy. (Courtesy of Brian Kim, MD, Burlington, VT.)

However, the ACCORD study failed to show that reducing blood pressure to less than 120 mm Hg offered further benefit.[29]

Retinal photocoagulation for the treatment of diabetic retinopathy was introduced in the 1960s. The effectiveness of photocoagulation in the treatment of diabetic retinopathy has been shown in several clinical trials. The Diabetic Retinopathy Study (DRS) concluded that retinal photocoagulation reduced the risk of severe vision loss to 6.4% of treated eyes compared with 15.9% of untreated eyes.[50] The Early Treatment Diabetic Retinopathy Study (ETDS) showed that focal retinal photocoagulation was effective in reducing macular edema.[50] Both the DRS and the ETDS showed the efficacy of retinal photocoagulation in the reduction of further vision loss from diabetic retinopathy, but did not show that photocoagulation could reverse retinopathy.

An active factor in the pathophysiology of diabetic retinopathy is inflammation, which leads to macular edema, ischemia, and neovascularization.[51] Vascular endothelial growth factor is one of many proinflammatory mediators that have been shown to induce angiogenesis and vascular permeability.[51] Treatment with vascular endothelial growth factor inhibitors (ranibizumab and bevacizumab) has been shown to improve vision and reduce further need for photocoagulation in patients with clinically significant diabetic macular edema.[52] These intravitreal drug therapies are typically injected every 4 to 6 weeks.

The EURODIAB controlled trial of lisionpril in insulin-dependent diabetes mellitus (EUCLID) study reported that use of an ACE inhibitor may reduce the progression of diabetic retinopathy and the incidence of proliferative diabetic retinopathy in normotensive patients with type 1 diabetes.[53] The more recent ADVANCE/the action in diabetes and vascular disease controlled evaluation retinal measurement (ADREM) trial seemed to show some protective effect of ACE inhibitors on the progression of retinopathy in patients with type 2 diabetes, although the data were not statistically significant.[54] The Diabetic Retinopathy Candesartan Trials (DIRECT) were a group of 3 multicenter, randomized, placebo-controlled studies design to determine whether pharmacologic blockade of the renin-angiotensin system by candesartan could prevent the onset (DIRECT-Prevent 1)[55] or progression (DIRECT-Protect 1)[55] of diabetic retinopathy in patients with type 1 diabetes or promote regression of diabetic retinopathy in type 2 diabetes (DIRECT-Protect 2).[56] The severity of retinopathy at the end of the study was significantly more favorable in patients treated with candesartan in DIRECT-Prevent 1, DIRECT-Protect 1, and DIRECT-Protect 2. The results of DIRECT-Protect 2 showed a statistically significant 34% increase in the probability of regression of diabetic retinopathy in patients with type 2 diabetes treated with candesartan.

Lipid level–lowering agents may also decrease the risk of vision loss in patients with diabetic retinopathy. The fenofibrate intervention and event lowering in diabetes (FIELD) study reported a 30% reduction in the need for laser treatment of diabetic macular edema and proliferative diabetic retinopathy in patients treated with a fenofibrate.[57] The ACCORD Eye Study Group also reported a reduction in the progression of diabetic retinopathy in patients with type 2 diabetes treated with a fenofibrate and statin compared with patients treated with statin alone.[49]

Diabetic Peripheral Neuropathy

Diabetic neuropathy is a common complication of both type 1 and type 2 diabetes. The term diabetic neuropathy encompasses a spectrum of clinical syndromes with differing anatomic distributions, clinical courses, and underlying pathogenic mechanisms.[58] Each clinical syndrome is characterized by diffuse or focal damage to peripheral somatic or autonomic nerve fibers resulting from hyperglycemia. Diabetic neuropathy is typically divided into diabetic peripheral neuropathy (DPN) and autonomic neuropathy. DPN has been defined as the presence of symptoms and/or signs of peripheral nerve dysfunction after the exclusion of other causes (ie, traumatic, compressive, neoplastic, metabolic, or other systemic illnesses).[58,59] The prevalence of diabetic neuropathy in newly diagnosed patients with diabetes is estimated to be 8% and greater than 50% in patients with long-standing disease.[60] Diabetic neuropathy remains the leading cause of nontraumatic limb amputations.[61] Several epidemiologic studies have shown that duration and severity of diabetes are significant risk factors for the development of diabetic neuropathy in patients with type 1 and type 2 diabetes.[62] Additional investigations have also shown that smoking, dyslipidemia, and hypertension increase an individual's risk of developing neuropathy.[63,64]

Symptoms such as burning, tingling, numbness, shooting (electric shock), and stabbing are present in 33% of patients with DPN.[65,66] Patients may first experience symptoms in their toes that gradually move proximally. These symptoms are most often worst at night and can disrupt sleep.[67] The high prevalence of diabetic neuropathy results in significant morbidity, including an increased risk of recurrent lower-extremity infections, ulcerations, depression, foot and ankle fractures, and lower-limb amputations.[68–71]

The pathogenesis of DPN is multifactorial and includes a combination of metabolic, vascular, and hormonal factors that shift the balance between nerve fiber damage and repair. The combination of direct nerve injury caused by hyperglycemia, endothelial injury, and microvascular dysfunction leads to nerve ischemia.[72] In addition to nerve ischemia and hypoxia, increased cytokine levels also play a role in the formation of DPN.[73–75]

Several questionnaires have been developed to assist clinicians in the diagnosis of DPN.[76] The douleur neuropathique 4 questions (DN4) questionnaire can be completed rapidly and is easy to use, with reported good specificity (83%) and sensitivity (90%).[77] There are several simple clinical tests that should be used to screen patients for DPN. Patients with type 1 and type 2 diabetes should be screened for DPN on an annual basis. Pinprick sensation and light touch perception should be assessed using a 10-g monofilament. In addition, vibratory threshold should be assessed using a 128-Hz tuning fork. The combined use of appropriate tools and clinical examination/inspection has been shown to provide greater than 87% specificity in the detection of DPN.[78–80]

Improved glycemic control has been shown to improve nerve function in patients with diabetes.[81–83] Intensive glycemic control has also been shown to reduce the risk of developing diabetic neuropathy in patients with type 1 diabetes and may reduce the risk in patients with type 2 diabetes.[84,85] The evidence for glycemic control and the prevention of neuropathy in patients with type 2 diabetes is not as strong. The UKPDS investigators reported a 25% risk reduction in microvascular complications after 10 years of intensive treatment. However, most of the risk reduction was driven by the reduction in retinopathy. Some studies have shown a slowing of the progression of diabetic neuropathy with improved glycemic control in patients with type 2 diabetes. Intensive glycemic control, particularly early in the disease, seems to provide a long-term benefit for the prevention of diabetic neuropathy. The EDIC trial followed approximately 95% of the subjects enrolled in the DCCT cohort for several years.[7] During the EDIC trial, the glycemic separation between the intensively treated group and the standard treatment group disappeared. Patients with previous intensive treatment of their type 1 diabetes had a decrease in the prevalence of neuropathy that persisted through the EDIC follow-up despite deterioration of their glycemic control.[78]

There are no treatments currently available to repair the underlying nerve damage in diabetic neuropathy; however, there are effective symptomatic treatments for the neuropathic pain associated with DPN. Patients with painful neuropathy should be treated with a systematic, stepwise approach. Treatments that may be beneficial include several antidepressants (eg, amitriptyline, duloxetine, venlafaxine) and anticonvulsants (eg, pregabalin, sodium valproate). Effective treatment of painful diabetic neuropathy includes a balance between pain relief and medication side effects (**Table 1**). General principles regarding pharmaceutical management include careful selection of initial drug therapy and titration based on efficacy and side effects.

Several randomized, placebo-controlled trials have shown the effectiveness of tricyclic antidepressant drugs in the treatment of painful diabetic neuropathy[86–89]; however, use is often limited by significant side effects. Serotonin-noradrenaline reuptake inhibitors have been shown to be effective treatments for painful diabetic neuropathy. Medications in this class include venlafaxine, milnacipran, and duloxetine. These drugs block reuptake of both serotonin and norepinephrine with differing selectivity. The extended-release version of venlafaxine (doses of 150–225 mg daily) was superior to placebo in nondepressed patients with diabetic neuropathy.[90] The most common side effects of venlafaxine were nausea and fatigue. Given reports of seizures with this medication it should be used with caution in patients with a history of frequent hypoglycemic seizures. Duloxetine has been licensed in the United States for treatment of painful diabetic neuropathy. The benefit of duloxetine was established in 3 separate 12-week randomized controlled investigations involving more than 1100 patients. In these 3 trials, pain control was better with duloxetine 60 or 120 mg daily than with placebo.[91–93]

Antiepileptic drugs have a long history of effectiveness in the treatment of neuropathic pain. Gabapentin is a anticonvulsant medication whose structure is similar to gamma-aminobutyric acid. The exact mechanism of action of gabapentin with regard to treatment of neuropathic pain is not fully understood. In an 8-week, multicenter,

Table 1
Treatment options for painful, diabetic neuropathy

Drug Class	Drug Name	Dose	Side Effects
TCAs	Amitriptyline	50–150 mg at bedtime	Sedation, anticholinergic effects, dry mouth, tachycardia
	Nortriptyline	50–150 mg at bedtime	Constipation, urinary retention, blurred vision
	Imipramine	25–150 mg at bedtime	Confusion
	Desipramine	25–150 mg at bedtime	—
SNRIs	Venlafaxine	75–225 mg daily	Nausea, fatigue
	Duloxetine	60–120 mg daily	Nausea, fatigue, decreased appetite, dizziness, constipation
Anticonvulsants	Gabapentin	300–1200 mg TID	Fatigue, dizziness, peripheral edema
	Pregabalin	50–150 mg TID	Fatigue, dizziness, peripheral edema
Opioids	Tramadol	50–100 mg BID	Nausea, constipation, dizziness, somnolence
	Oxycodone CR	10–30 mg BID	Nausea, constipation, dizziness, somnolence
Topical	Capsaicin	0.075% QID	Local irritation
	Lidocaine	0.04% daily	Local irritation

Abbreviations: BID, twice a day; QID, 4 times a day; SNRI, serotonin-noradrenaline reuptake inhibitor; TCAs, tricyclic antidepressants; TID, 3 times a day.

randomized controlled trial of 165 patients with diabetes gabapentin had moderate pain relief compared with placebo.[94] However, the overall evidence regarding gabapentin as an effective treatment of painful diabetic retinopathy has been described as weak.[95] Gabapentin has been shown to improve sleep, which is often disturbed in patients with chronic pain and particularly with diabetic neuropathy.[96] Lightheadedness and fatigue were the most common adverse events reported in approximately 23% patients in the randomized controlled trial. Weight gain has also been reported with use of gabapentin. Several clinical trials have investigated the effectiveness of pregabalin in the treatment of painful diabetic neuropathy.[97–100] In a pooled analysis from 7 randomized, placebo-controlled trials, pregabalin was shown to relieve pain and improve quality-of-life measures, social functioning, and mental health as well as improve sleep.[101] The most common adverse events seen in the clinical trials were dizziness, fatigue, and peripheral edema. Pregabalin has also been shown to cause vertigo, incoordination, ataxia, diplopia, blurred vision, sedation, and confusion.[102] Pregabalin may also be habit forming.

For patients who are unable to tolerate any of the pharmaceutical treatments for painful diabetic neuropathy, alternative treatments include capsaicin cream,[103,104] lidocaine patch,[105] alpha-lipoic acid,[106,107] and transcutaneous electrical nerve stimulation.[108] The use of opioids for chronic management remains controversial. Several trials have shown relief of symptoms following treatment with controlled-release oxycodone in patients whose pain was not well controlled on standard treatment.[109,110] However, opioid-related side effects were common among participants in these trials. Treatment of painful diabetic neuropathy with opioid medications should be reserved for patients who have failed to respond or cannot tolerate several first-line medications used in combination.

Diabetic Nephropathy

Nephropathy is a common complication of both type 1 and type 2 diabetes, occurring in 15% to 25% and 30% to 40% of patients, respectively.[111–113] In the analysis of patients enrolled in the UKPDS trial, 24.9% of patients with type 2 diabetes developed microalbuminuria, 5.3% developed microalbuminuria, and 0.8% showed increased creatinine levels or required dialysis within the first 10 years after diagnosis.[114] Diabetes is the leading cause of end-stage renal disease (ESRD) in both developed and emerging countries.[115] The clinical manifestations of diabetic nephropathy, including proteinuria, increased blood pressure, and decreased glomerular filtration rate (GFR), are the same in patients with type 1 and type 2 diabetes.[116] However, by the time the laboratory or clinical abnormalities of diabetic nephropathy become evident, significant pathologic changes are already present within the kidney. Glomerulosclerosis, thickening of the glomerular basement membrane, mesangial cell expansion, loss of podocytes, renal cell hypertrophy, and tubulointerstitial fibrosis are the major pathologic changes that occur during the progression of diabetic nephropathy.[116–119] These changes lead to progressive albuminuria, reduction in GFR, increase in blood pressure, and fluid retention. Chronic kidney disease is associated with a substantially increased risk for CVD that is independent of the traditional CVD risk factors.[120,121]

Screening for diabetic nephropathy should include the evaluation for increased urinary albumin excretion using an albumin/creatinine ratio on a random spot urine collection (**Fig. 2**). An albumin/creatinine ratio should be performed on patients with type 1 diabetes for more than 5 years and in all patients with type 2 diabetes at the time of diagnosis. There may be significant variability in urine albumin excretion. Exercise within 24 hours of collection, infection, fever, congestive heart failure, marked

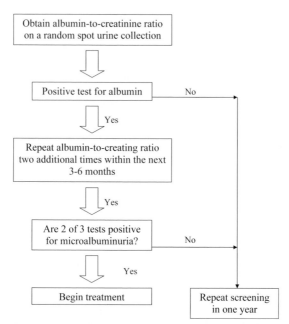

Fig. 2. Algorithm for screening and initiation of treatment in diabetic nephropathy.

hyperglycemia, menstrual blood, and hypertension have all been shown to increase urinary albumin excretion to more than baseline values. Therefore 2 of 3 specimens collected within a period of 3 to 6 months should be abnormal before diagnosing the patient with increased urinary albumin excretion. Clinicians should obtain a serum creatinine level with estimated GFR on a yearly basis in all patients with diabetes regardless of the degree of urine albumin excretion. Clinical studies have found decreased GFR in patients without evidence of increased urine albumin excretion (**Table 2**).[122,123] The role of continued annual assessment of urine albumin excretion after the diagnosis of albuminuria has been made remains unclear. The American Diabetes Association recommends continued monitoring of urine albumin excretion to assess both response to therapy and progression of disease. The development of complications from chronic kidney disease correlates with level of kidney function, particularly GFR. It is recommended that clinicians begin screening for complications of chronic kidney disease in patients with estimated GFR less than 60 mL/min/1.73 m².

The optimal approach to therapy in patients with diabetic nephropathy includes targeting multiple factors, such as hypertension, hyperglycemia, and dyslipidemia. Early

Table 2		
Stages of chronic kidney disease		
Stage	**GFR (mL/min/1.73 m²)**	**Description**
1	>90	Normal or high
2	60–89	Mildly decreased
3a	45–59	Mildly to moderately decreased
3b	30–44	Moderately to severely decreased
4	15–29	Severely decreased
5	<15	Renal failure

treatment of risk factors can delay or prevent diabetic nephropathy. In the UKPDS trial, intensive blood pressure control was associated with a 30% risk reduction for the development of microalbuminuria.[8] The optimal lower limit for systolic blood pressure for the prevention of diabetic nephropathy has not yet been established. Adequate blood pressure control with drugs that modulate the renin-angiotensin system has been shown to reduce the incidence and progression of diabetic nephropathy.[115] Among patients with type 1 diabetes and diabetic nephropathy, remission or regression may occur with control of systemic blood pressure, particularly with ACE inhibitors.[124] Several large, prospective, randomized trials in patients with type 1 diabetes have shown that reduction of systolic blood pressures (<140 mm Hg) as a result of treatment with an ACE inhibitor delayed the progression of microalbuminuria and slowed the reduction in GFR in patients with proteinuria.[125,126] The ADVANCE trial compared the use of an ACE inhibitor with placebo in 11,000 patients with type 2 diabetes. After 4.3 years of follow-up there was a significant reduction in blood pressure and in the rate of new-onset microalbuminuria.[12] The effects of ACE inhibitors and ARBs seem to be independent of blood pressure reduction, suggesting a direct renoprotective effect.[127,128]

Several large, randomized, clinical trials have shown that ARBs reduced the progression of albuminuria as well as ESRD in patients with type 2 diabetes and diabetic nephropathy.[129–136] Other classes of antihypertensive agents can be used in addition to ACE inhibitors and/or ARBs to further reduce blood pressure or in patients who cannot tolerate an ACE inhibitor or ARB.

Intensive glucose control has been shown to decrease the risk of development and delay or prevent progression of diabetic nephropathy. The DCCT and its long-term follow-up, the EDIC trial, showed that intensive glucose control prevented the development of microalbuminuria in patients with type 1 diabetes.[7,47] In patients with type 2 diabetes, the UKPDS showed that intensive glucose control reduced the risk of microalbuminuria or proteinuria by 33%.[137] More recently, the ADVANCE trial confirmed the benefits of intensive glucose control in the landmark clinical trials discussed earlier.[12]

Table 3
Screening recommendations for microvascular complications of diabetes mellitus

Microvascular Complication	Screening Method	Timing of Initial Screening	Frequency of Screening
Retinopathy	Dilated and comprehensive eye examination	T1DM: within 5 y of diagnosis	Annually
		T2DM: at the time of diagnosis	Annually
DPN	Pinprick sensation and light touch perception using a 10-g monofilament and vibratory threshold should be assessed using a 128-Hz tuning fork	At the time of diagnosis	Annually
Diabetic nephropathy	Albumin/creatinine ratio	T1DM: duration of disease >5 y	Annually
		T2DM: at the time of diagnosis	
	Serum creatinine for estimation of GFR	At the time of diagnosis	Annually

Abbreviation: T2DM, type 2 diabetes mellitus.

Clinicians should consider referral to a nephrologist if there are questions regarding the cause of the patient's kidney disease. Consultation with the nephrologist in patients with stage IV chronic kidney disease has been found to reduce cost, improve quality of care, and delay the need for dialysis.[123] Additional triggers for referral may include anemia, secondary hyperparathyroidism, or electrolyte disturbances (**Table 3**).

ACKNOWLEDGMENTS

The author would like to acknowledge Brian Kim, MD, for supplying the retinal photographs and Annis Marney, MD, for editorial support.

REFERENCES

1. American Diabetes Association. Economic costs of diabetes in the U.S. in 2012. Diabetes Care 2013;36(4):1033–46.
2. Emerging Risk Factors Collaboration, Sarwar N, Gao P, et al. Diabetes mellitus, fasting blood glucose concentration, and risk of vascular disease: a collaborative meta-analysis of 102 prospective studies. Lancet 2010;375(9733): 2215–22.
3. Anand DV, Lim E, Lahiri A, et al. The role of non-invasive imaging in the risk stratification of asymptomatic diabetic subjects. Eur Heart J 2006;27(8):905–12.
4. Ali MK, Bullard KM, Saaddine JB, et al. Achievement of goals in U.S. diabetes care, 1999-2010. N Engl J Med 2013;368(17):1613–24.
5. Buse JB, Ginsberg HN, Bakris GL, et al. Primary prevention of cardiovascular diseases in people with diabetes mellitus: a scientific statement from the American Heart Association and the American Diabetes Association. Diabetes Care 2007;30(1):162–72.
6. Gaede P, Lund-Andersen H, Parving HH, et al. Effect of a multifactorial intervention on mortality in type 2 diabetes. N Engl J Med 2008;358(6):580–91.
7. Nathan DM, Cleary PA, Backlund JY, et al. Intensive diabetes treatment and cardiovascular disease in patients with type 1 diabetes. N Engl J Med 2005; 353(25):2643–53.
8. Intensive blood-glucose control with sulphonylureas or insulin compared with conventional treatment and risk of complications in patients with type 2 diabetes (UKPDS 33). UK Prospective Diabetes Study (UKPDS) Group. Lancet 1998; 352(9131):837–53.
9. Holman RR, Paul SK, Bethel MA, et al. 10-year follow-up of intensive glucose control in type 2 diabetes. N Engl J Med 2008;359(15):1577–89.
10. Duckworth W, Abraira C, Moritz T, et al. Glucose control and vascular complications in veterans with type 2 diabetes. N Engl J Med 2009;360(2):129–39.
11. Action to Control Cardiovascular Risk in Diabetes Study Group, Gerstein HC, Miller ME, et al. Effects of intensive glucose lowering in type 2 diabetes. N Engl J Med 2008;358(24):2545–59.
12. ADVANCE Collaborative Group, Patel A, MacMahon S, et al. Intensive blood glucose control and vascular outcomes in patients with type 2 diabetes. N Engl J Med 2008;358(24):2560–72.
13. Chobanian AV, Bakris GL, Black HR, et al. The seventh report of the Joint National Committee on Prevention, Detection, Evaluation, and Treatment of High Blood Pressure: the JNC 7 report. JAMA 2003;289(19):2560–72.
14. Lewington S, Clarke R, Qizilbash N, et al. Age-specific relevance of usual blood pressure to vascular mortality: a meta-analysis of individual data for one million adults in 61 prospective studies. Lancet 2002;360(9349):1903–13.

15. Stamler J, Vaccaro O, Neaton JD, et al. Diabetes, other risk factors, and 12-yr cardiovascular mortality for men screened in the Multiple Risk Factor Intervention Trial. Diabetes Care 1993;16(2):434–44.

16. Tight blood pressure control and risk of macrovascular and microvascular complications in type 2 diabetes: UKPDS 38. UK Prospective Diabetes Study Group. BMJ 1998;317(7160):703–13.

17. Hansson L, Zanchetti A, Carruthers SG, et al. Effects of intensive blood-pressure lowering and low-dose aspirin in patients with hypertension: principal results of the Hypertension Optimal Treatment (HOT) randomised trial. HOT Study Group. Lancet 1998;351(9118):1755–62.

18. Adler AI, Stratton IM, Neil HA, et al. Association of systolic blood pressure with macrovascular and microvascular complications of type 2 diabetes (UKPDS 36): prospective observational study. BMJ 2000;321(7258):412–9.

19. Baigent C, Keech A, Kearney PM, et al. Efficacy and safety of cholesterol-lowering treatment: prospective meta-analysis of data from 90,056 participants in 14 randomised trials of statins. Lancet 2005;366(9493):1267–78.

20. Cholesterol Treatment Trialists Collaborators, Mihaylova B, Emberson J, et al. The effects of lowering LDL cholesterol with statin therapy in people at low risk of vascular disease: meta-analysis of individual data from 27 randomised trials. Lancet 2012;380(9841):581–90.

21. Knopp RH, d'Emden M, Smilde JG, et al. Efficacy and safety of atorvastatin in the prevention of cardiovascular end points in subjects with type 2 diabetes: the Atorvastatin Study for Prevention of Coronary Heart Disease Endpoints in Non-Insulin-Dependent Diabetes Mellitus (ASPEN). Diabetes Care 2006;29(7): 1478–85.

22. Colhoun HM, Betteridge DJ, Durrington PN, et al. Primary prevention of cardiovascular disease with atorvastatin in type 2 diabetes in the Collaborative Atorvastatin Diabetes Study (CARDS): multicentre randomised placebo-controlled trial. Lancet 2004;364(9435):685–96.

23. Cannon CP, Braunwald E, McCabe CH, et al. Intensive versus moderate lipid lowering with statins after acute coronary syndromes. N Engl J Med 2004; 350(15):1495–504.

24. de Lemos JA, Blazing MA, Wiviott SD, et al. Early intensive vs a delayed conservative simvastatin strategy in patients with acute coronary syndromes: phase Z of the A to Z trial. JAMA 2004;292(11):1307–16.

25. Nissen SE, Tuzcu EM, Schoenhagen P, et al. Effect of intensive compared with moderate lipid-lowering therapy on progression of coronary atherosclerosis: a randomized controlled trial. JAMA 2004;291(9):1071–80.

26. Stone NJ, Robinson JG, Lichtenstein AH, et al. 2013 ACC/AHA guideline on the treatment of blood cholesterol to reduce atherosclerotic cardiovascular risk in adults: a report of the American College of Cardiology/American Heart Association Task Force on Practice Guidelines. Circulation 2014;129(25 Suppl 2):S1–45.

27. Rubins HB, Robins SJ, Collins D, et al. Gemfibrozil for the secondary prevention of coronary heart disease in men with low levels of high-density lipoprotein cholesterol. Veterans Affairs High-Density Lipoprotein Cholesterol Intervention Trial Study Group. N Engl J Med 1999;341(6):410–8.

28. Keech A, Simes RJ, Barter P, et al. Effects of long-term fenofibrate therapy on cardiovascular events in 9795 people with type 2 diabetes mellitus (the FIELD study): randomised controlled trial. Lancet 2005;366(9500):1849–61.

29. ACCORD Study Group, Ginsberg HN, Elam MB, et al. Effects of combination lipid therapy in type 2 diabetes mellitus. N Engl J Med 2010;362(17):1563–74.

30. Antithrombotic Trialists Collaboration, Baigent C, Blackwell L, et al. Aspirin in the primary and secondary prevention of vascular disease: collaborative meta-analysis of individual participant data from randomised trials. Lancet 2009; 373(9678):1849–60.

31. Belch J, MacCuish A, Campbell I, et al. The Prevention of Progression of Arterial Disease and Diabetes (POPADAD) trial: factorial randomised placebo controlled trial of aspirin and antioxidants in patients with diabetes and asymptomatic peripheral arterial disease. BMJ 2008;337:a1840.

32. Ogawa H, Nakayama M, Morimoto T, et al. Low-dose aspirin for primary prevention of atherosclerotic events in patients with type 2 diabetes: a randomized controlled trial. JAMA 2008;300(18):2134–41.

33. Voulgari C, Katsilambros N, Tentolouris N. Smoking cessation predicts amelioration of microalbuminuria in newly diagnosed type 2 diabetes mellitus: a 1-year prospective study. Metabolism 2011;60(10):1456–64.

34. Klein R, Klein BE, Moss SE, et al. The Wisconsin Epidemiologic Study of Diabetic Retinopathy. IX. Four-year incidence and progression of diabetic retinopathy when age at diagnosis is less than 30 years. Arch Ophthalmol 1989;107(2): 237–43.

35. Klein R, Klein BE, Moss SE, et al. The Wisconsin Epidemiologic Study of Diabetic Retinopathy. III. Prevalence and risk of diabetic retinopathy when age at diagnosis is 30 or more years. Arch Ophthalmol 1984;102(4):527–32.

36. Progression of retinopathy with intensive versus conventional treatment in the Diabetes Control and Complications Trial. Diabetes Control and Complications Trial Research Group. Ophthalmology 1995;102(4):647–61.

37. Stratton IM, Kohner EM, Aldington SJ, et al. UKPDS 50: risk factors for incidence and progression of retinopathy in type II diabetes over 6 years from diagnosis. Diabetologia 2001;44(2):156–63.

38. Klein R, Sharrett AR, Klein BE, et al. The association of atherosclerosis, vascular risk factors, and retinopathy in adults with diabetes: the Atherosclerosis Risk in Communities Study. Ophthalmology 2002;109(7):1225–34.

39. Antonetti DA, Klein R, Gardner TW. Diabetic retinopathy. N Engl J Med 2012; 366(13):1227–39.

40. Klein R, Lee KE, Gangnon RE, et al. The 25-year incidence of visual impairment in type 1 diabetes mellitus the Wisconsin Epidemiologic Study of Diabetic Retinopathy. Ophthalmology 2010;117(1):63–70.

41. Hutchinson A, McIntosh A, Peters J, et al. Effectiveness of screening and monitoring tests for diabetic retinopathy–a systematic review. Diabet Med 2000; 17(7):495–506.

42. Javitt JC, Aiello LP, Chiang Y, et al. Preventive eye care in people with diabetes is cost-saving to the federal government. Implications for health-care reform. Diabetes Care 1994;17(8):909–17.

43. Singer DE, Nathan DM, Fogel HA, et al. Screening for diabetic retinopathy. Ann Intern Med 1992;116(8):660–71.

44. Hooper P, Boucher MC, Cruess A, et al. Canadian Ophthalmological Society evidence-based clinical practice guidelines for the management of diabetic retinopathy. Can J Ophthalmol 2012;47(Suppl 2):S1–30, S31–54.

45. Agardh E, Tababat-Khani P. Adopting 3-year screening intervals for sight-threatening retinal vascular lesions in type 2 diabetic subjects without retinopathy. Diabetes Care 2011;34(6):1318–9.

46. Bragge P, Gruen RL, Chau M, et al. Screening for presence or absence of diabetic retinopathy: a meta-analysis. Arch Ophthalmol 2011;129(4):435–44.

47. The effect of intensive treatment of diabetes on the development and progression of long-term complications in insulin-dependent diabetes mellitus. The Diabetes Control and Complications Trial Research Group. N Engl J Med 1993;329(14):977–86.

48. Effect of intensive blood-glucose control with metformin on complications in overweight patients with type 2 diabetes (UKPDS 34). UK Prospective Diabetes Study (UKPDS) Group. Lancet 1998;352(9131):854–65.

49. ACCORD Study Group, ACCORD Eye Study Group, Chew EY, et al. Effects of medical therapies on retinopathy progression in type 2 diabetes. N Engl J Med 2010;363(3):233–44.

50. Preliminary report on effects of photocoagulation therapy. The Diabetic Retinopathy Study Research Group. Am J Ophthalmol 1976;81(4):383–96.

51. Bandello F, Berchicci L, La Spina C, et al. Evidence for anti-VEGF treatment of diabetic macular edema. Ophthalmic Res 2012;48(Suppl 1):16–20.

52. Nguyen QD, Brown DM, Marcus DM, et al. Ranibizumab for diabetic macular edema: results from 2 phase III randomized trials: RISE and RIDE. Ophthalmology 2012;119(4):789–801.

53. Chaturvedi N, Sjolie AK, Stephenson JM, et al. Effect of lisinopril on progression of retinopathy in normotensive people with type 1 diabetes. The EUCLID Study Group. EURODIAB Controlled Trial of Lisinopril in Insulin-Dependent Diabetes Mellitus. Lancet 1998;351(9095):28–31.

54. Beulens JW, Patel A, Vingerling JR, et al. Effects of blood pressure lowering and intensive glucose control on the incidence and progression of retinopathy in patients with type 2 diabetes mellitus: a randomised controlled trial. Diabetologia 2009;52(10):2027–36.

55. Chaturvedi N, Porta M, Klein R, et al. Effect of candesartan on prevention (DIRECT-Prevent 1) and progression (DIRECT-Protect 1) of retinopathy in type 1 diabetes: randomised, placebo-controlled trials. Lancet 2008;372(9647):1394–402.

56. Sjolie AK, Klein R, Porta M, et al. Effect of candesartan on progression and regression of retinopathy in type 2 diabetes (DIRECT-Protect 2): a randomised placebo-controlled trial. Lancet 2008;372(9647):1385–93.

57. Keech AC, Mitchell P, Summanen PA, et al. Effect of fenofibrate on the need for laser treatment for diabetic retinopathy (FIELD study): a randomised controlled trial. Lancet 2007;370(9600):1687–97.

58. Edwards JL, Vincent AM, Cheng HT, et al. Diabetic neuropathy: mechanisms to management. Pharmacol Ther 2008;120(1):1–34.

59. Vinik AI, Park TS, Stansberry KB, et al. Diabetic neuropathies. Diabetologia 2000;43(8):957–73.

60. Boulton AJ, Vinik AI, Arezzo JC, et al. Diabetic neuropathies: a statement by the American Diabetes Association. Diabetes Care 2005;28(4):956–62.

61. Thomas PK. Diabetic peripheral neuropathies: their cost to patient and society and the value of knowledge of risk factors for development of interventions. Eur Neurol 1999;41(Suppl 1):35–43.

62. Genuth S. Insights from the Diabetes Control and Complications trial/Epidemiology of Diabetes Interventions and Complications study on the use of intensive glycemic treatment to reduce the risk of complications of type 1 diabetes. Endocr Pract 2006;12(Suppl 1):34–41.

63. Dyck PJ, Davies JL, Wilson DM, et al. Risk factors for severity of diabetic polyneuropathy: intensive longitudinal assessment of the Rochester Diabetic Neuropathy Study cohort. Diabetes Care 1999;22(9):1479–86.

64. Hanssen KF. Blood glucose control and microvascular and macrovascular complications in diabetes. Diabetes 1997;46(Suppl 2):S101–3.

65. Tesfaye S, Boulton AJ, Dyck PJ, et al. Diabetic neuropathies: update on definitions, diagnostic criteria, estimation of severity, and treatments. Diabetes Care 2010;33(10):2285–93.
66. Davies M, Brophy S, Williams R, et al. The prevalence, severity, and impact of painful diabetic peripheral neuropathy in type 2 diabetes. Diabetes Care 2006;29(7):1518–22.
67. Quattrini C, Tesfaye S. Understanding the impact of painful diabetic neuropathy. Diabetes Metab Res Rev 2003;19(Suppl 1):S2–8.
68. Athans W, Stephens H. Open calcaneal fractures in diabetic patients with neuropathy: a report of three cases and literature review. Foot Ankle Int 2008;29(10):1049–53.
69. Veves A, Backonja M, Malik RA. Painful diabetic neuropathy: epidemiology, natural history, early diagnosis, and treatment options. Pain Med 2008;9(6):660–74.
70. Obrosova IG. Diabetic painful and insensate neuropathy: pathogenesis and potential treatments. Neurotherapeutics 2009;6(4):638–47.
71. Gandhi RA, Marques JL, Selvarajah D, et al. Painful diabetic neuropathy is associated with greater autonomic dysfunction than painless diabetic neuropathy. Diabetes Care 2010;33(7):1585–90.
72. Singh R, Kishore L, Kaur N. Diabetic peripheral neuropathy: current perspective and future directions. Pharmacol Res 2014;80:21–35.
73. Yamakawa I, Kojima H, Terashima T, et al. Inactivation of TNF-alpha ameliorates diabetic neuropathy in mice. Am J Physiol Endocrinol Metab 2011;301(5):E844–52.
74. Cameron NE, Cotter MA. Pro-inflammatory mechanisms in diabetic neuropathy: focus on the nuclear factor kappa B pathway. Curr Drug Targets 2008;9(1):60–7.
75. Leininger GM, Vincent AM, Feldman EL. The role of growth factors in diabetic peripheral neuropathy. J Peripher Nerv Syst 2004;9(1):26–53.
76. Deli G, Bosnyak E, Pusch G, et al. Diabetic neuropathies: diagnosis and management. Neuroendocrinology 2013;98(4):267–80.
77. Hartemann A, Attal N, Bouhassira D, et al. Painful diabetic neuropathy: diagnosis and management. Diabetes Metab 2011;37(5):377–88.
78. Martin CL, Albers J, Herman WH, et al. Neuropathy among the diabetes control and complications trial cohort 8 years after trial completion. Diabetes Care 2006;29(2):340–4.
79. Pop-Busui R, Lu J, Brooks MM, et al. Impact of glycemic control strategies on the progression of diabetic peripheral neuropathy in the Bypass Angioplasty Revascularization Investigation 2 Diabetes (BARI 2D) Cohort. Diabetes Care 2013;36(10):3208–15.
80. Herman WH, Pop-Busui R, Braffett BH, et al. Use of the Michigan Neuropathy Screening Instrument as a measure of distal symmetrical peripheral neuropathy in type 1 diabetes: results from the Diabetes Control and Complications Trial/Epidemiology of Diabetes Interventions and Complications. Diabet Med 2012;29(7):937–44.
81. Graf RJ, Halter JB, Pfeifer MA, et al. Glycemic control and nerve conduction abnormalities in non-insulin-dependent diabetic subjects. Ann Intern Med 1981;94(3):307–11.
82. Holman RR, Dornan TL, Mayon-White V, et al. Prevention of deterioration of renal and sensory-nerve function by more intensive management of insulin-dependent diabetic patients. A two-year randomised prospective study. Lancet 1983;1(8318):204–8.

83. Pietri A, Ehle AL, Raskin P. Changes in nerve conduction velocity after six weeks of glucoregulation with portable insulin infusion pumps. Diabetes 1980;29(8): 668–71.

84. Callaghan BC, Hur J, Feldman EL. Diabetic neuropathy: one disease or two? Curr Opin Neurol 2012;25(5):536–41.

85. Peltier A, Goutman SA, Callaghan BC. Painful diabetic neuropathy. BMJ 2014; 348:g1799.

86. Max MB, Culnane M, Schafer SC, et al. Amitriptyline relieves diabetic neuropathy pain in patients with normal or depressed mood. Neurology 1987;37(4):589–96.

87. Max MB, Lynch SA, Muir J, et al. Effects of desipramine, amitriptyline, and fluoxetine on pain in diabetic neuropathy. N Engl J Med 1992;326(19):1250–6.

88. Kvinesdal B, Molin J, Froland A, et al. Imipramine treatment of painful diabetic neuropathy. JAMA 1984;251(13):1727–30.

89. Vrethem M, Boivie J, Arnqvist H, et al. A comparison a amitriptyline and maprotiline in the treatment of painful polyneuropathy in diabetics and nondiabetics. Clin J Pain 1997;13(4):313–23.

90. Simpson DA. Gabapentin and venlafaxine for the treatment of painful diabetic neuropathy. J Clin Neuromuscul Dis 2001;3(2):53–62.

91. Goldstein DJ, Lu Y, Detke MJ, et al. Duloxetine vs. placebo in patients with painful diabetic neuropathy. Pain 2005;116(1-2):109–18.

92. Raskin J, Pritchett YL, Wang F, et al. A double-blind, randomized multicenter trial comparing duloxetine with placebo in the management of diabetic peripheral neuropathic pain. Pain Med 2005;6(5):346–56.

93. Wernicke JF, Pritchett YL, D'Souza DN, et al. A randomized controlled trial of duloxetine in diabetic peripheral neuropathic pain. Neurology 2006;67(8):1411–20.

94. Backonja M, Beydoun A, Edwards KR, et al. Gabapentin for the symptomatic treatment of painful neuropathy in patients with diabetes mellitus: a randomized controlled trial. JAMA 1998;280(21):1831–6.

95. Vinik AI, Casellini CM. Guidelines in the management of diabetic nerve pain: clinical utility of pregabalin. Diabetes Metab Syndr Obes 2013;6:57–78.

96. Dworkin RH, Backonja M, Rowbotham MC, et al. Advances in neuropathic pain: diagnosis, mechanisms, and treatment recommendations. Arch Neurol 2003; 60(11):1524–34.

97. Lesser H, Sharma U, LaMoreaux L, et al. Pregabalin relieves symptoms of painful diabetic neuropathy: a randomized controlled trial. Neurology 2004;63(11): 2104–10.

98. Richter RW, Portenoy R, Sharma U, et al. Relief of painful diabetic peripheral neuropathy with pregabalin: a randomized, placebo-controlled trial. J Pain 2005;6(4):253–60.

99. Rosenstock J, Tuchman M, LaMoreaux L, et al. Pregabalin for the treatment of painful diabetic peripheral neuropathy: a double-blind, placebo-controlled trial. Pain 2004;110(3):628–38.

100. Freynhagen R, Strojek K, Griesing T, et al. Efficacy of pregabalin in neuropathic pain evaluated in a 12-week, randomised, double-blind, multicentre, placebo-controlled trial of flexible- and fixed-dose regimens. Pain 2005;115(3):254–63.

101. Freeman R, Durso-Decruz E, Emir B. Efficacy, safety, and tolerability of pregabalin treatment for painful diabetic peripheral neuropathy: findings from seven randomized, controlled trials across a range of doses. Diabetes Care 2008;31(7):1448–54.

102. Zaccara G, Gangemi P, Perucca P, et al. The adverse event profile of pregabalin: a systematic review and meta-analysis of randomized controlled trials. Epilepsia 2011;52(4):826–36.

103. Derry S, Lloyd R, Moore RA, et al. Topical capsaicin for chronic neuropathic pain in adults. Cochrane Database Syst Rev 2009;(4):CD007393.

104. Mason L, Moore RA, Derry S, et al. Systematic review of topical capsaicin for the treatment of chronic pain. BMJ 2004;328(7446):991.

105. Baron R, Mayoral V, Leijon G, et al. Efficacy and safety of combination therapy with 5% lidocaine medicated plaster and pregabalin in post-herpetic neuralgia and diabetic polyneuropathy. Curr Med Res Opin 2009;25(7):1677–87.

106. Ziegler D, Ametov A, Barinov A, et al. Oral treatment with alpha-lipoic acid improves symptomatic diabetic polyneuropathy: the SYDNEY 2 trial. Diabetes Care 2006;29(11):2365–70.

107. Ziegler D, Nowak H, Kempler P, et al. Treatment of symptomatic diabetic polyneuropathy with the antioxidant alpha-lipoic acid: a meta-analysis. Diabet Med 2004;21(2):114–21.

108. Abuaisha BB, Costanzi JB, Boulton AJ. Acupuncture for the treatment of chronic painful peripheral diabetic neuropathy: a long-term study. Diabetes Res Clin Pract 1998;39(2):115–21.

109. Watson CP, Moulin D, Watt-Watson J, et al. Controlled-release oxycodone relieves neuropathic pain: a randomized controlled trial in painful diabetic neuropathy. Pain 2003;105(1–2):71–8.

110. Gilron I, Bailey JM, Tu D, et al. Morphine, gabapentin, or their combination for neuropathic pain. N Engl J Med 2005;352(13):1324–34.

111. Steinke JM, Mauer M, International Diabetic Nephropathy Study Group. Lessons learned from studies of the natural history of diabetic nephropathy in young type 1 diabetic patients. Pediatr Endocrinol Rev 2008;5(Suppl 4):958–63.

112. Bogdanovic R. Diabetic nephropathy in children and adolescents. Pediatr Nephrol 2008;23(4):507–25.

113. Koro CE, Lee BH, Bowlin SJ. Antidiabetic medication use and prevalence of chronic kidney disease among patients with type 2 diabetes mellitus in the United States. Clin Ther 2009;31(11):2608–17.

114. Adler AI, Stevens RJ, Manley SE, et al. Development and progression of nephropathy in type 2 diabetes: the United Kingdom Prospective Diabetes Study (UKPDS 64). Kidney Int 2003;63(1):225–32.

115. Atkins RC, Zimmet P, International Society of Nephrology/International Federation of Kidney Foundations World Kidney Day Steering Committee, et al. Diabetic kidney disease: act now or pay later. Am J Med Sci 2010;339(2):102–4.

116. Mauer SM, Steffes MW, Ellis EN, et al. Structural-functional relationships in diabetic nephropathy. J Clin Invest 1984;74(4):1143–55.

117. Dalla Vestra M, Saller A, Bortoloso E, et al. Structural involvement in type 1 and type 2 diabetic nephropathy. Diabetes Metab 2000;26(Suppl 4):8–14.

118. Mason RM, Wahab NA. Extracellular matrix metabolism in diabetic nephropathy. J Am Soc Nephrol 2003;14(5):1358–73.

119. Ziyadeh FN. The extracellular matrix in diabetic nephropathy. Am J Kidney Dis 1993;22(5):736–44.

120. Go AS, Chertow GM, Fan D, et al. Chronic kidney disease and the risks of death, cardiovascular events, and hospitalization. N Engl J Med 2004;351(13):1296–305.

121. Wu AY, Kong NC, de Leon FA, et al. An alarmingly high prevalence of diabetic nephropathy in Asian type 2 diabetic patients: the MicroAlbuminuria Prevalence (MAP) Study. Diabetologia 2005;48(1):17–26.

122. National Kidney Foundation. KDOQI clinical practice guideline for diabetes and CKD: 2012 update. Am J Kidney Dis 2012;60(5):850–86.

123. Levinsky NG. Specialist evaluation in chronic kidney disease: too little, too late. Ann Intern Med 2002;137(6):542–3.
124. Steffes MW. Affecting the decline of renal function in diabetes mellitus. Kidney Int 2001;60(1):378–9.
125. Lewis EJ, Hunsicker LG, Bain RP, et al. The effect of angiotensin-converting-enzyme inhibition on diabetic nephropathy. The Collaborative Study Group. N Engl J Med 1993;329(20):1456–62.
126. Laffel LM, McGill JB, Gans DJ. The beneficial effect of angiotensin-converting enzyme inhibition with captopril on diabetic nephropathy in normotensive IDDM patients with microalbuminuria. North American Microalbuminuria Study Group. Am J Med 1995;99(5):497–504.
127. Mogensen CE. Microalbuminuria and hypertension with focus on type 1 and type 2 diabetes. J Intern Med 2003;254(1):45–66.
128. Viberti G, Wheeldon NM. MicroAlbuminuria Reduction With VSI. Microalbuminuria reduction with valsartan in patients with type 2 diabetes mellitus: a blood pressure-independent effect. Circulation 2002;106(6):672–8.
129. Lewis EJ, Hunsicker LG, Clarke WR, et al. Renoprotective effect of the angiotensin-receptor antagonist irbesartan in patients with nephropathy due to type 2 diabetes. N Engl J Med 2001;345(12):851–60.
130. Atkins RC, Briganti EM, Lewis JB, et al. Proteinuria reduction and progression to renal failure in patients with type 2 diabetes mellitus and overt nephropathy. Am J Kidney Dis 2005;45(2):281–7.
131. Brenner BM, Cooper ME, de Zeeuw D, et al. Effects of losartan on renal and cardiovascular outcomes in patients with type 2 diabetes and nephropathy. N Engl J Med 2001;345(12):861–9.
132. Parving HH, Lehnert H, Brochner-Mortensen J, et al. The effect of irbesartan on the development of diabetic nephropathy in patients with type 2 diabetes. N Engl J Med 2001;345(12):870–8.
133. Mogensen CE, Neldam S, Tikkanen I, et al. Randomised controlled trial of dual blockade of renin-angiotensin system in patients with hypertension, microalbuminuria, and non-insulin dependent diabetes: the Candesartan and Lisinopril Microalbuminuria (CALM) study. BMJ 2000;321(7274):1440–4.
134. Schjoedt KJ, Jacobsen P, Rossing K, et al. Dual blockade of the renin-angiotensin-aldosterone system in diabetic nephropathy: the role of aldosterone. Horm Metab Res 2005;37(Suppl 1):4–8.
135. Schjoedt KJ, Rossing K, Juhl TR, et al. Beneficial impact of spironolactone in diabetic nephropathy. Kidney Int 2005;68(6):2829–36.
136. Parving HH, Persson F, Lewis JB, et al. Aliskiren combined with losartan in type 2 diabetes and nephropathy. N Engl J Med 2008;358(23):2433–46.
137. Bilous R. Microvascular disease: what does the UKPDS tell us about diabetic nephropathy? Diabet Med 2008;25(Suppl 2):25–9.

Polycystic Ovarian Syndrome

Subbulaxmi Trikudanathan, MD, MRCP, MMSc

KEYWORDS

- Polycystic ovarian syndrome • Anovulation • Hyperandrogenism • Insulin resistance
- Infertility • Type 2 diabetes

KEY POINTS

- Polycystic ovarian syndrome (PCOS) is a heterogeneous endocrine disorder characterized by anovulation, hyperandrogenism, infertility, and metabolic dysfunction.
- Diagnosis of PCOS is made based on the presence of 2 of 3 criteria: chronic anovulation, clinical or biochemical evidence of hyperandrogenism, and polycystic ovaries on morphology.
- Management of PCOS should be tailored according to the patient's clinical presentation and desire for pregnancy.
- Long-term health implications for metabolic and cardiovascular health need to be addressed throughout the lifespan with an emphasis on prevention of cardiometabolic risks.

INTRODUCTION

Polycystic ovarian syndrome (PCOS) is the most common endocrine disorder in reproductive-aged women. The most recognized description for PCOS comes from Stein and Leventhal in 1935, who described obese women with amenorrhea, hirsutism, and infertility with enlarged and cystic ovaries.

PCOS is a heterogeneous condition with variable phenotypic expression leading to significant controversy on the diagnostic criteria. The prevalence of this disorder is from 6% to 15% depending on the diagnostic criteria used.[1] Every individual experiences a variable severity of the components of PCOS and management needs to be tailored according to the patient's preferences.

CLINICAL PRESENTATION

Key clinical features are anovulation with menstrual irregularities, hyperandrogenism, infertility, and metabolic abnormalities (**Fig. 1**).

Disclosures: None.
Division of Metabolism, Endocrinology and Nutrition, Department of Medicine, University of Washington Medical Center, 4245 Roosevelt Way Northeast, Seattle, WA 98105, USA
E-mail address: tsubbu@uw.edu

Med Clin N Am 99 (2015) 221–235
http://dx.doi.org/10.1016/j.mcna.2014.09.003   medical.theclinics.com

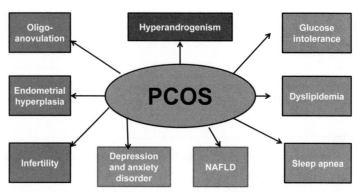

Fig. 1. Clinical components of PCOS. This figure illustrates the clinical features of PCOS that needs to be carefully assessed and addressed. NAFLD, non alcoholic fatty liver disease.

Menstrual Abnormalities

Oligoanovulation typically presents as oligomenorrhea (<9 cycles per year) or amenorrhea. Dysfunctional uterine bleeding is occasionally encountered from unopposed estrogen stimulation with lack of progesterone from anovulation. These menstrual irregularities develop peripubertally and are often noted after periods of weight gain. It is reported that women with PCOS may ovulate spontaneously, although the frequency of this is unknown.[1] Menstrual cycles in women with PCOS tend to become more regular as the women approach menopause.

Infertility

Women with PCOS have a higher risk for infertility from oligoanovulation. Additional mechanisms leading to infertility include diminished oocyte competence,[2] unfavorable endometrial changes, and obesity.

Endometrial Cancer Risk

Women with PCOS have chronic unopposed estrogen exposure resulting in endometrial hyperplasia from anovulation, which may increase the risk for endometrial cancer. Other factors that may compound this risk include chronic hyperinsulinemia, hyperandrogenemia, and obesity.

Hyperandrogenism

Hyperandrogenism is clinically manifested by hirsutism, acne, and androgenic alopecia. Hirsutism is defined as increased terminal (coarse, pigmented) hair in a male pattern distribution around the upper lip, chin, shoulders, chest, periareolar areas, along the linea alba of the abdomen, inner aspects of the thighs, and midline lower back area. The degree of hirsutism can be gauged by the Ferriman-Gallwey score,[3] a semiobjective quantitative method for recording the distribution and severity of excess body hair in 9 skin areas. Documenting these scores objectively helps in evaluating the response of hirsutism to treatment interventions (**Fig. 2**). Photographs before the patient shaves could help document hirsutism precisely.

Other hyperandrogenic signs in women with alopecia include acne and androgenic alopecia. Signs of virilization such as deepening of the voice, clitoromegaly, decreased breast size, and increased muscle mass should alert the clinician to more severe forms of androgen excess (discussed later, with examples).

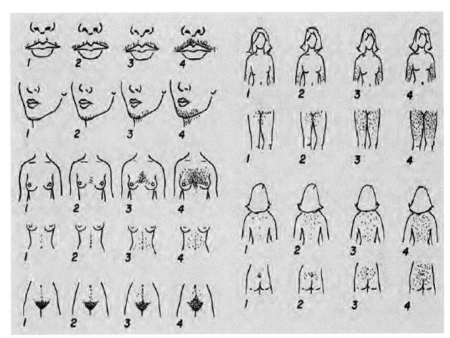

Fig. 2. Ferriman-Gallwey score. Each of the 9 areas receive a score from 0 (no hair) to 4 (frankly virile). These scores are finally added to obtain a total hormonal score. Total score greater than or equal to 8 indicates hirsutism. (*From* Hatch R, Rosenfield RL, Kim MH, et al. Hirsutism: implications, etiology, and management. Am J Obstet Gynecol 1981;140(7):815–30.)

Metabolic Components

Women with PCOS are frequently overweight or obese, particularly with visceral adiposity.[4] It has also been well recognized that most women with PCOS have hyperinsulinemia and insulin resistance, irrespective of obesity.[5,6] Women with PCOS should be examined for clinical signs of insulin resistance such as acanthosis nigricans, multiple skin tags,[7] and keratosis pilaris.[8] A 2-fold increase in the prevalence of metabolic syndrome has been noted in women with PCOS from retrospective studies.[9,10] Women with PCOS have a significantly increased risk for impaired glucose tolerance and type 2 diabetes. Large cross-sectional studies have found 23% to 35% prevalence for impaired glucose tolerance and 4% to 10% for diabetes. This finding accounts for a 3-fold higher prevalence rate of impaired glucose tolerance in women with PCOS compared with age-matched women from the National Health and Nutrition Survey (NHANES) II.[11,12] Approximately a 7.5-fold to 10-fold higher prevalence rate was noted for undiagnosed type 2 diabetes in women with PCOS compared with NHANES II women of similar age.[11,12] The risk of type 2 diabetes increased in women with PCOS in the presence of family history of diabetes.[13]

Women with PCOS are predisposed to hypertension and vascular endothelial dysfunction,[14] putting them at a higher risk for macrovascular diseases. Several studies have shown dyslipidemia, especially increases in small dense low-density lipoprotein cholesterol particles and triglyceride levels with decreased high-density lipoprotein cholesterol.[15] Although precise cardiovascular morbidity and mortality have not been established in long-term studies, the clustering of cardiometabolic risk factors predisposes women with PCOS to coronary heart disease.

Other Components

Sleep apnea is common in women with PCOS. Insulin resistance seems to be a more important predictor of the severity of obstructive sleep apnea[16,17] than obesity. The prevalence of nonalcoholic fatty liver disease has also been increased in women with PCOS with increased serum alanine aminotransferase concentrations in up to 30% of women with PCOS.[18] Women with PCOS are at higher risk to develop mood disorders, particularly depression and anxiety.[19]

PATHOPHYSIOLOGY

Multiple causal factors have emerged in the pathophysiology of PCOS (**Fig. 3**). It is unclear which of these abnormalities triggers the vicious cycle of anovulation, androgen excess, and hyperinsulinemia seen in PCOS. One of the primary neuroendocrine defects described is alterations in gonadotropin secretion. There is an underlying insensitivity of the hypothalamic gonadotropin-releasing hormone (GnRH) secretion to ovarian steroids leading to increased luteinizing hormone (LH) pulse amplitude and frequency.[20] Low progesterone levels have also been postulated to enhance the pulsatility of GnRH, leading to increased LH/follicle-stimulating hormone (FSH) ratio. The relative increase in LH stimulates the ovarian theca cells to secrete more androgenic precursors and androgens. The FSH regulates the aromatase activity of the ovarian granulosa cells. Impaired FSH synthesis and secretion leads to inadequate follicle development and reduced aromatase levels. Hence there is a relative inability to

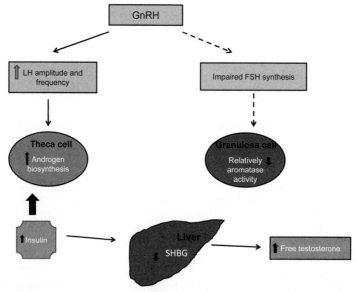

Fig. 3. Pathophysiology of PCOS. There is intrinsic abnormality in gonadotrophin-releasing hormone (GnRH) pulse generator leading to increased luteinizing hormone (LH) pulse amplitude and frequency with relative impairment in follicle-stimulating hormone (FSH) secretion. Augmented LH activity amplified by increased insulin drives the increased androgen production in the ovarian theca cells with reduced aromatase levels. Hyperinsulinemia further inhibits the production of sex hormone–binding protein (SHBG) in the liver, thereby increasing the proportion of free testosterone compared with total testosterone. (*Courtesy of* Dr Diane E. Woodford, Clinical Assistant professor, Reproductive Endocrinology and Infertility, University of Washington Medical Center, Seattle.)

aromatize androgenic precursors to estrogen, which in turn results in preferential increase of ovarian androgens.[21]

Women with PCOS have intrinsic abnormalities in ovarian theca cell steroidogenesis resulting in hyperandrogenemia. In the ovarian theca cells, androgen biosynthesis is mediated by cytochrome P-450c17 enzymes to form androstenedione. Androstenedione is then converted to testosterone by 17β-hydroxysteroid enzyme or aromatized to form estrone. In vivo and in vitro studies have shown that PCOS ovaries have an increased cytochrome P-450c17 enzymatic activity[22] leading to enhanced synthesis of androgenic precursors, and thereby testosterone.

Euglycemic clamp studies have shown insulin resistance in both obese and lean women with PCOS. Hyperinsulinemia augments androgen production in women with PCOS. Insulin plays both a direct role on the ovaries by amplifying LH activity to synthesize more androgens and an indirect role in increasing the amplitude of LH pulses.[21] Furthermore, insulin also inhibits hepatic synthesis of sex hormone–binding protein (SHBG), which binds to testosterone. Therefore, women with PCOS have an increased proportion of free or biologically active testosterone compared with total testosterone.

GENETICS OF POLYCYSTIC OVARIAN SYNDROME

Familial clustering of PCOS suggests a genetic basis for this disorder. Several susceptibility genes have been implicated, particularly in the region of the insulin receptor gene, insulin gene, follistatin, fibrillin-3, and other members of the transforming growth factor beta signaling family.[23] Reproductive phenotype of hyperandrogenism and metabolic abnormalities aggregates in families with PCOS. Some sisters have hyperandrogenism with regular menses and insulin resistance, whereas others have menstrual irregularities. Mothers of women with PCOS who had menstrual abnormalities had higher testosterone levels, dyslipidemia, and markers of insulin resistance.[24] Brothers of women with PCOS had increased dehydroepiandrosterone sulfate (DHEAS), suggesting defects in androgen steroidogenesis similar to their sisters with PCOS.[25] In another study, brothers of women with PCOS showed defects in the pancreatic beta-cell function with increased risk for type 2 diabetes.[26]

DIAGNOSIS OF POLYCYSTIC OVARIAN SYNDROME

There has been considerable controversy over the 3 different definitions that have been proposed by professional organizations for the diagnosis of PCOS.

The National Institutes of Health (NIH) in 1990 proposed the following diagnostic criteria for PCOS:

- Chronic anovulation
- Clinical and/or biochemical signs of hyperandrogenism
- Exclusion of other causes of hyperandrogenism, such as congenital adrenal hyperplasia, androgen-secreting tumors, and hyperprolactinemia

Rotterdam Criteria

The European Society of Human Reproduction and Embryology/American Society of Reproductive Medicine held a consensus meeting at Rotterdam in 2003 and developed revised criteria incorporating a wider spectrum of phenotypes in PCOS.[27] Two out of 3 criteria would be needed to make the diagnosis after exclusion of the other causes for hyperandrogenism.

- Oligoanovulation and/or anovulation
- Clinical and/or biochemical signs of hyperandrogenism
- Polycystic ovarian morphology by ultrasonography

Androgen Excess Society Criteria

The Androgen Excess Society (2006) recommended diagnosing PCOS by the presence of 3 features:

- Clinical and/or biochemical signs of hyperandrogenism
- Ovarian dysfunction (oligoanovulation and/or polycystic ovarian morphology)
- Exclusion of other causes of hyperandrogenism

These 3 diagnostic criteria identified different phenotypes of women with PCOS. Although the NIH criteria identified the hyperandrogenic women who are at higher metabolic risk, the Rotterdam criteria also identified women with ovulatory dysfunction and polycystic ovarian morphology. Most recently, in December 2012, the NIH sponsored an expert panel that endorsed the acceptance of the Rotterdam criteria because they encompass a broad spectrum of phenotypes representing PCOS.

EVALUATION

Serum total testosterone provides the best estimate of the androgen status because direct assays for free testosterone can be inaccurate unless the equilibrium dialysis method is used. Serum total testosterone can be measured at any point during the menstrual cycle. Liquid chromatography–tandem mass spectrometry accurately measures the testosterone levels in female patients. However, several clinical laboratories use direct immunoassays to minimize the cost and increase throughput. Because the direct immunoassays skip the extraction steps, there is considerable cross reactivity from other steroids, leading to inaccuracies.[28] Another factor to consider is low circulating levels of testosterone in women (15–20 times lower than in men). Other measurements to assess androgen excess in women with PCOS include free androgen index (FAI), androstenedione, and DHEAS.

FAI is defined as the ratio between total testosterone and SHBG and can also be used to evaluate hyperandrogenemia. Androstenedione, an immediate precursor of testosterone, is produced by the ovaries, adrenals, and peripheral tissues. A recent study reported that measuring both androstenedione and total testosterone better predicted metabolic risks in women with PCOS.[29] This study also revealed that androstenedione levels can be increased when total testosterone levels are normal in women with PCOS. The utility of androstenedione merits further investigation in longitudinal studies. Levels of DHEAS primarily derived from the adrenal glands, although not routinely measured, can also be increased in women with PCOS.

Other Biochemical Features

Antimüllerian hormone (AMH) produced by the granulosa cells of small antral follicles has recently been proposed as a marker for PCOS. Increased AMH level has been suggested as a good substitute for polycystic ovarian morphology.[30] Until there is standardization of assay techniques and larger studies, the diagnostic cutoff for AMH in PCOS will remain a research tool.

Low SHBG level reflects insulin resistance and predicts the susceptibility for developing metabolic syndrome.[4] Low SHBG also increases free testosterone levels in target tissues.

In the past, increased LH/FSH ratio has been used for diagnosis of PCOS. However, LH secretion is pulsatile and a single measurement of LH can miss the intrinsic variability. Hence an increased LH/FSH ratio contributes to the diagnosis of PCOS, but the absence does not rule out the diagnosis of PCOS.

Screening for Cardiometabolic Risks

All women with PCOS at the time of initial diagnosis should have a 75-g oral glucose tolerance test (OGTT) with fasting and 2-hour glucose levels. If OGTT is not feasible, then fasting glucose and hemoglobin A1c can be obtained. If OGTT is normal, rescreening every 3 to 5 years, or earlier in case of excessive weight gain, is advocated.[31] The gold standard for assessing insulin resistance is a euglycemic hyperinsulinemic clamp, which can be conducted only in a research setting. Routine assessment for insulin resistance in a clinical setting with calculated indices such as homeostasis model assessment of insulin resistance is not recommended because it has several limitations. Fasting lipid profile should also be measured at the time of initial diagnosis.

Ultrasonography Assessment of Polycystic Ovarian Morphology

The 2003 Rotterdam criteria for polycystic ovarian morphology recommends the presence of 12 or more follicles in each ovary measuring 2 to 9 mm in diameter and/or increased ovarian volume (>10 mL) (**Fig. 4**). Establishing threshold values for follicle number per ovary (FNPO) and ovarian volume has been a highly complex issue. A recent study showed that more than 50% of normal young ovulatory women[32] meet the FNPO criteria. Moreover, considerable interobserver variability exists in the technical methods used for counting and reporting FNPO. The transvaginal route allows precise measurement of the follicles. When not feasible, a transabdominal route can be used to measure ovarian volume. Women with PCOS show increased ovarian volume. Ovarian size reaches its maximum during adolescence and shrinks during and after menopause.[33] Other measurements such as ovarian stromal volume and ovarian blood flow have not been fully validated.

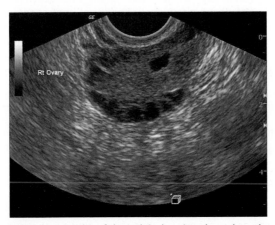

Fig. 4. Transvaginal ultrasonography of the pelvis showing the polycystic morphology of the right ovary. There is increased central ovarian stroma with the arrangement of subcapsular follicles in a string-of-pearls pattern. (*Courtesy of* Dr Diane E. Woodford, Clinical Assistant professor, Reproductive Endocrinology and Infertility, University of Washington Medical Center, Seattle.)

DIFFERENTIAL DIAGNOSIS

PCOS is considered a diagnosis of exclusion (**Box 1**). Therefore, it becomes important to screen for thyroid functions with thyroid-stimulating hormone, prolactin, and 17 hydroxyprogesterone (17OHP) levels. Thyroid disorders can present with menstrual irregularities. Hyperprolactinemia typically presents with oligomenorrhea or amenorrhea with minimal hyperandrogenemic symptoms. Mild increases in prolactin levels are sometimes noted in the setting of hyperandrogenism with no clear significance. Nonclassic congenital adrenal hyperplasia (CAH) caused by 21-hydroxylase deficiency should be excluded in women with hyperandrogenism. Some ethnic groups such as Ashkenazi Jews, and those of Italian or Slavic descent, have a high prevalence of this disorder. Nonclassic CAH can be ruled out with a measurement of early morning 17OHP. Values more than 200 to 400 ng/dL are considered abnormal. A cosyntropin test with stimulated 17OHP greater than 1000 ng/dL confirms the diagnosis. Women with amenorrhea and hirsutism with clinical signs of proximal muscle weakness, tendency to bruise easily, and purplish striae should be tested for Cushing syndrome.[31]

It is also important to rule out androgen-secreting ovarian or adrenal tumors when women present with a rapid onset and short duration of hirsutism. These women also have other signs of virilization such as frontal balding, severe acne, clitoromegaly, and a deepening of the voice. Serum testosterone and DHEAS are markedly increased. MRI of the adrenal glands or ultrasonography of the ovaries assists in the diagnosis.

MANAGEMENT OF POLYCYSTIC OVARIAN SYNDROME

Goals of treatment include minimizing hyperandrogenic symptoms, prevention of endometrial hyperplasia, and addressing the underlying metabolic risk factors to delay type 2 diabetes. Women desiring pregnancy may need assistance with ovulation induction therapy.

Hyperandrogenism

In women who do not desire pregnancy, hormonal contraceptives (estrogen/progestin combinations) remain the first line of treatment of hirsutism and acne. The progestin component in oral contraceptives (OC) inhibits LH secretion, thereby reducing the LH-dependent androgen production.[31] The estrogen component increases hepatic synthesis of SHBG, thus reducing free testosterone levels. OC pills

---

Box 1
Conditions to exclude before the diagnosis of PCOS

- Nonclassic congenital adrenal hyperplasia
- Primary hypothyroidism
- Hyperprolactinemia
- Virilizing adrenal or ovarian tumors[a]
- Cushing syndrome[b]

   [a] In case of extremely increased androgen levels or rapid and short duration of virilization.
   [b] In case of clinical signs such as proximal myopathy, purple striae, tendency to bruise easily, and hypertension.

also mildly reduce adrenal androgen production (the exact mechanism is unclear) and reduce the binding of androgen to its receptors. The progestin component of OC pills bind with progesterone and androgen receptors. The first-generation progestins, norethindrone and norethindrone acetate, are possible options in women with PCOS for hyperandrogenism. Levonorgestrel, a second-generation progestin, has the most androgenic properties with adverse metabolic effects and should be avoided. The third-generation progestins such as norgestimate, desogestrel, and gestodene have less androgenic activity and fewer metabolic effects; however, there are concerns about increased risk of venous thrombosis. Some progestins like drospirenone (a derivative of spironolactone) have antiandrogenic and antimineralocorticoid properties but need to be carefully prescribed in light of increased concerns about an increased risk of venous thromboembolism.[4] Note that the absolute risk for venous thromboembolism is minimal but may outweigh the overall benefits of OC pill in reducing androgen excess.

Screening for contraindications to hormonal contraceptives is similar in all users. Available data do not confer additional risk for venous thromboembolism (VTE) in women with PCOS. Risk factors for VTE, such as age, obesity, smoking, prior VTE, and family history of thromboembolism, should be carefully considered. A trial of at least 6 months of therapy should be given before changing the preparation or adding another antiandrogen.

Spironolactone, an aldosterone antagonist, inhibits androgen receptor and 5α-reductase activity. It is usually started at 50 mg once daily and increased to 100 mg twice daily. It rarely results in hyperkalemia, although menstrual irregularities are seen at higher doses, and it is usually used in combination with the OC pill. Potassium levels are usually measured 4 to 6 weeks after initiating therapy and after dose escalation. Spironolactone is teratogenic and causes feminization of male fetal genitalia. Therefore, it should be used with adequate contraceptive coverage in women of childbearing age.

Cyproterone acetate (CPA) has antiandrogen activity at the level of androgen receptor and suppresses serum gonadotropins and androgen levels. It is administered for the first 10 days of the menstrual cycle at a dose of 50 to 100 mg/d. CPA is currently unavailable in the United States but is widely used in Europe and Canada. Finasteride inhibits type 2 5α-reductase enzyme, thereby reducing hirsutism. It is commonly used at the 5-mg dose after ensuring safe contraception. Flutamide has significant antiandrogen effects but has potential hepatotoxicity resulting in liver failure and even death. Hence flutamide is not recommended in routine use. The addition of metformin has not been shown to be effective for hirsutism.

Eflornithine is an irreversible inhibitor of ornithine decarboxylase, an enzyme involved in hair follicle formation. Topical therapy with eflornithine hydrochloride cream helps to reduce the rate of hair growth. Patients need to be advised that the hair growth returns on discontinuing the treatment.

Some women choose temporary hair removal therapy such as plucking, waxing, and chemical depilation. Other methods of hair reduction include electrolysis and photoepilation therapy. Photoepilation therapy includes lasers and nonlaser light sources such as intense pulsed light (IPL). The ideal women for laser hair removal are light-skinned women with dark hair, whereas long-wavelength laser or IPL is used for dark-skinned women.[34] The laser energy is absorbed by melanin of the hair follicle rather than the surrounding tissue. In the presence of androgen excess, the remaining vellus hair follicles can be converted to terminal dark hair. Hence it becomes important to treat underlying hyperandrogenemia to prevent hair regrowth.

ENDOMETRIAL PROTECTION

Women with PCOS have an increased risk for endometrial hyperplasia and possible endometrial cancer. OC, transdermal patches, or vaginal rings provide endometrial protection and regulate menstrual cycles. Women who chose not to use combined estrogen and progesterone can use intermittent progestin therapy or a progestin-releasing intrauterine device. Medroxyprogesterone 5 to 10 mg for 10 days every 2 to 3 months is usually a good option to shed the endometrium and protect from endometrial hyperplasia.

INFERTILITY

Women with PCOS have anovulatory infertility. These women are also at a higher risk for developing gestational diabetes, preterm delivery, and preeclampsia. Therefore, women seeking fertility assistance should have prepregnancy evaluations of body mass index (BMI), blood pressure, and OGTT.

Weight loss is the first line of treatment in overweight and obese women with PCOS and should be initiated before fertility therapies. Even 5% to 10% weight loss can improve menstrual irregularities, enhance the response to ovulation induction, and reduce obstetric complications.[35]

Current guidelines recommend clomiphene citrate as the first line of therapy for ovulation induction in women with PCOS.[31] Clomiphene citrate is a selective estrogen receptor modulator that binds to the estrogen receptors in the hypothalamus, thus inhibiting the negative feedback of estrogen on the hypothalamus. There is a secondary increase in FSH that stimulates follicular formation and induces ovulation. Clomiphene citrate is typically administered at a dose of 50 mg for 5 days from days 2 to 5 after the onset of menstrual periods. A dose escalation of up to 150 mg/d can be reached for a total of 6 cycles. In a large randomized controlled trial comparing the efficacy of clomiphene citrate versus metformin in women with PCOS, women in the clomiphene citrate arm had significantly more live births compared with women given metformin alone (22.5% vs 7.2%).[36] The combination of clomiphene and metformin did not show any significant increase in live birth rates.[36] The rate of multiple births was 6% in the clomiphene group compared with 0% in the metformin group.[36] Metformin can be used to reduce multiple pregnancy rates because it has been thought to induce monofollicular ovulation. A Finnish study recently showed that women with BMI greater than 27 benefitted from 3 months' pretreatment with metformin in improving live birth rates.[37] Metformin (up to 1–2 g/d in divided doses)[38] is currently used as an adjuvant therapy to prevent ovarian hyperstimulation syndrome in women with PCOS undergoing in vitro fertilization.[31]

Aromatase inhibitors such as letrozole have also been used for ovulation induction. Letrozole blocks the conversion of androgens to estrogen. Therefore, there is less negative feedback on the hypothalamus leading to increased levels of GnRH and thereby FSH. Letrozole is usually used in women resistant to clomiphene citrate or who have side effects from clomiphene, such as vasomotor symptoms, headaches, and thin endometrium. A recent NIH-sponsored clinical trial showed a significant increase in live births with letrozole compared with clomiphene in women with PCOS, adding letrozole in the treatment armentarium.[39]

In clomiphene-resistant patients, gonadotropin therapy with FSH administration can be used for ovulation induction. This option has a higher risk for ovarian hyperstimulation syndrome and multiple pregnancies. Another procedure considered in clomiphene-resistant women who are not candidates for FSH therapy is laparoscopic ovarian drilling. This surgical procedure is performed with laser or electrocautery and involves perforation of 5 to 6 holes on the surface and stroma of the ovary.[35] Needle punctures induce thermal damage, thereby reducing ovarian stromal blood flow, which in turn decreases the androgen microenvironment. This procedure does not improve insulin sensitivity and therefore is not useful in obese patients seeking fertility. In addition, in vitro fertilization is offered for clomiphene-resistant women or in women with PCOS with coexisting reproductive issues such as tubal damage, endometriosis, or male factor infertility.[40]

CARDIOMETABOLIC RISK MANAGEMENT

Weight loss from dietary interventions and exercise forms the first line of management in obese women with PCOS. Several studies have attempted to use variations of the Diabetes Prevention Program[41] (DPP) to tailor lifestyle therapy in PCOS. One-hundred and fifty minutes per week in divided sessions of moderate to vigorous exercise along with a 500-calorie deficit per day promotes 450 g (1 pound) of weight loss per week. About 5% to 10% weight loss has a beneficial influence on metabolic risk factors and improved ovulation. Although there is a paucity of large randomized trials showing exercise benefits in PCOS populations, there is overall evidence of the benefits of exercise in reducing the risk of metabolic disease. In the DPP study, lifestyle modifications with exercise and diet reduced the progression of impaired glucose tolerance to T2 diabetes by 58% versus a 31% decrease with metformin. Current guidelines recommend metformin in women with PCOS who have impaired glucose tolerance and to prevent diabetes, especially in women who fail lifestyle modifications.[31] The unfavorable side effects of thiazolidinediones have discouraged their use in women with PCOS, especially in the childbearing age group. Other insulin-sensitizing agents that promote weight loss, such as glucagon like peptide -1 (GLP-1) analogues, have not been widely studied in women with PCOS. Newer weight loss medications, such as phenteramine/topiramate and locarserin, have shown promise in sustained weight loss and metabolic benefits in obese adults[42] but have not been studied in women with PCOS. Bariatric surgery has been used to treat morbid obesity with PCOS and some small studies have shown resolution of metabolic abnormalities[43] and improved fertility.[44]

Other cardiometabolic risks, such as dyslipidemia and obstructive sleep apnea, need appropriate treatment according to the standard of care.

POLYCYSTIC OVARIAN SYNDROME IN ADOLESCENTS

Oligomenorrhea with anovulatory cycles are common during the first 2 years after the onset of menarche. Persistence of menstrual irregularities beyond this period is indicates PCOS. Current guidelines[31] suggest that the diagnosis of PCOS in adolescents should be made based predominantly on hyperandrogenism (clinical or biochemical) in the presence of oligomenorrhea. However, there is a lack of normative cutoff values for androgen levels during puberty. The Rotterdam ultrasonography criteria for PCO morphology have not been validated for adolescents because multifollicular ovaries are seen in normal puberty.[31] Because transvaginal ultrasonography raises a practical concern in this age group, transabdominal ultrasonography is preferred, but may not be sensitive in evaluating ovarian follicles. OC pills are the first-line therapy for hirsutism and anovulatory symptoms. Although there is a lack of large randomized controlled trials, a few smaller studies have suggested the benefits of exercise in women with PCOS.[45] Lifestyle modifications with a calorie-restricted diet along with exercise are advocated for overweight and obese adolescents to improve their metabolic profile and regulate ovulation. Metformin can be used in the presence of metabolic syndrome or impaired glucose tolerance.

POLYCYSTIC OVARIAN SYNDROME IN PERIMENOPAUSE AND MENOPAUSE

It is unusual to develop PCOS for the first time during menopause; usually these women have symptoms of PCOS much earlier during adult life. There is paucity of data tracking the natural history of PCOS through menopause. Ovarian follicular count, AMH, and androgen levels decline with age[46] in women with and without PCOS. In the presence of very high androgen levels and rapid onset of virilization, it is pertinent to rule out androgen-secreting tumors.

Large longitudinal studies are needed to determine whether increased cardiovascular risks in women with PCOS persist after menopause.[47] There is an increased risk for endometrial cancer in women with PCOS. Assessment of the endometrial thickness by ultrasonography and prevention of endometrial hyperplasia with progesterone withdrawal bleed may reduce the risk for endometrial cancer. Despite the increased risk of endometrial cancer and PCOS, current guidelines do not recommend routine ultrasonography screening for endometrial thickness.[31,42] There is also a suggestion of increased risk for breast and ovarian cancer in women with PCOS.

SUMMARY

Women with PCOS present with signs of chronic anovulation, hyperandrogenism, and metabolic abnormalities. The NIH recently embraced the Rotterdam criteria to broadly identify all the phenotypes of PCOS. Women with PCOS are often obese with insulin resistance and hence have an increased susceptibility to glucose intolerance and type 2 diabetes. Future research should focus on the genetic, epigenetic, and environmental determinants of PCOS to develop new therapies to address the prevention of this disorder and its long-term complications.

ACKNOWLEDGMENTS

The ultrasonography image (see **Fig. 3**) was kindly provided by Dr Diane E. Woodford, Clinical Assistant professor, Reproductive Endocrinology and Infertility, University of Washington Medical Center, Seattle, Washington.

REFERENCES

1. Consensus on women's health aspects of polycystic ovary syndrome (PCOS). Hum Reprod 2012;27(1):14–24. http://dx.doi.org/10.1093/humrep/der1396.
2. Wood JR, Dumesic DA, Abbott DH, et al. Molecular abnormalities in oocytes from women with polycystic ovary syndrome revealed by microarray analysis. J Clin Endocrinol Metab 2007;92(2):705–13.
3. Ferriman D, Gallwey JD. Clinical assessment of body hair growth in women. J Clin Endocrinol Metab 1961;21:1440–7.
4. Conway GS, Dewailly D, Diamanti-Kandarakis E, et al. The polycystic ovary syndrome: an endocrinological perspective from the European Society of Endocrinology. Eur J Endocrinol 2014;171(4):489–98.
5. Dunaif A, Segal KR, Futterweit W, et al. Profound peripheral insulin resistance, independent of obesity, in polycystic ovary syndrome. Diabetes 1989;38(9): 1165–74.
6. DeUgarte CM, Bartolucci AA, Azziz R. Prevalence of insulin resistance in the polycystic ovary syndrome using the homeostasis model assessment. Fertil Steril 2005;83(5):1454–60.
7. Tamega Ade A, Aranha AM, Guiotoku MM, et al. Association between skin tags and insulin resistance. An Bras Dermatol 2010;85(1):25–31 [in Portuguese].

8. Plascencia Gomez A, Vega Memije ME, Torres Tamayo M, et al. Skin disorders in overweight and obese patients and their relationship with insulin. Actas Dermosi-filiogr 2014;105(2):178–85. http://dx.doi.org/10.1016/j.ad.2013.09.1008.

9. Apridonidze T, Essah PA, Iuorno MJ, et al. Prevalence and characteristics of the metabolic syndrome in women with polycystic ovary syndrome. J Clin Endocrinol Metab 2005;90(4):1929–35.

10. Dokras A, Bochner M, Hollinrake E, et al. Screening women with polycystic ovary syndrome for metabolic syndrome. Obstet Gynecol 2005;106(1):131–7.

11. Legro RS, Kunselman AR, Dodson WC, et al. Prevalence and predictors of risk for type 2 diabetes mellitus and impaired glucose tolerance in polycystic ovary syndrome: a prospective, controlled study in 254 affected women. J Clin Endocrinol Metab 1999;84(1):165–9.

12. Ehrmann DA, Barnes RB, Rosenfield RL, et al. Prevalence of impaired glucose tolerance and diabetes in women with polycystic ovary syndrome. Diabetes Care 1999;22(1):141–6.

13. Ehrmann DA, Kasza K, Azziz R, et al. Effects of race and family history of type 2 diabetes on metabolic status of women with polycystic ovary syndrome. J Clin Endocrinol Metab 2005;90(1):66–71.

14. Kelly CJ, Speirs A, Gould GW, et al. Altered vascular function in young women with polycystic ovary syndrome. J Clin Endocrinol Metab 2002;87(2):742–6.

15. Talbott E, Guzick D, Clerici A, et al. Coronary heart disease risk factors in women with polycystic ovary syndrome. Arterioscler Thromb Vasc Biol 1995;15(7):821–6.

16. Vgontzas AN, Legro RS, Bixler EO, et al. Polycystic ovary syndrome is associated with obstructive sleep apnea and daytime sleepiness: role of insulin resistance. J Clin Endocrinol Metab 2001;86(2):517–20.

17. Tasali E, Van Cauter E, Ehrmann DA. Relationships between sleep disordered breathing and glucose metabolism in polycystic ovary syndrome. J Clin Endocrinol Metab 2006;91(1):36–42.

18. Schwimmer JB, Khorram O, Chiu V, et al. Abnormal aminotransferase activity in women with polycystic ovary syndrome. Fertil Steril 2005;83(2):494–7.

19. Barry JA, Kuczmierczyk AR, Hardiman PJ. Anxiety and depression in polycystic ovary syndrome: a systematic review and meta-analysis. Hum Reprod 2011;26(9):2442–51. http://dx.doi.org/10.1093/humrep/der197.

20. McCartney CR, Eagleson CA, Marshall JC. Regulation of gonadotropin secretion: implications for polycystic ovary syndrome. Semin Reprod Med 2002;20(4):317–26.

21. Ehrmann DA. Polycystic ovary syndrome. N Engl J Med 2005;352(12):1223–36.

22. Tsilchorozidou T, Overton C, Conway GS. The pathophysiology of polycystic ovary syndrome. Clin Endocrinol (Oxf) 2004;60(1):1–17.

23. Diamanti-Kandarakis E, Dunaif A. Insulin resistance and the polycystic ovary syndrome revisited: an update on mechanisms and implications. Endocr Rev 2012;33(6):981–1030. http://dx.doi.org/10.1210/er.2011-1034.

24. Sam S, Legro RS, Essah PA, et al. Evidence for metabolic and reproductive phenotypes in mothers of women with polycystic ovary syndrome. Proc Natl Acad Sci U S A 2006;103(18):7030–5.

25. Legro RS, Kunselman AR, Demers L, et al. Elevated dehydroepiandrosterone sulfate levels as the reproductive phenotype in the brothers of women with polycystic ovary syndrome. J Clin Endocrinol Metab 2002;87(5):2134–8.

26. Sam S, Sung YA, Legro RS, et al. Evidence for pancreatic beta-cell dysfunction in brothers of women with polycystic ovary syndrome. Metabolism 2008;57(1):84–9.

27. Fauser BC, Tarlatzis BC, Rebar RW, et al. Consensus on women's health aspects of polycystic ovary syndrome (PCOS): the Amsterdam ESHRE/ASRM-Sponsored 3rd PCOS Consensus Workshop Group. Fertil Steril 2012;97(1):28–38.e25. http://dx.doi.org/10.1016/j.fertnstert.2011.1009.1024.

28. Keevil BG. How do we measure hyperandrogenemia in patients with PCOS? J Clin Endocrinol Metab 2014;99(3):777–9. http://dx.doi.org/10.1210/jc.2014-1307.

29. O'Reilly MW, Taylor AE, Crabtree NJ, et al. Hyperandrogenemia predicts metabolic phenotype in polycystic ovary syndrome: the utility of serum androstenedione. J Clin Endocrinol Metab 2014;99(3):1027–36. http://dx.doi.org/10.1210/jc.2013-3399.

30. Eilertsen TB, Vanky E, Carlsen SM. Anti-Mullerian hormone in the diagnosis of polycystic ovary syndrome: can morphologic description be replaced? Hum Reprod 2012;27(8):2494–502. http://dx.doi.org/10.1093/humrep/des213.

31. Legro RS, Arslanian SA, Ehrmann DA, et al. Diagnosis and treatment of polycystic ovary syndrome: an Endocrine Society clinical practice guideline. J Clin Endocrinol Metab 2013;98(12):4565–92. http://dx.doi.org/10.1210/jc.2013-2350.

32. Johnstone EB, Rosen MP, Neril R, et al. The polycystic ovary post-Rotterdam: a common, age-dependent finding in ovulatory women without metabolic significance. J Clin Endocrinol Metab 2010;95(11):4965–72. http://dx.doi.org/10.1210/jc.2010-0202.

33. Dewailly D, Lujan ME, Carmina E, et al. Definition and significance of polycystic ovarian morphology: a task force report from the Androgen Excess and Polycystic Ovary Syndrome Society. Hum Reprod Update 2014;20(3):334–52. http://dx.doi.org/10.1093/humupd/dmt061.

34. Martin KA, Chang RJ, Ehrmann DA, et al. Evaluation and treatment of hirsutism in premenopausal women: an endocrine society clinical practice guideline. J Clin Endocrinol Metab 2008;93(4):1105–20. http://dx.doi.org/10.1210/jc.2007-2437.

35. Usadi RS, Legro RS. Reproductive impact of polycystic ovary syndrome. Curr Opin Endocrinol Diabetes Obes 2012;19(6):505–11. http://dx.doi.org/10.1097/MED.0b013e328359ff92.

36. Legro RS, Barnhart HX, Schlaff WD, et al. Clomiphene, metformin, or both for infertility in the polycystic ovary syndrome. N Engl J Med 2007;356(6):551–66.

37. Morin-Papunen L, Rantala AS, Unkila-Kallio L, et al. Metformin improves pregnancy and live-birth rates in women with polycystic ovary syndrome (PCOS): a multicenter, double-blind, placebo-controlled randomized trial. J Clin Endocrinol Metab 2012;97(5):1492–500. http://dx.doi.org/10.1210/jc.2011-3061.

38. Palomba S, Falbo A, Carrillo L, et al. Metformin reduces risk of ovarian hyperstimulation syndrome in patients with polycystic ovary syndrome during gonadotropin-stimulated in vitro fertilization cycles: a randomized, controlled trial. Fertil Steril 2011;96(6):1384–90.e4.

39. Legro RS, Brzyski RG, Diamond MP, et al. The pregnancy in polycystic ovary syndrome II study: baseline characteristics and effects of obesity from a multicenter randomized clinical trial. Fertil Steril 2014;101(1):258–69.e8. http://dx.doi.org/10.1016/j.fertnstert.2013.08.056.

40. Perales-Puchalt A, Legro RS. Ovulation induction in women with polycystic ovary syndrome. Steroids 2013;78(8):767–72. http://dx.doi.org/10.1016/j.steroids.2013.05.005.

41. Knowler WC, Barrett-Connor E, Fowler SE, et al. Reduction in the incidence of type 2 diabetes with lifestyle intervention or metformin. N Engl J Med 2002;346(6):393–403.

42. Bates GW, Legro RS. Longterm management of polycystic ovarian syndrome (PCOS). Mol Cell Endocrinol 2013;373(1–2):91–7. http://dx.doi.org/10.1016/j.mce.2012.1010.1029.

43. Escobar-Morreale HF, Botella-Carretero JI, Alvarez-Blasco F, et al. The polycystic ovary syndrome associated with morbid obesity may resolve after weight loss induced by bariatric surgery. J Clin Endocrinol Metab 2005;90(12):6364–9.

44. Eid GM, Cottam DR, Velcu LM, et al. Effective treatment of polycystic ovarian syndrome with Roux-en-Y gastric bypass. Surg Obes Relat Dis 2005;1(2):77–80.

45. Harrison CL, Lombard CB, Moran LJ, et al. Exercise therapy in polycystic ovary syndrome: a systematic review. Hum Reprod Update 2011;17(2):171–83.

46. Winters SJ, Talbott E, Guzick DS, et al. Serum testosterone levels decrease in middle age in women with the polycystic ovary syndrome. Fertil Steril 2000;73(4):724–9.

47. Welt CK, Carmina E. Clinical review: lifecycle of polycystic ovary syndrome (PCOS): from in utero to menopause. J Clin Endocrinol Metab 2013;98(12):4629–38.

Index

Note: Page numbers of article titles are in **boldface** type.

Med Clin N Am 99 (2015) 237–248
http://dx.doi.org/10.1016/S0025-7125(14)00186-2
0025-7125/15/$ – see front matter © 2015 Elsevier Inc. All rights reserved.

medical.theclinics.com

Moving?

Make sure your subscription moves with you!

To notify us of your new address, find your **Clinics Account Number** (located on your mailing label above your name), and contact customer service at:

Email: journalscustomerservice-usa@elsevier.com

800-654-2452 (subscribers in the U.S. & Canada)
314-447-8871 (subscribers outside of the U.S. & Canada)

Fax number: 314-447-8029

Elsevier Health Sciences Division
Subscription Customer Service
3251 Riverport Lane
Maryland Heights, MO 63043

*To ensure uninterrupted delivery of your subscription, please notify us at least 4 weeks in advance of move.